Clinical Documentation Improvement for Outpatient Care

Clinical Documentation Improvement for Outpatient Care

Design and Implementation

Pamela Carroll Hess, MA, RHIA, CCS, CDIP, CPC

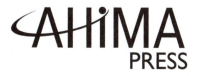

Copyright ©2018 by the American Health Information Management Association. All rights reserved. Except as permitted under the Copyright Act of 1976, no part of this publication may be reproduced, stored in a retrieval system, or transmitted, in any form or by any means, electronic, photocopying, recording, or otherwise, without the prior written permission of AHIMA, 233 North Michigan Avenue, 21st Floor, Chicago, Illinois, 60601-5809 (http://www.ahima.org/reprint).

ISBN: **978-1-58426-584-9**
AHIMA Product No.: AB121717

AHIMA Staff:
Jessica Block, MA, Production Development Editor
Chelsea Brotherton, MA, Assistant Editor
Colton Gigot, MA, Production Development Editor
Megan Grennan, Managing Editor

Cover image: ©from2015, iStockphoto

Limit of Liability/Disclaimer of Warranty: This book is sold, as is, without warranty of any kind, either express or implied. While every precaution has been taken in the preparation of this book, the publisher and author assume no responsibility for errors or omissions. Neither is any liability assumed for damages resulting from the use of the information or instructions contained herein. It is further stated that the publisher and author are not responsible for any damage or loss to your data or your equipment that results directly or indirectly from your use of this book.

The websites listed in this book were current and valid as of the date of publication. However, webpage addresses and the information on them may change at any time. The user is encouraged to perform his or her own general web searches to locate any site addresses listed here that are no longer valid.

CPT® is a registered trademark of the American Medical Association. All other copyrights and trademarks mentioned in this book are the possession of their respective owners. AHIMA makes no claim of ownership by mentioning products that contain such marks.

For more information, including updates, about AHIMA Press publications, visit **http://www.ahima.org/education/press.**

American Health Information Management Association
233 North Michigan Avenue, 21st Floor
Chicago, Illinois 60601-5809
ahima.org

Contents

Detailed Contents — vii
About the Author — xv
Preface — xvii
Acknowledgments — xxi

Part I Fundamentals of Outpatient Clinical Documentation

Chapter 1 The Case for High-Quality Outpatient Clinical Documentation — 3

Chapter 2 Sources and Types of Outpatient Clinical Documentation — 21

Chapter 3 The Translation of Clinical Documentation into Coded Data — 49

Chapter 4 Regulation of Outpatient Healthcare and Compliant CDI Practice — 81

Chapter 5 Outpatient CDI Assessment — 117

Chapter 6 Analyzing Clinical Documentation Data — 137

Chapter 7 Assessing Outpatient CDI Program Technology Options — 159

Part II Implementing an Outpatient Clinical Documentation Improvement Program

Chapter 8 Moving Forward with a CDI Program — 191

Chapter 9 Creating Interdisciplinary CDI Leadership Teams in the Outpatient Healthcare Setting — 209

Chapter 10 Project Management Using a CDI Workplan — 223

Chapter 11 Program Staffing Options — 245

Chapter 12	Training the Outpatient Clinical Documentation Specialist	259
Chapter 13	Provider and Clinical Staff CDI Education in the Outpatient Setting	289
Chapter 14	Educational Programs for Outpatient Coders	309
Chapter 15	Physician Queries in the Outpatient Setting	333
Chapter 16	Expanding the Outpatient CDI Program	347
Glossary		369
Index		381

Detailed Contents

About the Author	xv
Preface	xvii
Acknowledgments	xxi

Part I Fundamentals of Outpatient Clinical Documentation

Chapter 1 The Case for High-Quality Outpatient Clinical Documentation 3

The Rationale for Clinical Documentation Improvement in the Outpatient Setting	4
Selected Benefits of High-Quality Outpatient Clinical Documentation	7
Meeting Regulatory Requirements	7
Maximizing Reimbursement	8
Preventing and Detecting Fraud, Waste, and Abuse in Healthcare	10
Measuring and Marketing Quality of Care	10
Promoting Evidence-Based Medicine	11
Improving Population Health	12
The Challenges of Outpatient Clinical Documentation	12
Seven Criteria for Quality in Clinical Documentation	14
Legibility	15
Reliability	15
Precision	16
Completeness	16
Consistency	17
Clarity	17
Timeliness	17

Chapter 2 Sources and Types of Outpatient Clinical Documentation 21

Sources of Clinical Documentation	22
EHRs	22
Other Sources of Clinical Documentation	23
Types of Clinical Documentation	24
Designated Record Sets and Legal Records	24
Protected Patient Information and Deidentified Records	25

Categorizing Record Types in Clinical Documentation	26
Clinical Record Contents	28
Emergency Department Record	28
Glasgow Coma Scale	29
Anesthesia Record	29
Consultation Reports	30
Diagnostic Test Results	30
Encounter Summary	31
Patient History and Physical Examination	31
Medication Administration Record	32
Operative and Procedure Reports	32
Physician Orders	33
Problem List	33
Progress Notes	34
Vital Signs Flowsheet	35
Outpatient Records by Settings	35
Authors of Clinical Documentation	37
Attending Physicians	37
Consultants	37
House Staff	37
Surgeons	37
Diagnosticians	38
Physician Executives	38
Nonphysician Practitioners	39
Clinical Documentation Challenges in the Outpatient Setting	40
Outpatient Coding and Reimbursement Systems	40
Outpatient-Specific Coding and Billing Guidelines	41
Limited Supply of Outpatient Coding Experts	42
Establishing the Medical Necessity of Brief Encounters	43

Chapter 3 The Translation of Clinical Documentation into Coded Data — 49

The Coding Process	50
Interoperability	52
Relationship between Clinical Documentation and Coding	54
Basic Coding Guidelines	56
ICD-10-CM	56
CPT and HCPCS	57
Coding in the Physician Practice	63
E/M Coding	63
RVUs and the Physician Fee Schedule	65
HCC Codes for Risk-Adjusted Payment	68
Coding in the Facility Ambulatory Care Setting	71
OPPS and APCs	72
The Hospital Chargemaster	74
Coding in the ED	74

Chapter 4 Regulation of Outpatient Healthcare and Compliant CDI Practice — 81

Ambulatory CDI Compliance	82
Federal Compliance Guidance for CDI Programs	83
OIG Guidance	83

	Guidance from CMS	87
	DOJ Compliance Memorandum	87
	AHIMA Standards of Ethical Coding and Coding Compliance	92
	Operationalizing Program Compliance	93
	Government Agencies Regulating Healthcare	94
	Public Data and Quality Reporting	98
	Hospital Outpatient Quality Reporting Program	99
	Quality Payment Program	102
	MIPS	102
	Advanced APMs	105
	Advancing Care Information Performance Measure	107
	Privately Held Hospital Compare Organizations	108
Chapter 5	**Outpatient CDI Assessment**	**117**
	Assessing the Feasibility of CDI	118
	Benefits of Outpatient CDI	119
	Potential Barriers to an Outpatient CDI Program	120
	Steps in the Outpatient CDI Assessment Program	121
	Step 1: Gather Data and Identify Areas of Focus	122
	Step 2: Establish an Outpatient CDI Taskforce	124
	Step 3: Conduct Focused Case Review	124
	Step 4: Analyze Results of Case Review	127
	Step 5: Estimate the Return on Investment	129
	Step 6: Create a High-Level Workplan	131
	Executive and Key Stakeholder Buy-in	134
Chapter 6	**Analyzing Clinical Documentation Data**	**137**
	Selecting Clinical Documentation Data for Analysis	138
	Chargemaster	138
	Claims Edits	141
	Denials Trends and Reports	143
	Coding Audit Reports	143
	HCC Reports and Audits	143
	Quality Measure Scores	144
	Outpatient Research Identifiable Files	144
	Other HCPCS Code Utilization Files	145
	Preparing to Implement the Pilot CDI Plan	147
	Step 1: Identify the Pilot Sites	147
	Step 2: Review Data	148
	Step 3: Select Focus Areas	148
	Step 4: Review HCPCS/CPT Frequency Reports	149
	Step 5: Monitor HCC Capture	149
	Step 6: Audit a Sample of Cases from Each Group of Diagnoses and Procedures Identified in Steps 2 and 3	149
	Step 7: Conduct Key Stakeholder Interviews	150
	Step 8: Identify the Root Cause	150
	Step 9: Discuss Findings and Recommendations	150
	Step 10: Implement the Solution	151
	Focused Clinical Record Review Process	151
	Pre-encounter and Concurrent Case Review	151
	Postencounter Case Review	153
	Reporting on Program Data	153

Chapter 7	**Assessing Outpatient CDI Program Technology Options**	**159**
	The Outpatient Clinical Documentation Technology Landscape	160
	EHR Functionality	161
	Uses of EHRs for Clinical Documentation Improvement	161
	Clinical Documentation Risks Potentially Associated with EHRs	163
	Communication Tools in the EHR	165
	Natural Language Processing	165
	NLP Applications for CDI	167
	CAC Applications	167
	HCC Suspecting	168
	Patient HCC Capture Report	169
	Patient HCC Profile Report	171
	Physician HCC Capture Report	171
	Personal Mobile Device Query Options	172
	Denials Tracking	176
	Clinical Editors	179

Part II Implementing an Outpatient Clinical Documentation Improvement Program

Chapter 8	**Moving Forward with a CDI Program**	**191**
	Key Decision Makers	192
	Governance Structure	193
	Responsibilities of the Steering Committee	194
	Responsibilities of the Outpatient CDI Taskforce	196
	CDI Program Vision, Mission, Goals, and Objectives	197
	Vision Statement	197
	Mission Statement	198
	Goals and Objectives	199
	Organizational Communication	201
	Outpatient CDI Program Implementation Strategies	203
	Customization of an Existing CDI Program	203
	Implementation of a Redesigned Outpatient CDI Program	205

Chapter 9	**Creating Interdisciplinary CDI Leadership Teams in the Outpatient Healthcare Setting**	**209**
	Making the Case for an Interdisciplinary Team	210
	Identifying CDI Team Leaders in the Outpatient Healthcare Organization	211
	Team Member Selection and Roles	215
	Selecting Steering Committee Members	215
	Selecting CDI Taskforce Members	216
	Fostering Collaborative Team Dynamics	218

Chapter 10   Project Management Using a CDI Workplan   223

    Project Management for the Outpatient CDI Program   224
    The Project Workplan   225
    Example of an Outpatient CDI Program Workplan   227
        Phase I, Task 1: Data Analytics   227
        Phase I, Task 2: On-Site Kickoff Meeting and Interviews   228
        Phase I, Task 3: CDI Program Governance and Oversight   231
        Phase I, Task 4: Outpatient and Professional Practice Case Review   231
        Phase I, Task 5: High-Level Technology Assessment   234
        Phase I, Task 6: Outpatient Clinical Documentation Assessment   234
        Phase II, Task 7: Rapid Redesign of Clinical Documentation Workflow at Pilot Clinics   234
        Phase II, Task 8: Physician Collaboration and Education during Outpatient CDI Program Implementation   237
        Phase II, Task 9: Rapid Redesign of Clinical Documentation Workflow in Remaining Clinics   239
        Phase III, Task 10: Ongoing Program Monitoring   239

Chapter 11   Program Staffing Options   245

    Organizational Considerations   246
        Example 1: Integrated Inpatient and Outpatient CDI Programs   247
        Example 2: Separate Inpatient and Outpatient CDI Programs   247
    Selecting a Program Staffing Model   248
        Availability of Qualified Program Staff   248
        Cash Flow Issues   249
        Physician Leaders   249
        Outsourcing and Employed Staff Options   251

Chapter 12   Training the Outpatient Clinical Documentation Specialist   259

    CDS Skills in the Outpatient Setting   261
    Pretraining CDS Assessment   262
    Job Description for the Outpatient CDS   263
    CDS Self-Evaluation   265
    Training Topics and Resources   266
        CDI Program Process and Design   266
    CDS Training Programs and Topics   267
        Query Process   269
        Role of Physician Advisor   270
        Metrics and Trending   270
        Maintaining Program Visibility   273
    Posttraining Evaluation   274
    Critical Thinking Defined   275
    Why Is Critical Thinking Necessary in Healthcare?   276

Critical Thinking and the Learning Process	277
Problem Resolution without Critical Thinking	279
Problem Resolution with Critical Thinking	280
Using Critical Thinking to Surmount Barriers to Success	282
First Barrier: Historical Patient Data Unavailable to the Provider at the Time of the Visit	283
Second Barrier: Lack of CDS Interaction with Providers to Help Ensure Diagnostic Specificity in the Clinical Record	283
Third Barrier: Ineffective or Absent Query Communication Process	284
Fourth Barrier: Absence of an EHR In-line Documentation Process	284
Integrating Effective Communication	285

Chapter 13 Provider and Clinical Staff CDI Education in the Outpatient Setting — 289

Trends in Physician Education	290
Recommended Approaches to Physician Education about CDI	291
Nonphysician Providers	292
Nonprovider Clinicians	294
Establishing Group Educational Sessions	295
Selecting Instructors for Nonprovider Clinician CDI Educational Programs	296
Selecting Instructors for Physician CDI Educational Programs	296
Maximizing Educational Program Attendance	296
CME Presentation Content	297
Educational Session Content	297
How to Use the Sample Presentation	297
Suggested Slide Presentation	298

Chapter 14 Educational Programs for Outpatient Coders — 309

Medical Coding Professionals in the Outpatient Setting	310
Required Competencies	310
Educational and Training Background	311
Job Responsibilities	312
Preparing for and Running CDI Educational Sessions	312
Educational Session Content	313
Introduction (Title Slide)	313
Clinical Documentation Improvement: Team Approach	314
Outpatient CDI Defined	314
CDI in the Outpatient Setting	314
Outpatient Facility and Professional Practice Components	315
HCC Shadowing Process	316
HCC Shadowing Process Drill-Down	316
Physician Query Process in the Outpatient Setting	317
When to Query	317
Who to Query	318
Growing Demand for CDI to Support Risk Adjustment	318
Common HCCs	318

	Risk Score Example	319
	Return on Investment for the MA Plan	319
	OIG Risk-Adjustment Data Validation Audit	319
	Clinical Data Requirements	320
	Conduct an HCC Audit	320
	Example Scenario: HCC Case Review	321
	Incorporate Other Focus Areas	321
	Example 1: Outpatient CDI Focus Area	321
	Example 2: Outpatient CDI Focus Area	321
	Provider Program Adoption	322
	Technology for Outpatient CDI	322
	Technology for HCC Capture	323
	More on Workflow Redesign	323
	Outpatient CDI Mastery for Coders	324
	Credentials for Outpatient Coders	324
	Outpatient Coding and CDI Resources	324
	Knowledge Base for Outpatient Coders	324
	Knowledge Base for Coders: Making the Case for CDI	325
	Knowledge Base for Coders: Physician Fee Schedules	325
	Knowledge Base for Coders: Hospital Chargemaster	326
	Knowledge Base for Coders: Claims Editors	326
	Knowledge Base for Coders: Denials Management	326
	Knowledge Base for Coders: CMS Quality Programs in the Outpatient Setting	327
	Knowledge Base for Coders: HCC and Outpatient Code Assignment	328
	Knowledge Base for Coders: Data Analytics, Metrics, and Trending	328
Chapter 15	**Physician Queries in the Outpatient Setting**	**333**
	When to Submit a Query	334
	Criteria for Query Submission	334
	Query Process	335
	Metrics for Query Submission and Response	337
	Improving the Physician Query Process	339
	Specialty-Specific Diagnosis Queries	340
Chapter 16	**Expanding the Outpatient CDI Program**	**347**
	Organizational and Stakeholder Adoption	348
	Emergency Department	349
	Admission Documentation	350
	Critical Care Documentation	351
	Charge Capture	352
	E/M Levels	353
	E/M Level Benchmarking	355
	Observation Services	358
	Observation Services Dates and Times	359
	Provider Orders and Documentation in Observation Services	360
	Other Observation Services Documentation	363
Glossary		369
Index		381

About the Author

Pamela Carroll Hess, MA, RHIA, CCS, CDIP, CPC, is a health information management (HIM) professional with extensive healthcare experience in revenue cycle operations, electronic health record (EHR) applications, healthcare informatics, data analytics, revenue integrity, HIM operations, compliance, quality control, clinical documentation programs, and provider education. Ms. Hess has served in consulting, administrative, and interim management capacities within large academic and urban community hospitals. Her experience in the healthcare industry has focused on improving operational and financial performance in a variety of healthcare settings. Ms. Hess has assisted her clients with regulatory issues related to accurate claims submission, reimbursement reviews, fraud and abuse, corporate integrity agreements, and Joint Commission accreditation. In addition, Ms. Hess has led numerous large clinical documentation improvement projects, clinical appeals department redesigns, revenue cycle projects, and provider education programs. She has also provided consulting services at Deloitte & Touché, LLC; Navigant Consulting, Inc.; Himagine Solutions, Inc.; and Accretive Health (R1 RCM). She is currently vice president of strategy and operations with MedASTUTE Consulting, LLC, a consulting firm focused on leveraging analytics for performance improvement with healthcare providers and health plans. Areas of focus include clinical documentation improvement, data analytics, compliance, revenue integrity, cost management, service line management, network management and contracting, and pharmacy benefit management, among other healthcare disciplines. Ms. Hess appreciates the opportunity to speak with you about outpatient CDI. She may be reached at Pam.Hess@MedASTUTE.com.

Preface

Clinical documentation improvement specialists (CDSs) are a valuable resource for hospital outpatient clinics and departments as well as professional practices throughout the continuum of care. The CDS assists these organizations to ensure high-quality clinical documentation that supports provider-to-provider collaboration, quality patient care, reimbursement, and accurate healthcare data. The clinical documentation improvement (CDI) profession is based on guiding principles established by the American Health Information Management Association (AHIMA), the Centers for Medicare and Medicaid Services (CMS), the American Hospital Association (AHA), and the American Medical Association (AMA). This textbook is a resource that guides the reader through a discussion of fundamental knowledge needed to assess clinical documentation in the outpatient setting and methodologies for implementing a comprehensive CDI program in outpatient hospital clinics, departments, and professional practices.

The text is designed as a reference and guide to CDI activities in outpatient settings and is a general CDI resource for health information management (HIM), health informatics, nursing, healthcare administration, and other allied health programs. Readers of this text will have a variety of backgrounds, skill sets, and skill levels. Some may be credentialed CDI practitioners through AHIMA (CDIP). Others may be noncredentialed practitioners already working in the clinical documentation field. Yet others may be seasoned healthcare professionals new to CDI or healthcare students learning about CDI for the first time. A basic knowledge of the following topics will be beneficial to the readers of this textbook. This knowledge base can be obtained through HIM courses at colleges and universities or via online training through AHIMA:

- Fundamentals of ICD-10-CM, CPT, HCPCS, and evaluation and management (E/M) coding for disease and treatment classification and reimbursement
- Reimbursement methodologies used in the outpatient setting: Ambulatory payment classifications (APC), Hierarchical Condition Categories (HCC), Relative Value Units (RVU) and Medicare Physician Fee Schedule (MPFS), fee-for service, and risk-based reimbursement
- Quality measurement program methodologies, including the Quality Payment Program (QPP), the Medicare Access and CHIP Reauthorization Act of 2015 (MACRA), and the Merit-based Incentive Payment System (MIPS)

- Basic understanding of insurance company plans such as Medicare Advantage, Medicare Parts B and C, commercial payers, and risk-adjusted plans
- Medical claims processing and insurance company (payer) preauthorization, payment, and claims-denial processes
- Fundamentals of database management
- Basic electronic health record (EHR) and encoder functionality
- Basic HIPAA guidelines and use of deidentified healthcare data for quality measurement
- Basic job functions of medical coders

The organization of this text is based around two major content areas. Part I conveys fundamental knowledge related to high-quality clinical documentation as well as the sources and users of clinical data. Also discussed are classification and reimbursement systems as well as healthcare regulations around quality measures and the corresponding monitoring of quality metrics. Methodology for initial feasibility assessments of outpatient CDI programs is also discussed in detail.

Part II addresses the necessary information and methodologies for implementing an outpatient CDI program. This portion of the text starts with a discussion on key stakeholders as well as the creation and functionality of an interdisciplinary team. The steps for implementing an effective program are presented along with options for CDI program management and staffing. The physician shadowing and query processes are outlined and highlighted through query examples. Educational programs for providers, nonprovider clinicians, CDSs, and coders are also presented in this section.

The book is designed to help the reader convert basic principles into practice. Each chapter includes the following features and pedagogy

- Basic knowledge required for CDI program assessment and implementation.
- Review questions to check your understanding of the chapter content.
- Case examples based around the chapter content for the reader to consider and develop appropriate solutions.

An outline of chapters for parts I and II is provided below.

Part I Fundamentals of Outpatient Clinical Documentation

Chapter 1 The Case for High-Quality Outpatient Clinical Documentation establishes a case for the high-quality clinical record in the outpatient setting by presenting the need for more specific documentation throughout the continuum of care. The chapter discusses the seven criteria for high-quality documentation, users of clinical information and data, and the corresponding uses and benefits of clinical data.

Chapter 2 Sources and Types of Outpatient Clinical Documentation presents the various sources and types of clinical documentation in the outpatient setting. Challenges to producing high-quality clinical documentation, such as multiple reimbursement methodologies, multiple coding classification systems, and a lack of qualified clinical documentation specialists, are presented and discussed throughout the chapter.

Chapter 3 The Translation of Clinical Documentation into Coded Data highlights the classification systems used to code diagnoses and procedures in the outpatient setting. These include ICD-10-CM, HCPCS, and CPT. The differences between payment methodologies in the outpatient facility and professional practice setting are also discussed.

Chapter 4 Regulation of Outpatient Healthcare and Compliant CDI Practice explains the organizations, agencies, and government programs that regulate and monitor hospital coding, billing, reimbursement, quality, and safety. The government-mandated quality reporting programs and private-organization quality programs are explained, and the CDS's role in the compliance process is outlined.

Chapter 5 Outpatient CDI Assessment presents methods for assessing the initial state and ongoing feasibility of an outpatient clinical documentation program. The steps for completing such an assessment, along with the resources and executive-level support needed to conduct the assessment and implement the program, are outlined in this chapter.

Chapter 6 Analyzing Clinical Documentation Data discusses the various data sets used by clinical documentation programs. Steps for the CDS case review process, along with the key elements for reporting the results of the case reviews, are presented throughout the chapter.

Chapter 7 Assessing Outpatient CDI Program Technology Options offers an overview of the technology in the healthcare marketplace as well as insight into how to effectively use the technology to bring the outpatient CDI program to the next level.

Part II Implementing an Outpatient Clinical Documentation Improvement Program

Chapter 8 Moving Forward with a CDI Program describes the importance of key executive decision makers' buy-in to the new outpatient CDI program. The importance of effective organizational communication as well as various strategies for CDI program implementation are addressed throughout the chapter. The importance of—and methodologies for creating—program vision, mission, goals, and objectives are also presented.

Chapter 9 Creating Interdisciplinary CDI Leadership Teams in the Outpatient Healthcare Setting outlines the need for an interdisciplinary team approach to the outpatient CDI program. The role of program stakeholders is addressed, along with methods for creating a collaborative team and the team's primary functions.

Chapter 10 Project Management Using a CDI Workplan explains the value of a workplan for effective project management. The tasks required in the workplan, along with the stakeholder responsibilities, are outlined. A discussion on how to keep the project on track through the use of a workplan follows.

Chapter 11 Program Staffing Options explains where to find qualified CDI program staff. Various outsourcing models are discussed, and conversion methodology to an internal staffing model is presented. The chapter also explores the skill set requirements for the outpatient CDS. The importance and challenges of the physician advisor role are highlighted.

Chapter 12 Training the Outpatient Clinical Documentation Specialist identifies the need for the self-evaluation and assessment process for the outpatient CDS. Topics included in the outpatient CDS training program are detailed. Metrics for tracking and trending the program are also presented. The concepts and need for critical thinking in the outpatient CDI setting are discussed in detail.

Chapter 13 Provider and Clinical Staff CDI Education in the Outpatient Setting explains methods for teaching physicians and clinical staff the relationship between clinical documentation and the translation of data into ICD-10-CM, CPT, and HCPCS codes. Content for these training sessions are presented in detail.

Chapter 14 Education Programs for Outpatient Coders explains the recommended attendees for the outpatient CDI medical coder educational program and illustrates methodologies to engage the medical coder in the CDI program. The content and recommended instructors for a comprehensive CDI educational program are presented, and the challenges and interaction between the CDS and coder are highlighted.

Chapter 15 Physician Queries in the Outpatient Setting explains the need for physician queries in the outpatient setting. The process of physician shadowing and query submission is outlined, along with the components of a compliant query. Examples of specialty-specific queries are included.

Chapter 16 Expanding the Outpatient CDI Program describes the expansion of the outpatient CDI program into the emergency and observation services departments. The process for the CDI program case review in the emergency department and observation areas are outlined in detail. Guidelines for high-quality clinical documentation are presented.

Student Workbook

This textbook includes a student workbook featuring chapter-by-chapter key terms and definitions, comprehensive student activities, and additional articles and resources on essential CDI topics.

Acknowledgments

Writing a technical textbook such as *Clinical Documentation Improvement for Outpatient Care* is a daunting task even before the added complexities of family, work, and day-to-day life. Ms. Hess would like to acknowledge and thank her husband, Chaplain Dave Hess, for his commitment to this project, his personal support, and his creativity in graphic design that has made the book more fun to read while adding clarity to the subject matter. Through Chaplain Hess's faith, devotion, and contributions to the Hess family and many others, he has kept Ms. Hess going, kept her eye on the ball, and made life better. Without him, this book would not be possible.

The author would also like to acknowledge the contributions of Michael Marron-Stearns, MD, CPC, CFPC, to this textbook. Dr. Marron-Stearns is a physician informaticist, health information technology (HIT), and healthcare compliance consulting professional. He has 18 years of experience in the areas of electronic health records, quality reporting, health information exchange, clinical terminology development, standards, and billing and coding compliance. He is the CEO and founder of Apollo HIT, LLC, a company that provides HIT and compliance consulting services to the healthcare industry. Dr. Marron-Stearns has provided leadership to informatics and terminology projects at the National Library of Medicine, the National Cancer Institute, and the College of American Pathologists. He served as the international director of SNOMED International, where he played a central role in the design and development of SNOMED CT. Dr. Marron-Stearns is a leading national authority on protecting the integrity of digital health information in electronic health records and health information exchange.

AHIMA Press would like to thank Leslie Gordon, MS, RHIA, FAHIMA; Lauree Handlon, RHIA, CCS, MS, CPC-H, FAHIMA; Kathleen Kirk, Ph.D., RHIA; and Donna Wilson, RHIA, CCS, CCDS, for their review of, feedback on, and contributions to this textbook and instructor materials.

PART I
Fundamentals of Outpatient Clinical Documentation

The Case for High-Quality Outpatient Clinical Documentation

1

Learning Objectives

- Explain the rationale for high-quality clinical documentation in the outpatient setting.
- Describe how high-quality clinical documentation is used to maximize reimbursement.
- Learn the role of clinical documentation in evidence-based medicine and population health.
- Identify challenges to establishing a clinical documentation improvement program in the outpatient setting.
- Describe and apply the seven criteria for high-quality clinical documentation in the outpatient setting.

Key Terms

Clarity
Clinical documentation
Completeness
Conditions for Coverage (CfCs)
Conditions of Participation (CoPs)
Consistency
Electronic health record (EHR)
Evidence-based clinical practice guidelines
Evidence-based medicine (EBM)
Fee-for-service payment methodology
Healthgrades

Hierarchical Condition Category (HCC)
Hybrid health record
The Joint Commission
Leapfrog Group
Legibility
Population health
Precision
Reliability
Risk-based payment methodologies
Timeliness

The US healthcare delivery system is currently being transformed by the expansion of health information technology and government policies that promote its use (Middleton et al. 2013). In particular, the **electronic health record (EHR)** has changed the way that healthcare is delivered. An EHR is an electronic record of health-related information about an individual that conforms to nationally recognized interoperability standards and that authorized clinicians and staff across more than one healthcare organization can create, manage, and consult. According to the Centers for Medicare and Medicaid Services (CMS), an EHR

> is maintained by the provider over time, and may include all of the key administrative clinical data relevant to that person's care under a particular provider, including demographics, progress notes, problems, medications, vital signs, past medical history, immunizations, laboratory data, and radiology reports. The EHR automates access to information and has the potential to streamline the clinician's workflow. The EHR also has the ability to support other care-related activities directly or indirectly through various interfaces, including evidence-based decision support, quality management, and outcomes reporting. (CMS 2012)

As CMS makes clear in this description, EHRs offer opportunities to improve the quality of patient care across the continuum of care. When providers use high-quality documentation to collaborate, the continuity of care is strengthened. Specific and complete clinical information supports the timely and proper payment for services rendered. Also, the sharing of detailed health information about patient diagnoses and treatments can help us identify epidemiological trends, implement new payment models for healthcare, assess cutting-edge treatment outcomes, evaluate pharmaceutical efficacy, carry out further research to cure catastrophic illnesses, and prevent fraud and abuse.

However, the use of the EHR has risks, many of which are related to the quality of clinical documentation. For example, user errors, such as entering the wrong dose of a medication into the record, may result in undue harm to patients, or the documentation about the patient in the EHR may be incomplete, which could affect medical decision making (Middleton et al. 2013). Also, system interoperability issues abound, and valuable healthcare data needed for provider collaboration are therefore unavailable because systems do not "talk" to each other. In recent decades, the healthcare industry and peer-reviewed research have established the importance of accurate, timely, and complete health information in all settings (Hess 2015). Although much has been accomplished in the inpatient setting to improve clinical documentation, high-quality clinical documentation is unfortunately still frequently lacking in the ambulatory setting in hospitals, as well as in many clinics, diagnostic and treatment centers, and physician practices. This chapter sets out arguments for improving clinical documentation in these settings, reviews some of the challenges involved in such improvements, and addresses the basic criteria for high-quality clinical documentation.

The Rationale for Clinical Documentation Improvement in the Outpatient Setting

Inpatient clinical documentation improvement (CDI) programs implemented in recent decades offer evidence that organizations that focus on clinical documentation and provider education can achieve more specific clinical records relevant to provider-to-provider collaboration, health research, improved patient care, and accurate reimbursement (Hess 2015). **Clinical documentation** refers to any manual or electronic notation (or recording) made by a physician or other healthcare clinician related to a patient's medical condition or treatment. Like inpatient clinical documentation, outpatient and professional fee documentation are important to the quality of care for individual patients, reimbursement, population health, and the success of the healthcare industry. Among the parties that use such clinical data are the following:

- Providers aiming to identify disease processes and treatment options and collaborating on patient care
- Public health agencies tracking information about infectious diseases and other public health issues
- Research institutions developing and implementing evidence-based treatment protocols
- Pharmaceutical companies assessing the efficacy of medications
- Healthcare organizations developing strategies to manage future health challenges
- Government agencies charged with preventing and detecting potential fraud and abuse
- Payers that allocate funds based on fee schedules, cost- or charge-based payment, risk adjustment, or prospective payment systems, such as CMS's Inpatient Prospective Payment System (IPPS) and Outpatient Prospective Payment System (OPPS)
- Health systems and facilities aiming to ensure their strategic use of resources and operational efficiency

The relationship among the aforementioned parties is shown in figure 1.1.

Figure 1.1. Users of outpatient clinical documentation

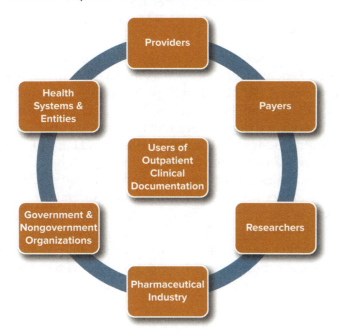

The rationale for high-quality clinical records in the outpatient setting can be easily communicated to providers and other stakeholders using the following categories of need:

- *Clinical records to facilitate provider collaboration via the EHR across the continuum of patient care:* Continuity of care is essential as patients move back and forth among inpatient, ambulatory, rehabilitation, and home care settings. Incomplete and incompatible records hinder provider communication and may adversely affect the patient's progress to wellness or increase the cost of care.
- *Clinical data to demonstrate an organization's or practitioner's quality of care:* Accurate, consistent, and specific documentation about diagnoses and treatments generates coded data about the quality of care, which can be used to rank providers and facilities and help the public select the best in class.
- *Clinical and claims data to improve strategic planning and operational efficiencies at the health system and facility level:* For example, healthcare organizations can analyze data such as procedure and diagnosis volumes by specialty to determine profitable areas for future expansion, and data that help identify the root causes of payer denials for medical necessity and inaccurate coding can be used to improve accounts receivable targets and educate providers about best practices in clinical documentation processes.
- *Clinical outcomes data to select service lines for future expansion and market these success stories:* To attract patients in an increasingly competitive marketplace, health system marketing teams can publicize data about successful treatments for specific diagnostic categories.
- *Clinical data to generate evidence-based treatment guidelines:* **Evidence-based clinical practice guidelines** are explicit statements that guide clinical decision making and have been systematically developed from scientific evidence and clinical expertise to answer clinical questions; systematic use of these guidelines is termed evidence-based medicine (EBM).
- *Coded sets of high-quality clinical data for government and healthcare industry research:* Federal agencies, such as the Centers for Disease Control and Prevention (CDC), CMS, and the National Institutes of Health, as well local, state, and international healthcare organizations, and representatives of the pharmaceutical, medical supply, and healthcare equipment industries are all interested in using clinical data sets for research. For example, such data sets can be used by epidemiologists to study epidemics, by drug manufacturers to find evidence about the efficacy of medications, or by insurance companies to evaluate the cost-effectiveness of new medical technology and procedures.

Figure 1.2 identifies selected focus areas for the CDI program. CDI professionals can emphasize these areas during discussions with providers and other stakeholders to support the need for improved high-quality clinical documentation in the outpatient setting.

Figure 1.2. Selected uses of high-quality clinical documentation

- Quality of Care
- Provider Collaboration
- High-Quality Data
- Strategy & Operations
- Patient Outcomes
- Evidence-Based Treatments

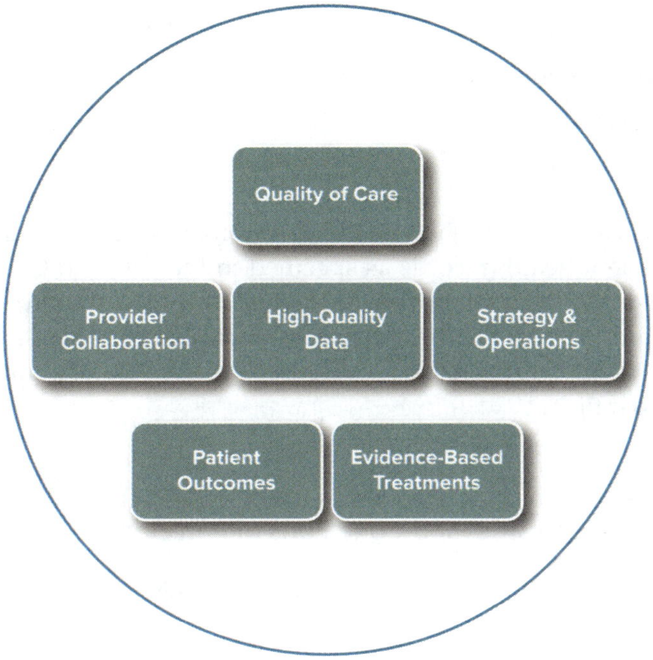

Selected Benefits of High-Quality Outpatient Clinical Documentation

The rationale for CDI in the outpatient setting touches on a variety of benefits associated with high-quality clinical documentation. Some of these benefits are further explored here.

Meeting Regulatory Requirements

High-quality clinical documentation helps healthcare entities and providers meet the regulatory requirements of the government and accreditation agencies. Among the most important US requirements are the **Conditions for Coverage (CfCs)** and **Conditions of Participation (CoPs)** issued by CMS to regulate the participation of healthcare entities in the Medicare and Medicaid programs. These health and safety standards, which are the foundation for improving quality and protecting the health and safety of beneficiaries, include guidelines for the continuum of care in the following outpatient settings (CMS 2013):

- Hospital swing beds
- Psychiatric hospitals
- Intermediate care facilities for individuals with intellectual disabilities
- Programs for all-inclusive care for the elderly
- Clinics, rehabilitation agencies, and public health agencies as providers of outpatient physical therapy and speech-language pathology services

- Religious nonmedical healthcare institutions
- Rural health clinics
- Long-term care facilities
- Organ procurement organizations
- Transplant centers
- Portable x-ray suppliers

Figure 1.3 provides an overview of the requirements for comprehensive and complete outpatient health records as specified in the CfC and CoP guidelines (CMS 2013). Overall, the components of the health record should be available, be consistent, and support the diagnoses and treatment provided to the patient (Cassidy 2012; CMS 2013). Chapter 4 discusses the regulatory framework for CDI in greater detail.

Figure 1.3. Health record–related Medicare and Medicaid Conditions for Coverage (CfCs) and Conditions of Participation (CoPs)

1. The medical record must contain information to justify the admission and continued hospitalization (in the outpatient setting, the outpatient encounter), support the diagnosis, and describe the patient's progress and response to medications and services.

2. All patient medical record entries must be legible, complete, dated, timed, and authenticated in written or electronic form by the person responsible for providing or evaluating the service provided, consistent with hospital outpatient clinic policies and procedures.

3. All records must document the following, as appropriate:

   - ✓ A medical history (in the outpatient setting, a chief complaint and history of present and chronic illnesses) and physical examination. A history and physical exam must be documented prior to surgery or a procedure requiring anesthesia services.
   - ✓ Admitting diagnosis (in the outpatient setting, a primary diagnosis for the encounter).
   - ✓ Results of all consultative evaluations of the patient and appropriate findings by clinical and other staff involved in the care of the patient.
   - ✓ Documentation of complications, hospital-acquired infections, and unfavorable reactions to drugs and anesthesia.
   - ✓ Properly executed informed consent forms for procedures and treatments specified by the medical staff, or by federal or state law if applicable, to require written patient consent.
   - ✓ All practitioners' orders, nursing notes, reports of treatment, medication records, radiology, laboratory reports, vital signs, and other information necessary to monitor the patient's condition.
   - ✓ Discharge summary with the outcome of hospitalization, disposition of case, and provisions for follow-up care (in the outpatient setting, a progress note for the outpatient visit and a summary progress note prior to release from outpatient surgery).
   - ✓ Final diagnosis.

Source: Adapted from CMS 2013

Maximizing Reimbursement

Improved documentation in outpatient and ambulatory settings can help providers maximize reimbursement under the payment models that have emerged in recent decades. Historically, US providers were reimbursed based on the volume of services they performed for patients (a **fee-for-service payment methodology**). For example, payers would reimburse providers for any diagnostic test as long as the clinical record included documentation that justified the medical necessity of the test. This arrangement increased the financial incentive to order multiple tests. In contrast, **risk-based payment methodologies** are more widely used today. Under risk-based payment plans, providers are reimbursed based on treatment outcomes, which increases their financial incentive to use the most effective and cost-efficient services and decreases their incentive to provide services that are less likely to improve outcomes. Examples of risk-based contracts range are (1) capitated payments based on a monthly payment covering enrollee care; (2) bundled payments that include services for a specific set of treatments, such as surgical and postoperative care for joint replacements; (3) Medicare contracts that offer shared savings; and (4) quality-based reimbursement that include quality-based bonuses and penalties (Barkholz 2016). Thus, as government and private risk-based incentive payment programs expand in the ambulatory setting, providers, patients, and payers all seek high-quality clinical documentation data to support the diagnoses and treatments provided in this setting.

Each insurance plan, including government plans, establishes rules for submitting reimbursement claims. To ensure that outpatient clinical documentation supports reimbursement, clinical documentation specialists (CDSs) should be familiar with the requirements of the major plans used by their health system. The specific insurance plan's guidelines for documentation can typically be found on the payer's website. For example, CMS publishes the Medicare Claims Processing Manual to govern the Medicare claims submission process, and the claims processing requirements for each state Medicaid program are found in the State Medicaid Provider Manual (CMS 2017a). These CMS manuals are updated annually around the start of the federal government's fiscal year (October 1), to correspond with changes in the *International Classification of Diseases, Tenth Revision, Clinical Modification* (ICD-10-CM), *International Classification of Diseases, Tenth Revision, Procedure Coding System* (ICD-10-PCS), Current Procedural Terminology (CPT), Healthcare Common Procedure Coding System (HCPCS), and **Hierarchical Condition Category (HCC)** code sets.

HCC coding is a payment model that identifies individuals with a serious or chronic illness and assigns a risk factor score to the person based upon a combination of the individual's health conditions and demographic details. The individual's health conditions are identified via ICD-10-CM diagnoses that are submitted by providers on incoming claims.

CDSs should keep abreast of changes to all applicable classification systems used in reimbursement, as they affect the correct claims process and prevent denials. Further details on the claims submission process are discussed in chapters 6 and 7 of this text.

The American Health Information Management Association (AHIMA) has published guidance for documenting a complete ambulatory record from a coding and reimbursement perspective (Cassidy 2012). The following are general examples of clinical documentation that may need to be included in an outpatient coding compliance policy:

- Emergency department records
- Medical history and physical examination findings (such as from outpatient or observation services)

- Procedure reports (such as from same-day surgery, gastrointestinal laboratory tests, interventional radiology, cardiac catheterization interventions)
- Progress notes
- Diagnostic testing results (such as pathology, laboratory, and imaging)
- Anesthesia records
- Authenticated physician orders for the services provided
- Diagnosis or reason for service
- Medication list
- Problem list
- Therapies

More specific information about these types of documentation are covered in chapter 2 and elsewhere in this textbook.

Preventing and Detecting Fraud, Waste, and Abuse in Healthcare

The federal government, healthcare entities, payers, and consumer watchdog groups are all interested in preventing and detecting fraud, waste, and abuse in healthcare. For example, the Office of Inspector General (OIG) of the US Department of Health and Human Services (HHS) is charged with oversight of Medicare, Medicaid, and other HHS programs. As part of its mission, OIG conducts independent audits of HHS programs, grantees, and contractors; investigates possible criminal, civil, and administrative cases of fraud and misconduct related to HHS programs, operations, and beneficiaries; and provides tools and education to help healthcare entities comply with OIG requirements (OIG n.d.). High-quality clinical documentation can minimize billing mistakes and help deter fraud, lower the risk for OIG audits, and allow healthcare entities to self-monitor for unnecessary services, unethical behavior in billing, and other problems related to waste and abuse (OIG 2000).

Measuring and Marketing Quality of Care

The federal government has established measures that will improve the quality of care by creating programs to make providers accountable through publicly available data (CMS 2017b). These quality measures are used for quality improvement, public reporting, and pay-for-performance programs. Data coded with ICD-10-CM, ICD-10-PCS, CPT, HCPCS, and HCC code sets are used to measure and report quality of care through online dashboards.

Private sector organizations also monitor the quality and safety of healthcare services, and their reports are used both by healthcare entities to publicize the quality of care they offer and by patients to identify the best providers for the services they seek. Examples of private organizations that measure quality and publish web-based comparisons of provider quality include the following:

- **The Joint Commission**, a not-for-profit organization that uses sets of standards to evaluate the quality of service delivery from healthcare entities such as hospitals, home care agencies, nursing care centers, behavioral healthcare centers, ambulatory care centers, and laboratory service providers. Healthcare entities may become accredited by the Joint Commission and earn certifications for specific programs and services. Accredited organizations are held to specific, self-reported quality performance measures, which are closely aligned with measures used by CMS (Joint Commission 2017).

- **Healthgrades**, an organization that provides online information on hospitals, physicians, and other healthcare providers to help consumers search for and select providers based on the providers' experience and their ratings for patient satisfaction and quality of care (Healthgrades 2017).
- The **Leapfrog Group**, a nonprofit organization that aims to promote healthcare quality and safety by collecting and reporting data about hospital performance (Leapfrog Group 2017). The organization also grades hospitals based on patient safety performance. Leapfrog Group survey results for specific hospitals are published for the following categories: inpatient care management, medication safety, maternity care, high-risk surgeries, and infections and injuries.

Promoting Evidence-Based Medicine

Evidence-based medicine (EBM) is the practice of medicine informed by the best scientific data available. It pursues optimal outcomes by relying on three key types of knowledge: research-based evidence (knowledge learned through research), clinical expertise (knowledge gained through practical experience), and the patient's values and preferences (knowledge learned through patient interactions) (Haughom n.d.). It aims to create and test standards in medical care, emphasizes peer-reviewed research, and operates within the framework of healthcare laws and regulations.

Patient-centered health record keeping and the evolving standards in CDI are closely tied to the practice of EBM (Hess 2015; Timmermans and Berg 2003). There are several ways that EBM advances healthcare, and, notably, CDI is involved in each:

- EBM generates current, standardized, evidence-based protocols. Clinical documentation supports evidence-based practice through the use of templates and standardized documentation processes that follow such protocols.
- EBM supports the use of up-to-date data to make clinical decisions. EHRs give providers immediate access to the patient's clinical history and help them follow clinical documentation guidelines and standards.
- EBM promotes transparency, accountability, and value in healthcare. Information available through EHR systems can help providers and CDSs understand the reasoning behind healthcare standards and policies, including those related to clinical documentation and reimbursement.
- EBM elevates the quality of healthcare. High-quality documentation facilitates collaboration among providers by helping them rapidly access and share the patient's clinical information and relevant evidence-based protocols.
- EBM improves healthcare outcomes. Clinical documentation systems not only give providers access to information on successful treatment methodologies but also can collect accurate and specific clinical data for future research on outcomes-based options. (Haughom n.d.)

Improving Population Health

Population health refers to the capture and reporting of healthcare data that are used for public health purposes, such as the tracking and trending of data on infectious diseases, immunizations, cancer, and other reportable conditions. Improving population health can therefore be understood as increasing positive health outcomes (for example, longevity of life) and decreasing adverse health outcomes (for example, incidence of a chronic disease) in the group. A population may be very large (such as all residents of the United States), or it may be more narrowly defined by specific characteristics (such as older adults living in skilled nursing facilities, employees of a particular company, or homeless people with mental illnesses who live in Chicago).

Population health research often focuses on which factors explain why some people in a population are healthy, while others in the same group are not. For example, researchers may look at whether certain dietary choices are associated with good health or whether access to affordable public transportation correlates with better health outcomes. Population health studies may also point to ways to reduce health risks, improve healthcare delivery, and lower the costs of healthcare throughout the population. The evolution of population health in the future depends on establishing benchmarks that can encourage change in the continuum of care (Kindig 2015). This focus on benchmarks requires accurate healthcare data, including from outpatient settings, about the population being studied. For example, CMS and other payers designing risk-based reimbursement methodologies are interested in learning about incentives that will encourage more people to make healthy lifestyle choices (such as exercising or quitting smoking), thereby lowering the costs of medical interventions. High-quality clinical data from primary care physicians, emergency departments, rehabilitation centers, and home care agencies could provide invaluable information about which incentives work for a given population.

The Challenges of Outpatient Clinical Documentation

Throughout the healthcare industry, CDI professionals often express concern when faced with the prospect of implementing and improving outpatient clinical documentation. Outpatient CDI covers a broad area of the continuum of care and involves many moving parts. The ambulatory record includes data from facility outpatient clinics, emergency departments, physician practices, urgent care facilities, rehabilitation centers, treatment centers, ambulatory surgery centers, home healthcare, and hospice. Given the range of providers and settings, the development of a best-in-class outpatient CDI program that provides consistent, reliable clinical records involves a multiplicity of challenges, including the following:

- *Physicians may be unaware of the need for improving clinical records in the outpatient setting.* This problem stems in part from the fact that medical school and residency programs do not typically teach clinical documentation practices (Hess 2015). Refer to chapter 13 for more information on physician training in clinical documentation requirements.
- *The quality of the outpatient clinical record may not be a top priority for leadership in the outpatient setting.* Chief financial officers and other leaders in

health systems and facilities may not recognize a return on investment (ROI) for CDI in an outpatient program. Therefore, the CDI leader must gather data and present a convincing argument for the ROI on outpatient CDI. Also, key clinic and physician practice leaders may need to be convinced that a governance model for outpatient CDI has value. It is important to identify formal and informal leaders in an organization to ensure "buy-in" and ownership of the process. A pilot project involving a large, high-profile service line and the corresponding physician practice is an excellent way to begin. Refer to chapters 5, 8, and 9 for more information on CDI program ROI and executive leader CDI program buy-in.

- *The clinical information in the outpatient setting may be spread across a variety of systems, which may not interface with each other.* To recommend system improvements and streamline accurate EHR documentation, the CDI team must assess the functionality of all related systems. Refer to chapter 7 for an overview of systems used to support CDI programs.

- *Multiple providers document in the clinical record in a variety of settings.* The CDI team can help these providers understand that a CDI program can lower the risk of inconsistent documentation of the diagnoses and treatments provided to the patient, thereby improving the quality of patient care and the accuracy of reimbursement. Refer to chapter 13 for a discussion of clinical documentation requirements for physicians and clinical staff.

- *Unstructured or inconsistent processes for EHR documentation and collection of patient data are prevalent.* CDI review of documentation practices as they relate to the EHR can help ensure accurate documentation practices among the providers. Refer to chapters 2 and 6 for further discussion on EHR documentation and its importance to CDI program goals and objectives.

- *CDI requires a skillful CDS team.* Figure 1.4 lists areas of expertise required of outpatient CDS teams, and chapter 9 discusses team-building in greater detail. Refer to chapter 12 for more information on the skill set requirements for CDS teams.

Although the challenges outlined here are substantial, they can be overcome. For example, relationship building and collaboration between CDI professionals and physicians can help address the physicians' knowledge gaps about CDI practices (see chapter 13). Selection of the right outpatient CDI program leader is the starting point for this project. The ideal leader will have extensive knowledge of industry and regulatory best practices for clinical documentation; health informatics and health information system functionality; outpatient reimbursement systems; coding in ICD-10-CM, CPT, HCPCS, and HCC; charge capture processes; physician communication and education; and project management. Because buy-in and program ownership by the executive and medical staff leadership are essential to program success, the selection of an outpatient CDI program leader who is known to the medical staff or the organization is recommended. After a comprehensive data analytics study is conducted and the ROI is determined, the CDI leader will be the one to develop a convincing argument for CDI and communicate it to health system leaders. Other CDI team members should also be selected carefully to ensure that their skills support those of the program leader. Refer to chapter 9 for additional information on building the CDI team.

Figure 1.4. Required areas of expertise for clinical documentation specialist teams in the outpatient setting

- Functionality of the health information systems' clinical and billing systems
- Best practices for clinical documentation in the ambulatory setting
- ICD-10-CM, CPT, HCPCS, and HCC coding
- Physician collaboration and communication
- Project management
- Documentation workflow
- Charge capture workflow
- Ambulatory reimbursement
- Quality scoring systems such as OPPS
- Risk adjustment
- Medicare Access and CHIP Reauthorization Act of 2015 (MACRA) and Quality Payment Program (QPP) framework for the Merit-Based Incentive Payment System (MIPS) and alternative payment models
- Hospital quality initiatives
- Critical thinking and root-cause determination related to coding and billing errors and claims denials
- Charge master description and fee-schedule development and evaluation

An outpatient CDI leader will be expected to manage the process, keep the spotlight on the project within the facility, and ensure that project goals and objectives are met. If there is a CDI program leader in the health information management organization who is already established within the facility, that person is recommended for this position. A secondary manager will also be needed to manage the day-to-day project and new workflows and processes established by the outpatient CDI taskforce.

Seven Criteria for Quality in Clinical Documentation

Requirements for quality clinical documentation in the outpatient setting are similar to the requirements in the inpatient setting. As illustrated in figure 1.5, the seven criteria used to evaluate clinical documentation are legibility, reliability, precision, completeness, consistency, clarity, and timeliness (Russo and Fitzgerald 2008; Russo 2007). These are fundamental expectations for clinical documentation in any setting and in any type of facility or professional practice. When these criteria are used to assess and improve the quality of documentation, the quality of other aspects of healthcare, such as reimbursement, quality indicators, research data, and patient care, will also improve. Research has proven that the use of the seven criteria during resident physician training directly correlates with the quality of resident physician documentation (Russo 2008). The criteria are further described in the following sections.

Figure 1.5. Criteria for high-quality clinical documentation

- Legibility
- Reliability
- Precision
- Completeness
- Consistency
- Clarity
- Timeliness
- Quality (center)

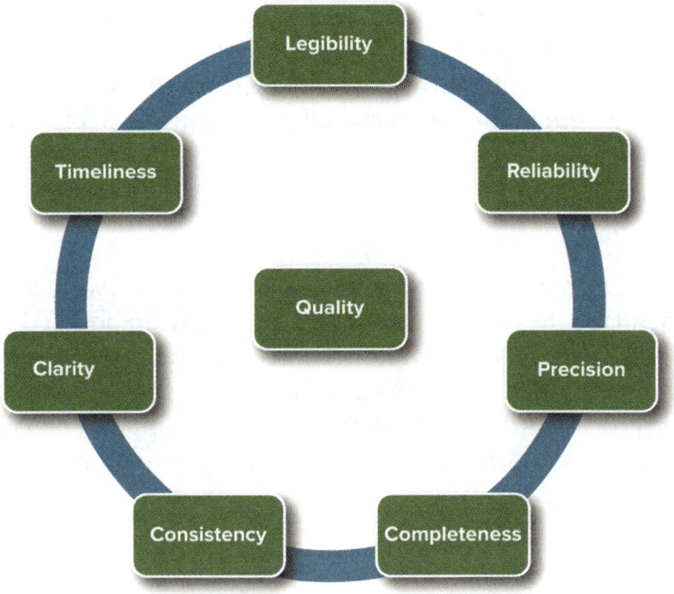

Source: Russo and Fitzgerald 2008; Russo 2007

Legibility

In clinical documentation, **legibility** means that provider entries and notations are readable. Illegible handwriting was a serious challenge to quality clinical documentation prior to the EHR. The issue is no longer as widespread, but many facilities and professional practices continue to handwrite documents. **Hybrid health records**, the combination of paper and electronic records, are used in many inpatient facilities. Where hybrid records exist, the handwritten notes are often scanned and added to the EHR. The Health Information Portability and Accountability Act of 1996 addresses illegible clinical records by stating that patients may request a clarification of information that is unreadable (Hess 2015).

Case Example

> A patient with Hunter syndrome visits a rural outpatient clinic for an infusion of idursulfase, a recombinant form of the human lysosomal enzyme iduronate-2-sulfatase. The date and time on the handwritten physician order for the medication are illegible. An audit by the payer results in a denial of reimbursement for this expensive therapeutic drug because proper documentation for the physician order is lacking.

Reliability

Reliability means the content of a record is trustworthy and safe and will yield the same result when repeated. A reliable record is an excellent tool for collaboration among providers to ensure high-quality patient care. A reliable record provides evidence of the patient's status at the time of the encounter.

Case Example

A patient is seen in the physician practice setting, and the documentation includes "history of cancer." However, the patient currently has cancer and is being treated at the hospital for chemotherapy and radiation therapy. Therefore, the "history of cancer" diagnosis is unreliable and could lead to denial of reimbursement to the physician practice for services related to cancer care.

Precision

Precision refers to a clinical record that is accurate and well defined so that the detail is available to support the clinical picture from both a diagnostic and a treatment perspective. An accurate record is essential when reporting clinical detail such as test results, vital signs, and other clinical indicators used in the diagnostic process. Adequate detail is critical to support such clinical information as vital sign patterns and trends, cardiology monitor data, medication records, and respiratory therapy data.

Case Example

A patient presents at the physician practice with shortness of breath and a history of chronic obstructive pulmonary disease (COPD). The physician notes that the patient's signs and symptoms include cough; thick, yellow-green sputum; stabbing chest pain that worsens with cough; sudden onset of chills; and a temperature of 104°F. The physician documents pneumonia in the record, and the coding professional codes the diagnosis as pneumonia, unspecified, and chronic COPD. However, an outpatient CDS hired to ensure capture of all HCCs reviews the record after the patient visit and identifies a potential HCC (bacterial pneumonia) based on the clinical documentation. The CDS queries the provider, who then documents the precise diagnosis of streptococcal pneumonia, based on a rapid strep test that was noted in the record, and the corresponding HCC is captured.

Completeness

Completeness refers to a clinical record that has the required content to provide a complete clinical picture of the patient encounter. The record must include the patient's chief complaint, the diagnostic test results, a record of the physician orders and reasons for them, therapy and procedure notes, nursing notes, and consultant provider and clinician notes. Examples of consulting clinician and provider notes include wound care clinic nursing notes, nutritionist consultations, and cardiology consultant physician notes.

Case Example

A patient presents at the outpatient clinic for treatment of multiple minor injuries related to an auto accident. The provider documents contusions, abrasions, and an abdominal laceration with repair. The patient reports severe pain in his ankle, and the physician orders a right ankle x-ray. However, the provider omits documentation of the severe ankle pain and possible right ankle fracture. Therefore, the payer denies the claim because the diagnoses required to demonstrate the medical necessity of the x-ray were not documented in the record and were not submitted in the final bill.

Consistency

Consistency refers to clinical documentation in which there are no contradictory statements from providers. For example, when the emergency department physician documents a diagnosis that is further refined and made more specific by another physician later in the encounter, the final diagnosis after study must be reinforced (made consistent) by documenting an explanation for the revised diagnosis. That can be done by documenting the initial diagnosis and reason for further specificity or alternate diagnosis.

Case Example

The patient presents to her primary care physician (PCP) for an annual checkup. The PCP documents hypertension and provides a refill prescription for lisinopril 10 mg orally once a day. The patient had also been recently seen by a cardiologist, who documented hypertensive heart disease with congestive heart failure (CHF). The PCP did not add the additional information to the progress note, and the coder submitted the claim with a diagnosis of hypertension. Therefore, the cardiologist's documentation and the primary care physician's record were inconsistent.

Clarity

Clarity refers to a clinical record that is comprehensible and distinct. Clinical documentation that is vague can be said to be ambiguous and therefore is often unclear. High-quality patient care relies in part on a clearly stated historical clinical record. The patient history is an important part of the provider's medical decision-making process.

Case Example

A patient presents to his family physician with chest pain. The physician is concerned and suggests that the patient go to the local emergency department for treatment. The diagnosis recorded on the progress note is "chest pain." The CDS reviews the record and queries the physician for the reason for the chest pain. The family practitioner documents that the patient had "unstable angina," which codes to HCC 87.

Timeliness

Timeliness refers to a clinical record that is available at the time it is needed for patient care delivery. Timeliness is one criterion that cannot be corrected after the fact—the legibility, reliability, precision, completeness, consistency, and clarity of a record can be addressed when a record is reviewed; however, once an entry is late, it remains late. The EHR helps improve the timeliness of documentation because the clinical record is often created at the time of patient care delivery.

Case Example

An observation admission summary is not documented until a week after the encounter. In the meantime, the patient is transferred to a nursing facility. The lack of availability of a timely admission summary might have implications for the continuity of care if the summary included information the nursing facility staff would need about the patient, such as diagnosis, ongoing therapies, current medications, and details related to activities of daily living.

Chapter 1 Review Exercises

1. Clinical documentation for inpatient, outpatient, and professional services are important to all of the following *except*:
    a. Interoperability
    b. Quality of patient care
    c. Efficacy of medications
    d. Tracking information on infectious diseases

2. Which users of clinical documentation focus on collaborating on patient care and aim to identify diseases, processes, and treatment options?
    a. Payers
    b. Providers
    c. Public health agencies
    d. Pharmaceutical companies

3. The success of the healthcare industry depends in part on clinical documentation efforts. The parties that use clinical data to assist in detecting and preventing potential fraud, waste, and abuse are:
    a. Health systems
    b. Research institutions
    c. Healthcare organizations
    d. Government organizations

4. Which of the following organizations provides certification for specific programs and services and grants accreditation for healthcare entities based on quality of service delivery?
    a. Healthgrades
    b. The Leapfrog Group
    c. The Joint Commission
    d. The Office of Inspector General

5. Implementing and improving outpatient clinical documentation presents challenges throughout the healthcare industry. Which of the following challenges involves issues related to knowledge of project management, clinical coding with ICD-10, CPT/HCPCS, and HCC coding, as well as documentation workflow?
    a. The need for a skillful CDS team
    b. Leadership not prioritizing the quality of the outpatient clinical record
    c. Multiple providers documenting in the clinical record in a variety of settings
    d. Physicians being unaware of the need for improving clinical records in the outpatient setting

6. Which of the criteria for evaluating clinical documentation is related to the accuracy of test results, vital signs, and other clinical indicators used to support the diagnostic and treatment pathway?
   a. Precision
   b. Reliability
   c. Consistency
   d. Completeness

7. The benefits of high-quality clinical documentation include meeting regulatory requirements; maximizing _____; preventing and detecting fraud, waste, and abuse in healthcare; measuring and marketing quality of care; promoting evidence-based medicine; and improving population health.
   a. Access
   b. Accuracy
   c. Efficiency
   d. Reimbursement

8. The seven criteria for high-quality clinical documentation in the outpatient setting are legibility, reliability, precision, completeness, consistency, clarity, and _____.
   a. Security
   b. Timeliness
   c. Availability
   d. Conciseness

9. When a health record is not contradictory, which of criteria for high-quality documentation does it meet?
   a. Clarity
   b. Precision
   c. Reliability
   d. Consistency

10. Pharmaceutical companies are interested in high-quality clinical documentation to gather information about the _____ of drugs.
    a. Efficacy
    b. Popularity
    c. Fraudulent usage
    d. Cost effectiveness

References

Barkholz, D. 2016 (June 18). Under construction: Risk-based reimbursement. *Modern Healthcare.* http://www.modernhealthcare.com/article/20160618/MAGAZINE/306189982.

Cassidy, B.S. 2012. Defining the core clinical documentation set for coding compliance. American Health Information Management Association (AHIMA). http://library.ahima.org/PdfView?oid=105782.

Centers for Medicare and Medicaid Services (CMS). 2017a. Manuals. https://www.cms.gov/Regulations-and-Guidance/Guidance/Manuals/index.html.

Centers for Medicare and Medicaid Services (CMS). 2017b. Quality Payment Program. https://qpp.cms.gov.

References

Centers for Medicare and Medicaid Services (CMS). 2013. Conditions for Coverage (CfCs) & Conditions of participation (CoPs). https://www.cms.gov/Regulations-and-Guidance/Legislation/CFCsAndCoPs/index.html?redirect=/CFCsAndCoPs.

Centers for Medicare and Medicaid Services (CMS). 2012. Electronic health records. https://www.cms.gov/Medicare/E-Health/EHealthRecords/index.html.

Haughom, J. n.d. 5 reasons the practice of evidence-based medicine is a hot topic. HealthCatalyst. https://www.healthcatalyst.com/5-reasons-practice-evidence-based-medicine-is-hot-topic.

Healthgrades. 2017. https://www.healthgrades.com.

Hess, P.C. 2015. *Clinical Documentation Improvement: Principles and Practice.* Chicago: AHIMA.

The Joint Commission. 2017. http://www.jointcommission.org.

Kindig, D. 2015. From health determinant benchmarks to health investment benchmarks. *Preventing Chronic Disease* 12:150010. DOI: 10.5888/pcd12.150010.

The Leapfrog Group. 2017. http://www.leapfroggroup.org.

Middleton, B., M. Bloomrosen, M.A. Dente, B. Hashmat, R. Koppel, J.M. Overhage, T.H. Payne, S.T. Rosenbloom, C. Weaver, and J. Zhang. 2013. Enhancing patient safety and quality of care by improving the usability of electronic health record systems: recommendations from AMIA. *Journal of Informatics in Health and Biomedicine* 20(e1): e2–e8.

Office of Inspector General (OIG), US Department of Health and Human Services. 2000. OIG compliance program for individual and small group physician practices. *Federal Register* 65(194): 59434–59452. https://oig.hhs.gov/authorities/docs/physician.pdf.

Office of Inspector General (OIG), US Department of Health and Human Services. n.d. About us. https://oig.hhs.gov/about-oig/about-us/index.asp.

Russo, R., and S. Fitzgerald. 2008. "Physician Clinical Documentation: Implications for Healthcare Quality and Cost." Presented at the Academy of Management annual meeting, Anaheim, CA.

Russo, R. 2008. *A Compelling Case for Clinical Documentation*, vol. 1. Bethlehem, PA: D J Iber Publishing.

Russo, R. 2007. *Improving Self-Efficacy and Organizational Performance: Identifying the Differences that May Exist from Educational Interventions Crafted to Utilize Two versus All Four Self-Efficacy Constructs* [dissertation]. Cypress, CA: Touro University International.

Timmermans, S., and M. Berg. 2003. *The Gold Standard: The Challenge of Evidence-Based Medicine and Standardization in Health Care.* Philadelphia: Temple University Press.

Sources and Types of Outpatient Clinical Documentation

2

Learning Objectives

- Discuss the sources of clinical documentation in the outpatient setting.
- Describe the types of clinical documentation in the outpatient setting.
- Identify the authors of clinical documentation in the outpatient setting.
- Discuss specific challenges to high-quality clinical documentation in the outpatient setting.
- Learn the knowledge-base requirements for the outpatient clinical documentation specialist.

Key Terms

Certified coding associate (CCA)
Certified coding specialist (CCS)
Certified coding specialist–physician-based (CCS-P)
Clinical documentation improvement practitioner (CDIP)
Current Procedural Terminology (CPT)
Deidentification
Designated record set
Encounter summary
Glasgow coma scale
Health Information Technology for Economic and Clinical Health (HITECH) Act
Health IT Standards Committee (HITSC)

Health Level Seven (HL7)
Healthcare Common Procedure Coding System (HCPCS)
Legal health record
Medication administration record (MAR)
Office of the National Coordinator for Health Information Technology (ONC)
Physician orders
Progress notes
Protected health information (PHI)
Relative value units (RVUs)
Treating providers
Virtual private network (VPN)
Vital signs flowsheet

Many of the sources of clinical documentation in the outpatient setting are similar to those of the inpatient setting, such as the patient history and physical examination, progress notes, procedure note, medication administration record, and physician orders, and are captured in the electronic health record (EHR). This chapter covers the sources and types of clinical information, clinical record contents, and authors of clinical information. The chapter will also discuss challenges in maintaining a high-quality outpatient clinical record and the role of the outpatient clinical documentation specialist (CDS).

Sources of Clinical Documentation

Clinical documentation is usually found in the EHR, a paper record, or a hybrid health record (a combination of EHR documentation and paper and scanned records). The EHR is generally the primary source for clinical documentation; however, CDSs are required to use *all* sources that are found in the health record or other documents about the care given to the patient.

EHRs

The use of EHRs was mandated as part of the **Health Information Technology for Economic and Clinical Health (HITECH) Act** of 2009, which was created to promote the adoption and Meaningful Use of health information technology in the United States. Subtitle D of HITECH provides for additional privacy and security requirements that will develop and support electronic health information, facilitate information exchange, and strengthen monetary penalties. Under HITECH, the principal federal entity charged with coordinating nationwide efforts to implement and use the most advanced health information technology and the electronic exchange of health information is the **Office of the National Coordinator for Health Information Technology (ONC)** (Charles et al. 2015).

EHRs have dramatically changed the ways that providers document in the clinical record. Rather than writing clinical information by hand in a paper chart at the hospital or physician practice, providers dictate or type documentation to create digital records. The Health Information Portability and Accountability Act of 1996 (HIPAA) has imposed requirements to make EHR data secure (HHS 2017). For example, a **virtual private network (VPN)** allows users to securely access a facility's or a practice's clinical records through a facility intranet, and the VPN must include security levels to satisfy HIPAA requirements. This technology allows providers to use laptops and other personal "smart" devices for clinical documentation from their offices, the patient examination room, their homes, or even the hospital cafeteria.

The **Health IT Standards Committee (HITSC)** makes recommended changes to the standards, implementation specifications, and certification criteria related to electronic healthcare data exchange. These recommendations are made to the Office of the National Coordinator for Health Information Technology (HITSC 2017).

Health Level Seven (HL7) is a set of standards for the exchange, integration, sharing, and retrieval of electronic health information (HL7 2017). Health Level Seven International, the organization, has grouped the HL7 standards into seven categories, as shown in table 2.1.

Table 2.1. Health Level Seven International's seven categories of HL7 standards

Section 1: Primary Standards	Primary standards are considered the most popular standards integral for system integrations, interoperability, and compliance. Our most frequently used and in-demand standards are in this category.
Section 2: Foundational Standards	Foundational standards define the fundamental tools and building blocks used to build the standards, and the technology infrastructure that implementers of HL7 standards must manage.
Section 3: Clinical and Administrative Domains	Messaging and documentation of standards for clinical specialties and groups are found in this section. These standards are usually implemented once primary standards for the organization are in place.
Section 4: EHR Profiles	These standards provide functional models and profiles that enable the constructs for management of electronic health records.
Section 5: Implementation Guides	This section is for implementation guides and/or support documents created to be used in conjunction with an existing standard. All documents in this section serve as supplemental material for a parent standard.
Section 6: Rules and References	Technical specifications, programming structures, and guidelines for software and standards development.
Section 7: Education and Awareness	Find HL7's Draft Standards for Trial Use (DSTUs) and current projects here, as well as helpful resources and tools to further supplement understanding and adoption of HL7 standards.

Source: HL7 2017

HL7 standardizes government specifications related to the development, adoption, use, and adherence of healthcare data exchange (HL7 2017). The standards are dynamic, and a process is in place to facilitate exchange of health information through a community of participants in the public and private sectors focused on tools, services, and guidance (ONC 2017).

Other Sources of Clinical Documentation

The use of paper records adds a workflow challenge for the CDS and others using the clinical record for patient care or business purposes. Paper records may be lost or illegible, or they may not be in one location. For example, the oncology clinic treatment records may be kept in the oncology department whereas the remaining outpatient records for the patient may be in the health information management department. If outpatient records are not in one location, it is difficult to make sure that all pertinent records are reviewed when evaluating clinical record quality and specificity. Facilities may also face this challenge during a payer audit of coding and billing compliance, which could result in denials of part or all of the audited claims due to missing information.

The existence of a hybrid health record may erroneously lead to the perception that all clinical records are included in the EHR. However, the CDS or a payer may review the EHR before all documents have been scanned. For example, if the cardiology diagnostic testing records are initially done on paper and not promptly entered into the EHR, the CDS or a payer may not know that the diagnostic test was performed. Thus, delays in scanning can result in payer denials or an ineffective clinical documentation workflow.

Types of Clinical Documentation

As discussed in chapter 1, the seven criteria for high-quality clinical documentation (the gold standard) must be met for each entry in the outpatient clinical record. Peer-reviewed research conducted on the quality of the patient record identified significant problems with the quality of the patient record in every type of health record studied (Hess 2015). CDSs play an important role is the improvement of the clinical record through collaboration with providers and through provider education on industry standards for clinical records.

The health record contains two types of information (Sayles 2014):

- *Clinical* information documents the patient's diagnoses and treatment provided.
- *Administrative* information documents demographic and financial information, as well as consents and authorizations.

Standards for healthcare records are established from the following four primary sources (Sayles 2014):

- *Facility-specific standards:* Developed and published in facility policies and procedures, these standards are established by the medical staff and are included in the medical staff bylaws, rules, and regulations.
- *Licensure requirements:* These are developed by the state or federal government entities that govern the licenses of practicing providers within their jurisdictions.
- *Certification standards:* These are established by government reimbursement programs, such as Medicare and Medicaid, and published in their Conditions of Participation or Conditions for Coverage.
- *Accreditation standards:* These are established by independent accrediting organizations, such as the Joint Commission, that develop standards for quality of care in the healthcare industry.

Designated Record Sets and Legal Records

Clinical record information is categorized into two types: the designated record set and the legal health record (AHIMA 2011). The **designated record set** includes the medical diagnostic and treatment information as well as the billing information related to enrollment, payment, and claims adjudication by the insurance payer. The **legal health record** is the official record of healthcare services delivered by a provider. This portion of the record is the business record for the healthcare institution; as a record of health status and documentation of care given, it facilitates business decision making and addresses the legal needs of the institution (AHIMA 2011). Table 2.2 elaborates on the definitions, purpose, content, and uses for the two types of clinical records.

Table 2.2. Comparison of the designated record set and the legal health record

	Designated Record Set	Legal Health Record
Definition	A group of records maintained by or for a covered entity that includes the medical and billing records about individuals; enrollment, payment, claims adjudication, and case or medical management record systems maintained by or for a health plan; information used in whole or in part by or for the HIPAA-covered entity to make decisions about individuals.	The business record generated at or for a healthcare organization. It is the record that would be released upon receipt of a request. The legal health record is the officially declared record of healthcare services provided to an individual delivered by a provider.
Purpose	Used to clarify the access and amendment standards in the HIPAA privacy rule, which provide that individuals generally have the right to inspect and obtain a copy of protected health information in the designated record set.	The official business record of healthcare services delivered by the entity for regulatory and disclosure purposes.
Content	Defined in organizational policy and required by the HIPAA privacy rule. The content of the designated record set includes medical and billing records of covered providers; enrollment, payment, claims, and case information of a health plan; and information used in whole or in part by or for the covered entity to make decisions about individuals.	Defined in organizational policy and can include individually identifiable data in any medium collected and directly used in documenting healthcare services or health status. It excludes administrative, derived, and aggregate data.
Uses	Supports individual HIPAA right of access and amendment.	Provides a record of health status as well as documentation of care for reimbursement, quality management, research, and public health purposes; facilitates business decision making and education of healthcare practitioners as well as the legal needs of the healthcare organization.

Source: AHIMA 2011

Protected Patient Information and Deidentified Records

Rules for releasing or sharing clinical records are established in the standards of the HIPAA privacy rule, which protects "individually identifiable health information transmitted or maintained by a covered entity or its business associates in any form or medium" (OCR 2015). According to the Office of Civil Rights (OCR) of the US Department of Health and Human Services (HHS), **protected health information (PHI)** is

> information, including demographic information, which relates to the individual's past, present, or future physical or mental health or condition, the provision of health care to the individual, or the past, present, or future payment for the provision of health care to the individual, and that identifies the individual or for which there is a reasonable basis to believe can be used to identify the individual. Protected health information includes many common identifiers (e.g., name, address, birth date, Social Security number) when they can be associated with the health information listed above. (OCR 2015)

As discussed in chapter 1, data from clinical documentation are used for wide-ranging purposes, such as population health research and analysis of risk-based payer plans. **Deidentification** of records allows for such uses of data without revealing the PHI of patients. When creating data sets, the following identifiers of the individual or of relatives, employers, or household members of the individual are types of PHI that are to be deidentified (OCR 2015):

- Names
- All geographic subdivisions smaller than a state, including street address, city, county, precinct, ZIP code, and their equivalent geocodes, except for the initial three digits of a ZIP code if, according to the current publicly available data from the Bureau of the Census:
  - The geographic unit formed by combining all ZIP codes with the same three initial digits contains more than 20,000 people; and
  - The initial three digits of a ZIP code for all such geographic units containing 20,000 or fewer people is changed to 000.
- All elements of dates (except year) for dates directly related to an individual, including birth date, admission date, discharge date, date of death; and all ages over 89; and all elements of dates (including year) indicative of such age, except that such ages and elements may be aggregated into a single category of age 90 or older
- Telephone numbers
- Fax numbers
- Electronic mail addresses
- Social Security numbers
- Medical record numbers
- Health plan beneficiary numbers
- Account numbers
- Certificate/license numbers
- Vehicle identifiers and serial numbers, including license plate numbers
- Device identifiers and serial numbers
- Web Universal Resource Locators (URLs)
- Internet Protocol (IP) address numbers
- Biometric identifiers, including fingerprints and voice prints
- Full face photographic images and any comparable images
- Any other unique identifying number, characteristic, or code, except as permitted by [HIPAA regulations]

Additional information on the HIPAA regulations related to PHI may be found on the HHS website (OCR 2015).

Categorizing Record Types in Clinical Documentation

Within the clinical record, there are a variety of record types, such as the patient history and physical examination, provider orders, diagnostic test results, progress notes, vital signs flowsheets, consultation reports, and procedure reports.

Figure 2.1. Types of records in clinical documentation

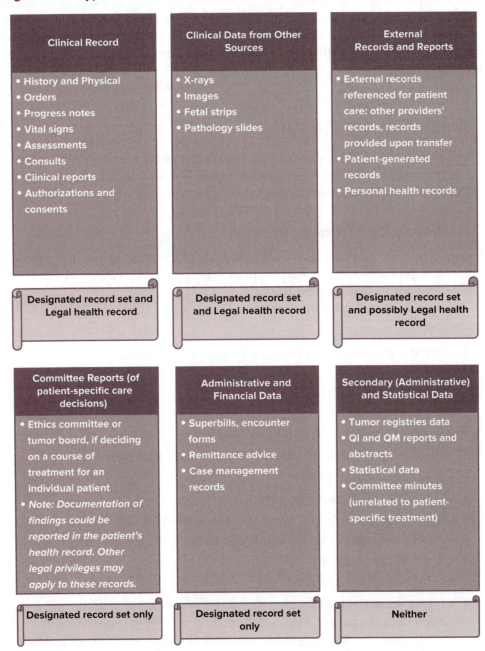

Source: AHIMA 2011

Figure 2.1 offers a visual depiction of the various record types and their categorization as a designated record set or legal health record. Categorizing record types can help organizations develop policies for each type of documentation.

Certain clinical records are found in both designated record sets and legal health records. Others are included in the designated record sets only. There are two points of view regarding the categorization of external records and reports. Some people contend that the external record set is part of the legal health record when the external records are used to make decisions. Those who hold the other view suggest that the organization should consult with internal legal counsel to determine how the external record should be categorized. At each facility, the health record committee responsible for clinical content and making decisions about categorizing records should discuss this matter. This committee is typically a medical staff committee with a functioning medical staff member as chair and the health information management director as the coordinator of the committee activities.

Clinical Record Contents

The clinical record includes a series of standard reports generated in most facilities and physician practices. The specific report format will vary depending on the EHR software and customization at each facility or practice.

Emergency Department Record

Emergency care documentation is limited to information about the patient's presenting problem and the diagnostic and therapeutic services provided during the episode of care (Sayles 2014).

The clinical record from the emergency department (ED) should include the following:

- Patient identification (or reason why it is not obtained)
- Time and means of the patient's arrival at the facility
- Pertinent history of the illness or injury and physician findings, including the patient's vital signs
- Diagnosis (or diagnoses) and procedures
- Emergency care given to the patient prior to or after arrival
- Presenting condition and initial assessment
- Diagnostic and therapeutic orders
- Clinical observations, including the results of treatment
- Reports and results of procedures and tests
- Diagnostic impressions
- Medication administered
- Conclusion at the termination of evaluation or treatment, including final disposition; the patient's condition on discharge or transfer; and any instructions given to the patient, the patient's representative, or another healthcare facility for follow-up care
- Documentation of cases when the patient left the facility against medical advice

The ED record is important for the identification of signs and symptoms as well as definitive diagnoses for ED patients, observation patients, and even ambulatory surgical patients in the outpatient setting. When signs and symptoms or less-specific diagnoses are found in the ED record, the CDS should clarify the information to determine the most specific diagnosis known at the time of the visit. When ED, observation, and ambulatory clinical records document diagnoses inconsistently, the CDS should clarify the diagnoses with the attending physician. For example, the CDS might find that the ED physician recorded a preliminary diagnosis of sepsis, but further details from the record do not provide clinical indicators for sepsis, and the treating physicians documented pneumonia as the primary diagnosis without recording sepsis in any other part of the record. In this case, a query should be submitted to the attending physician regarding the diagnosis of sepsis (Hess 2015).

Glasgow Coma Scale

The **Glasgow coma scale**, which may be part of a neurological assessment, provides an objective review of a patient's level of consciousness. The scale uses a point system to qualify responses from three categories: eye opening response, verbal response, and motor response. Examples of the point values for each of the three response areas are as follows:

Eye opening

- Spontaneous: 4
- To sound: 3
- To pressure: 2
- None: 1

Verbal response

- Oriented: 5
- Confused: 4
- Words: 3
- Sounds: 2
- None: 1

Motor response

- Obeys commands: 6
- Localizing: 5
- Normal flexion: 4
- Abnormal flexion: 3
- Extension: 2
- None: 1

Points from each category are added together for a total score. Brain injury is classified as severe for scores of 3 through 8, moderate for scores of 9 through 12, and minor for scores of 13 through 15 (Glasgow Coma Scale 2014). Where scores are beyond the normal ranges and no corresponding neurological diagnosis is present, the CDS should query the physician for clarification of the report findings.

Anesthesia Record

The anesthesiologist, midlevel practitioners (MLPs), and nursing staff create the anesthesia record, often by using a template. Diagnostic information that should be documented in the record includes any chronic conditions that the patient has, as well as any acute problems that have occurred during the current visit or during the surgery itself. Thus, the anesthesia record may capture distinctive details about the patient's history and complications occurring during the surgical procedure. For example, prior to surgery, the anesthesiologist discusses the patient's history with the patient and could add diagnoses not included in the patient history and physical examination documentation. These diagnoses may be coded and used to support the *International Classification of Diseases, Tenth Revision, Clinical Modification* (ICD-10-CM) and Current Procedural Terminology (CPT) codes as well as the medical necessity for services provided.

Anesthesiologists are considered treating physicians. Therefore, their documentation may be used for coding purposes. This point is clarified in *Coding Clinic*, the newsletter that is published by the American Hospital Association, the American Health Information Management Association (AHIMA), the Centers for Disease Control and Prevention National Center for Health Statistics (NCHS), and the Centers for Medicare and Medicaid Services (CMS) to provide advice on using the ICD-10-CM/PCS code sets. Where there may be conflicting information between the anesthesiologist and the attending or consulting physicians, the CDS should query for further clarification of the diagnostic information (AHA Second Quarter 2000, 15). In the outpatient setting, the anesthesiologist's documentation may be used for coding purposes and does not need to be clarified by the attending or other consulting physicians unless the information is conflicting (AHA Second Quarter 2000, 15).

Consultation Reports

Consultation reports document the opinions and findings of providers other than the attending physician. Consultations are normally requested by the attending physician and often related to a medical specialty–specific illness or condition. The *Coding Clinic* states that that the clinical record documented by any of the treating physicians may be used for coding purposes as long as there is no conflicting information from another physician. In those cases, a query should be submitted for clarification of the diagnostic information (AHA First Quarter 2004, 18–19).

In the inpatient setting, consultation reports are usually dictated into a standard format designed by the particular hospital. In the outpatient or physician office setting, the reports are provided in a letter format from the consulting physician to the requesting physician. Regardless of the format, all consultations must meet the seven criteria for high-quality clinical documentation (see chapter 1). Most consultations are requested to provide clarity and precision in a patient's diagnosis. Therefore, these two criteria are essential components in consultation documentation (Hess 2015).

Diagnostic Test Results

Diagnostic tests are performed in a variety of settings, including imaging, interventional radiology and cardiology, laboratory, respiratory therapy, and neurology. The results are important clinical indicators used by physicians for diagnostic medical decision making. When CDSs review clinical documentation, they can query the provider for clarification if they identify abnormal clinical indicators without a corresponding diagnosis.

In both the outpatient and inpatient settings, diagnostic tests with corresponding interpretations and final report from the treating physician may be used for coding purposes. The key phrase is "treating physician." If the test result is documented by a practitioner other than a treating physician, such as a diagnostic cardiologist or pathologist, diagnostic information must be clarified by an attending or other treating physician before the information may be used for coding purposes. In outpatient settings, rule-out and suspected conditions are not coded as definitive diagnoses. Instead, the sign or symptom must be coded as the final diagnosis (CMS and NCHS 2018, 107). As explained later in this chapter, this rule for coding signs and symptoms does not apply in the inpatient setting (see Patient History and Physical Examination section).

Encounter Summary

An **encounter summary** includes information related to the diagnosis, treatment, prognosis, and instructions for follow-up care. In this way, the content in an encounter summary in outpatient care is similar to the information found in a discharge summary in the inpatient setting. However, the discharge summary presents the diagnoses, treatment, and medical decision-making process during the entire inpatient stay, whereas an encounter summary is a briefer record of a short stay. This type of report is often created in the ambulatory surgery or observation setting and is less commonly used for a physician practice or urgent care visit.

Patient History and Physical Examination

The patient's history includes information about the patient's chief complaint and history of present illness, past medical diagnoses, and treatments. Physical examination information for the history and physical report may be taken and documented by house staff or midlevel practitioners, but the attending physician has a signature and ultimate responsibility for the quality of this document (42 CFR 412.46). The timeliness and legibility of the patient history and physical are essential in clinical documentation because all clinicians treating the patient rely on this content.

Other criteria of high-quality clinical documentation that may be an issue in the patient history and physical examination include clarity and completeness. If the author of the patient history and physical examination records knows or believes that a diagnosis is present, that diagnosis should be documented. If the diagnoses are differential, ruled out, probable or possible, or not established at the time of the writing, the author should document these points as well (Hess 2015). In the outpatient setting, probable, possible, suspected, and rule-out conditions are coded using the signs and symptoms listed in the clinical documentation. This coding rule is not used in the inpatient setting, where probable, possible, suspected, and rule-out conditions are coded as definitive diagnoses. For example, in the inpatient setting, a patient presenting with chest pain, "rule-out acute myocardial infarction" would be coded as an acute myocardial infarction. The same patient seen in the outpatient setting would be coded as having a final diagnosis of chest pain. This information is clarified in the *ICD-10-CM Official Guidelines for Coding and Reporting* (CMS and NCHS 2018, 107).

Medication Administration Record

The **medication administration record (MAR)** documents all medications given to a patient during the patient encounter. Figure 2.2 includes data from an example MAR. It lists the medications currently being given (benazepril) and medication that has been discontinued (esomeprazole). For the CDS, the report is a useful tool for identifying possible physician queries. The CDS and coding staff should be familiar with the common medications given and their purposes. When medications are given but do not have a corresponding diagnosis in the record, a physician query may be required. For example, vancomycin, cefuroxime, ceftriaxone, clindamycin, and gentamicin are antibiotic medications used to fight infections, including those related to sepsis. If the record shows that any of these drugs were administered intravenously but a corresponding diagnosis related to infection is not documented by the physician, a clarification should be submitted to the provider to determine the reason why the antibiotic was ordered. Further discussions of the physician query process are found in chapters 12, 15, and 16 of this textbook.

Figure 2.2. Medical administration record (MAR) example

Current Medications										
Medication Orders	11/11	11/12	11/13	11/14	11/15	11/16	11/17	11/18	11/19	11/20
benazepril (Lotensin) Dose: **40 mg** Freq: **Daily** Route: **Oral** Associated Diagnosis: **Hypotension** Start: **11/12 18:30** End: **11/20 18:30**		18:25	18:15	18:31	18:23	18:24	18:26	18:27	18:22	18:20
Discontinued										
Medication Orders	11/11	11/12	11/13	11/14	11/15	11/16	11/17	11/18	11/19	11/20
esomeprazole sodium (Nexium) Dose: **20 mg** Freq: **Daily** Route: **Oral** Associated Diagnosis: **Gastroesophageal Reflux Disease** Start Date/Time: **11/11 12:00** End Date/Time: **11/12 12:00**	12:00	11:55								

Operative and Procedure Reports

Complete documentation for a surgical procedure includes operative progress notes and an operative report. The surgeon documents brief operative notes in the patient record immediately before and after surgery. The complete operative report should be dictated within 24 hours of the procedure by the surgeon or a house staff physician who assisted in the surgery (42 CFR 412.46; Joint Commission 2017).

Common documentation problems in operative notes are lack of clarity and precision. In some cases, the operative note provides greater specificity than is found in the patient history and physical examination documentation. For example, the history and physical exam records might list a diagnosis of hip fracture whereas the operative note documents a subcapital neck fracture, right hip (Hess 2015). In this case, the CDS would query the physician for the specificity related to the site of the hip fracture or subcapital neck fracture versus other possible femoral fracture sites.

Physician Orders

Physician orders document the specific instructions for patient interventions, such as medications, diagnostics tests, therapies, or other treatments (Sayles 2014). Today, many hospitals use computerized provider order entry systems to ensure the accuracy and reliability of orders. In organizations that still use manual systems, physicians can enter orders themselves, but most physicians give verbal or telephone orders to a member of the nursing staff. Most facilities require that a verbal order is signed within 24 hours. Chapter 3, Section 3.3.2.4, "Signature Requirements" of the *Medicare Program Integrity Manual* provides the CMS guidelines on signature requirements (CMS 2017a). Documentation concerns include completeness; the record must include a diagnosis or reason for the test, medication, or other treatment being ordered (Hess 2015). With regard to Medicare reimbursement, CMS (2017b) advises that

> If admission order language used to specify inpatient or outpatient status is ambiguous, the best course of action would be to obtain and document clarification from the ordering practitioner before initial Medicare billing (ideally before the beneficiary is discharged). Under this policy, CMS will continue to treat orders that specify a typically outpatient or other limited service (e.g., admit "to ER [emergency room]," "to Observation," "to Recovery," "to Outpatient Surgery," "to Day Surgery," or "to Short Stay Surgery") as defining a non-inpatient service, and such orders will not be treated as meeting the inpatient admission requirements.

Problem List

The problem list is a list of illnesses, injuries, and other factors that affect the health of an individual patient, usually identifying the time of occurrence or identification and resolution. Problem lists can be a useful tool in inpatient, outpatient facility, and physician office clinical records for facilitating continuity of care between patient visits, providing a comprehensive list of patient problems for use in patient care and secondary data reporting, and serving as a communication vehicle during transitions of care and between care providers (Acker et al. 2011). The problem list also standardizes and provides structure to clinical documentation in the outpatient setting by presenting an easy-to-locate list of historical diagnoses that should be considered during concurrent encounters. The list creates structured data rather than free-text documentation of historical diagnoses and can be more easily used for data analytics queries and reporting.

Some healthcare entities have not adopted a facility-specific clinical record standard for including problem lists. However, when problem lists are used, they must be reliable. Documentation in a problem list that is inconsistent with entries in the patient's record makes the list unreliable and, more importantly, can result in quality-of-care concerns for the patient. The advent of the EHR has resulted in the overuse of the copy/paste functionality in clinical documentation. Often, the entire problem list is copied into the final progress note or visit summary, which creates the appearance that all the diagnoses on the list are pertinent to the current admission. During the coding process, diagnoses in the problem list should be validated by the remaining clinical record for the specific encounter.

When health systems use a comprehensive EHR system for all settings, careful consideration should be given to the structure and location of the problem lists used for documentation within each setting. Providers should be educated in the proper use of the problem list within each setting and how the list should be used as it relates to coding and billing.

The American Recovery and Reinvestment Act of 2009 provides specific guidance regarding the use of problem lists as part of the Meaningful Use incentive program. Stage 1 Meaningful Use requirements state that the provider must document an up-to-date list of current diagnoses with associated ICD-10-CM codes (ARRA 2009). Figure 2.3 lists each Stage 1 Meaningful Use requirement for the EHR. The Medicare Access and CHIP Reauthorization Act of 2015 (MACRA) has incorporated the Meaningful Use of health information technology regulations. MACRA repeals the sustainable growth rate methodology for determining updates to the Medicare Physician Fee Schedule. It establishes annual positive or flat fee updates for 10 years and institutes a two-track fee update beginning in 2019, and it establishes the Merit-based Incentive Payment System that consolidates existing Medicare quality programs. It also establishes a pathway for physicians to participate in an Alternative Payment Model (APM) (MACRA 2015). MACRA will be discussed further in chapter 4 of this text.

Figure 2.3. Problem list requirements for EHRs

Stage 1 Meaningful Use final rule requirements for EHR systems
Capable of electronically exchanging key clinical information (e.g., **problem list**, medication list, allergies, and diagnostic test results) among care providers and patient-authorized entities.
Provides patients with an electronic copy of their health information (including diagnostic test results, **problem list**, medication lists, and allergies) upon request.
Provides patients with timely electronic access to their health information (including lab results, **problem list**, medication lists, and allergies).
Provides clinical summaries, including patient **problems**, for each office visit.
Generates lists of patients by specific conditions for quality improvement, reduction of disparities, research, and outreach. The user will be able to electronically select, sort, retrieve, and generate lists of patients according to, at a minimum, the data elements included in the **problem list**, medication list, demographics, and laboratory test results.
Sends reminders to patients per patient preference for preventive or follow-up care based on data elements included in the **problem list**.

Source: Acker et al. 2011

These Meaningful Use requirements should be used by the clinical documentation improvement (CDI) team as guidance for the development of a compliant problem list. Where facilities identify issues related to inconsistent problem list documentation, a redesign of the documentation model with corresponding education should be considered so that the problem list will be effective for care planning and effective provider communication.

Progress Notes

Progress notes include clinical observations related to the patient diagnosis and subsequent treatments. The notes are documented by clinicians such as physicians, nurses, and allied health professionals. Today, most progress notes are integrated into the health record so that caregivers can reference the progress notes of other caregivers before and after their own entries. Primary concerns about the quality of documentation in progress notes include legibility, precision, clarity, and timeliness. CDSs often review the progress notes to connect ancillary report findings to a diagnosis. For example, if a patient's radiology film is positive for pneumonia, the attending physician must document the type of pneumonia (such as lower lobe) and the planned treatment (such as a course of intravenous antibiotics).

Vital Signs Flowsheet

The **vital signs flowsheet** documents the patient's height, weight, temperature, pulse, respiration, oxygen level (SpO_2), blood pressure (BP), and position, over time. The data captured in this document are applicable to the entire patient record and are especially important when reviewing the ED provider documentation. The flowsheet helps identify symptoms related to conditions such as infections (above-normal temperatures), hypertension (high BP), hypotension (low BP), and respiratory insufficiency or failure, and can be used for tracking a patient's response to treatment over time. Figure 2.4 is an example of a vital signs flowsheet. Note that the flowsheet records an above-normal BP reading at 4:30 a.m. (130/95 mmHg) and normal BP readings at 12:30 p.m. (119/78 mmHg) and 8:30 p.m. (116/75 mmHg). The morning BP is flagged in red to highlight the abnormal results. This flowsheet provides valuable clinical information related to the patient's temperature, blood pressure, and weight change. When vital signs are outside the normal range or there is an unusual increase or decrease in weight, the CDS should query the physician if these clinical findings are not associated with a definitive diagnosis already recorded in the clinical record.

Figure 2.4. Vital signs flowsheet example

Vital Signs Flowsheet (12/18/17)					
Vitals	12/18/17 04:30	12/18/17 08:30	12/18/17 12:30	12/18/17 16:30	12/18/17 20:30
Height	5'10"	5'10"	5'10"	5'10"	5'10"
Weight	175	173	169	170	173
Temperature	36.7 C (98.1 F)	37.0 C (98.6 F)	36.9 C (98.5 F)	36.4 C (97.5 F)	36.3 C (97.3 F)
Temperature source	Oral	Oral	Oral	Oral	Oral
Pulse Rate	67	80	78	73	65
Respiratory Rate	13	20	19	17	12
SpO_2	95%	94%	95%	97%	96%
Blood Pressure	130/95 mmHg		119/78 mmHg		116/75 mmHg
Blood Pressure Location		Right arm		Left arm	
Patient Position		Prone		Sitting	

Outpatient Records by Settings

Outpatient clinical records are found in a variety of settings. The types of content in these records tend to be similar across settings but may vary somewhat among various facilities and physician practices. The format of each record type will vary depending on the EHR software and individual facility or practice customization of each record type. Table 2.3 provides a list of possible document types. A check is placed in the corresponding column to indicate the outpatient site where the record is typically found. For example, the anesthesiology record may be found in all five settings.

Table 2.3. Outpatient record categories by type of setting

	Outpatient Clinic	Emergency Department	Ambulatory Surgery	Urgent Care Center	Physician Practice
Anesthesiology record	✔	✔	✔	✔	✔
Consultation report	✔	✔			
Diagnostic test results	✔	✔	✔	✔	✔
Encounter summary (final progress notes)		✔	✔		
External provider records	✔		✔		✔
Patient history and physical examination	✔	✔	✔	✔	✔
Medication administration record	✔	✔	✔	✔	✔
Operative or procedure report	✔	✔	✔	✔	✔
Physician orders	✔	✔	✔	✔	✔
Problem list	✔				✔
Progress notes	✔	✔	✔	✔	✔
Vital signs flowsheet	✔	✔	✔	✔	✔

The CDS plays an important role in the customization of the EHR to support clinical CDI program initiatives in outpatient settings. The following case example presents a possible improvement to the documentation of diabetes-related conditions.

Case Example

A CDI program was focusing on the implementation of an outpatient CDI initiative for a primary care practice when an audit of practice records identified a clinical documentation gap trend for patients with diabetes: Providers were not specific when recording a diagnosis of diabetes related to a secondary condition such as diabetic retinopathy, diabetic peripheral neuropathy, diabetic peripheral vascular disease, or diabetic pressure ulcers. The CDI physician collaboration team met to discuss options for EHR functionality that would resolve the documentation gap. The team included the information technology department's health informaticist in the discussion. After the meeting, a feature was added to the EHR to launch a pop-up menu to help prompt providers to document diabetes, if appropriate, along with any of the aforementioned secondary conditions. When providers used the menu, the EHR recorded the link between the two diagnoses in the clinical record. This change in EHR functionality resulted in an improved Hierarchical Condition Category (HCC) payment rate because a diagnosis of diabetes was more often linked to the secondary conditions in the documentation. The Balanced Budget Act of 1997 enacted and CMS implemented the risk-adjusted payment methodology to include HCC codes (CMS 2017c). The HCC risk-adjusted payment system uses chronic illness ICD-10-CM codes and a corresponding HCC code and weight table to establish a payment to the Medicare Advantage Plans. Additional information on HCC risk adjustment may be found in chapters 5 and 6 of this textbook.

Authors of Clinical Documentation

Many types of healthcare practitioners and clinicians can contribute to outpatient clinical documentation. The following sections provide information about their roles in the documentation process.

Attending Physicians

In the outpatient setting, the attending physician is the physician of record who is responsible for the care and treatment of the patient. For example, in the ED setting, the attending physician may be called in at the request of the ED physician after the initial triage, diagnosis, and urgent treatment is completed. The care of the patient is then transferred to the attending physician. If there is any inconsistency in documentation from the different physicians treating a patient, the attending physician is responsible for providing the final documented response (Hess 2015).

Consultants

As noted earlier in this chapter, the attending physician can ask physician specialists (such as oncologists, cardiologists, or infectious disease specialists) to act as consultants for a patient case. Under these circumstances, the physician consultant is responsible for documenting and authenticating the consultation report. If the consultant is asked to continue to follow the patient, the consultant is also responsible for documenting progress notes in the patient's record (Hess 2015). Diagnoses documented by the consultant may be used for coding purposes. Where there is a conflict between the consultant and the attending physician documentation, a clarification should be submitted to the attending physician, who is the person charged with making the final decision on the diagnosis used for coding purposes.

House Staff

House staff physicians, also known as *interns, residents,* and *fellows,* are treating physicians, but they have less accountability than other physicians because they cannot serve as attending physicians in the inpatient setting. Nevertheless, house staff physicians have the same level of responsibility as all physicians for consistently documenting patient care with high-quality clinical documentation criteria. House staff physicians often have the primary responsibility for documenting the patient history and physical examination, operative reports (for surgical house staff), and the discharge summary on behalf of the attending physician. They are also responsible for documenting a progress note for each patient visit that they conduct (Hess 2015).

Surgeons

If a patient undergoes surgery during the hospital visit, the patient will have an attending surgeon. That surgeon, often referred to as the *primary surgeon*, is responsible for documenting the pre- and postoperative progress notes as well as the operative report. In a teaching hospital, a surgical house staff physician who assists during surgery may dictate the operative report, but the attending surgeon is responsible for reviewing, approving, and signing the report.

Sometimes, the attending surgeon will also be the attending physician for the patient. In this case, the surgeon has the same responsibility and accountability for documentation as the attending physician. In other instances, the patient is treated by a primary care physician or other medical specialist who serves as the patient's attending physician, and the surgeon's documentation responsibilities and accountability are limited to the surgical care of the patient (Hess 2015).

Diagnosticians

Diagnosticians are typically not involved in the direct treatment of a patient. These professionals include radiologists, nuclear medicine physicians, and other diagnostic specialists whose primary role is to review film and test results of patients, interpret the information, and provide a diagnosis. In this role, the diagnostician's primary documentation responsibility is to document the test results and provide a diagnosis consistent with the criteria for high-quality clinical documentation. On its own, documentation from diagnosticians cannot be used for diagnostic coding purposes because diagnosticians are not treating physicians. In other words, if the physician does not have direct, "hands-on" contact with the patient, the documentation must be validated by the treating providers. **Treating providers** are those individuals licensed to practice medicine in the specific state and authorized by the medical staff bylaws. Types of treating providers include doctors of medicine, doctors of osteopathy, nurse practitioners, and physician assistants. (Refer to the discussion of nonphysician practitioners later in this chapter for more information.)

If diagnosticians become involved in direct patient care, they are considered to be consultants and held to the same level of documentation responsibility and accountability as other consulting physicians. For example, when interventional radiologists, interventional cardiologists, and anesthesiologists provide hands-on care of a patient, their documentation is acceptable for final diagnosis code assignment (Hess 2015).

Physician Executives

Physician executives in hospitals may or may not provide patient care. When physician executives admit and treat patients, their documentation responsibilities are consistent with those of an attending physician. Many physician executives serve as the physician leader for their hospital's clinical documentation program. If physician executives are also admitting or treating patients, they can serve as examples to their fellow physicians regarding how to practice high-quality clinical documentation.

However, it is imperative that physician executives limit their documentation only to patients they are treating. In their role as clinical documentation leaders, physician executives may be reviewing the records of fellow physicians and querying physicians when the records do not meet the criteria for high-quality clinical documentation. To help with CDI, they can ask other providers open-ended questions that are based on the criteria of high-quality clinical documentation, but executives must not tell or ask a treating physician to document something specifically in the patient's record (Hess 2015).

Nonphysician Practitioners

As explained in the following sections, several types of nonphysician practitioners may be authors of clinical documentation, although coding regulations limit the use of their documentation for coding diagnoses and procedures.

Midlevel Practitioners

MLPs such as nurse practitioners and physician assistants can play an important independent role in the delivery of care as well as a role supporting physicians in the delivery of care. State laws define the scope of an MLP's independent activities. In general, most states require physician supervision of the MLP. Because of the important role MLPs play in patient care, their training in clinical documentation is an essential part of an organization's clinical documentation program (Hess 2015).

Nurses

Nurses document extensively in a patient's clinical record. Much of the nurse's documentation involves recording data such as body temperature, input and output, and other objective or subjective indicators of the patient's current status. Nurses enter progress note data, usually in integrated progress notes with other caregivers. They may also review other portions of the patient's record and are aware of all activity involving the patient. Nurses may, therefore, be in one of the best positions to identify problems related to deficiencies in clinical documentation. However, the nurse's responsibilities are focused on giving care to the patient, not evaluating documentation across the continuum of care. Because of their unique position in giving care and providing clinical documentation, nurses should be trained in the principles of clinical documentation to ensure that their records are complete and specific for each encounter with the patient.

Wound care nurses document details of the diagnosis and treatment for patients with diagnoses such as decubitus ulcer, cellulitis, and wound infection. The stage of the decubitus ulcer documented in the bedside nurse's, wound care nurse's, or physical therapist's note may be used for final coding purposes (Ericson 2014). To reinforce this concept, the 2018 *Official Guidelines for Coding and Reporting* verify that pressure ulcer stage is among the types of information documented by nonprovider clinicians such as a nurse or a wound care nurse (CMS and NCHS 2018).

Nutritionists

Even healthcare professionals may not know that many patients receive consultations from state-licensed nutritionists (also known as *dietitians*) during their hospital stay (Hess 2015). In general, these consultations are reserved for more complex cases, such as a patient with uncontrolled diabetes, morbid obesity, or severe malnutrition. Nutrition staff members have a unique opportunity to document patient nutrition–related and metabolic disorders with great precision. However, unless they are trained in the principles of high-quality clinical documentation, they may document a patient simply with malnutrition instead of documenting severe protein-calorie malnutrition or other diagnosis that more precisely represents the patient's condition.

A nutritionist's documentation cannot be used to translate patient health record documentation into coded data, but it can be used to ask a physician whether the clinical evidence supports a more precise diagnosis. A nutritionist's note may be used to identify the patient's body mass index for coding purposes; however, the physician must be the one to diagnose and document obesity (AHA Fourth Quarter 2005, 96–98). From a compliance perspective, it is vitally important to review the latest HHS Office of Inspector General guidance regarding the coding of severe malnutrition as a secondary diagnosis based solely on the nutritionist's documentation (OIG 2017).

Therapists

The list of types of therapists practicing in healthcare is quite long, and, depending on the patient's condition, different therapists play essential roles in the healing process. All therapists who care for patients (such as respiratory, physical, and occupational therapists) should be identified and trained in the principles of clinical documentation. Like nutritionists, therapists have an opportunity to document the patient's condition in a precise manner. However, unless therapists are trained in the principles of clinical documentation, they are unlikely to document in a manner that consistently results in high-quality clinical documentation (Hess 2015).

Complementary and Integrative Medicine Practitioners

Complementary and integrative medicine (CIM) practitioners include acupuncturists, naturopathic doctors, and chiropractors, among others. CIM practitioners are responsible for documenting progress notes that detail the care they provide to the patient. They may also be asked to provide an initial consult and assessment, in which case they will document a report of their findings and recommendations, similar to the report of a consultant. These practitioners have the same responsibility and accountability for documentation as other caregivers, and they must meet the criteria for high-quality clinical documentation (Hess 2015).

Clinical Documentation Challenges in the Outpatient Setting

Outpatient clinical records offer specific challenges for the CDS, including the coding and reimbursement systems used in outpatient settings; unique coding guidelines for outpatient encounters; the scarcity of CDSs skilled in outpatient clinical documentation; and requirements to document the medical necessity of services performed in brief encounters.

Outpatient Coding and Reimbursement Systems

Outpatient services can involve coding and reimbursement systems unlike those used for inpatient services. For example, physician fee schedules may be based on **relative value units (RVUs)**, which are numbers assigned to a procedure that describe its relative difficulty and expense (compared with other procedures) by weighting such factors as personnel, time, and level of skill. Other examples include the Outpatient Prospective Payment System (OPPS), which is based on ambulatory payment classifications (APCs), and risk-based payer methodologies based on HCCs. Each coding and reimbursement system requires specific clinical documentation to support medical necessity, accurate coding, and claims submission.

Outpatient-Specific Coding and Billing Guidelines

The guidelines for coding applied in the outpatient setting are different from those applied in the inpatient setting. This fact is relevant because the use of documentation from different providers will vary depending on the differences in coding guidelines that apply to their services. Given the volume and briefness of outpatient visits, the levels of uncertainty and lack of clarity in coding requirements are greatly increased in the outpatient setting. Therefore, both management and clinical teams must be highly proactive to ensure accurate and timely documentation (Hess 2015). Refer to table 2.4 for a list of classification systems used to code patient care in outpatient settings.

Table 2.4. Outpatient classification systems

Classification System	Clinical Data Coded	Maintained By	Clinical Setting
ICD-10-CM	Clinical documentation related to diagnoses	Cooperating Parties: American Health Information Management Association, the American Hospital Association, the Centers for Medicare and Medicaid Services, and the National Center for Health Statistics	Outpatient facility and medical practice
HCPCS Level I: Current Procedural Terminology (CPT) Codes	Clinical documentation related to procedures	American Medical Association (AMA)	Outpatient facility and medical practice
Healthcare Common Procedure Coding System (HCPCS) Level II: CPT Codes	Various items and services that are not included in the CPT medical code set, such as medical supplies	CMS, Blue Cross Blue Shield Association (BCBSA), Health Insurance Association of America (HIAA)	Outpatient facility and medical practice
Ambulatory payment classification (APC)	HCPCS codes are crosswalked to APC groups as part of the Outpatient Prospective Payment System (OPPS)	CMS	Outpatient facility
Relative value units (RVUs)	HCPCS codes are crosswalked to RVUs as part of the Medicare Physician Fee Schedule	CMS, AMA	Medical practice
Hierarchical Condition Categories (HCCs)	Clinical documentation related to chronic illness diagnoses	CMS	Outpatient facility and medical practice

ICD-10-CM is the industry standard coding system for diagnoses in the outpatient setting. The CPT and Healthcare Common Procedure Coding System (HCPCS), as updated by CMS, are the standard coding systems for classifying procedures in the outpatient setting. **Current Procedural Terminology (CPT)** is a comprehensive, descriptive list of terms and associated numeric and alphanumeric codes used for reporting diagnostic and therapeutic procedures and other medical services performed by physicians; it is published and updated annually by the American Medical Association. **Healthcare Common Procedure Coding System (HCPCS)** is a healthcare code set that identifies healthcare procedures, equipment, and supplies for claims submission purposes. It has been selected for use in transactions regulated by HIPAA. HCPCS Level I contains numeric CPT codes, which are maintained by the AMA. HCPCS Level II contains alphanumeric codes used to identify various items and services that are not included in the CPT medical code set. These codes are maintained by CMS, the Blue Cross Blue Shield Association, and the Health Insurance Association of America. HCPCS Level III contains alphanumeric codes that are assigned by Medicaid state agencies to identify additional items and services not included in levels I or II. These are usually called "local codes" and must have W, X, Y, or Z in the first position. HCPCS Procedure Modifier Codes can be used with all three levels of HCPCS codes, with the WA–ZY range used for locally assigned procedure modifiers (CMS 2017d).

As noted previously, OPPS is based on APC codes and is used by CMS in the outpatient setting for Medicare reimbursement based on CPT codes that correspond to an APC code payment. APC groups are the basic units of the APC system. Within an APC group, the diagnoses and procedures are similar in terms of resources used, complexity of illness, and conditions represented. A single payment is made for the outpatient services provided. APC groups are based on HCPCS/CPT codes. A single visit can result in multiple APC groups. APC groups consist of five types of service: significant procedures, surgical services, medical visits, ancillary services, and partial hospitalization. The APC group was formerly known as the Ambulatory Visit Group (AVG) and Ambulatory Patient Group (APG) (CMS 2017e).

RVUs are weights established by CMS to calculate the payment for physician practices under the Medicare Physician Fee Schedule. RVUs are assigned to each CPT and HCPCS code and are multiplied by a conversion factor updated annually by CMS (AMA 2017). (These payment systems will be discussed in further detail in chapter 3.) As noted above, CMS also uses HCCs to risk-adjust payments for claims from Medicare Advantage patients based on the treatment of chronic conditions.

Limited Supply of Outpatient Coding Experts

One of the best investments any healthcare entity can make is to identify and cultivate internal outpatient coding experts capable of translating the documentation in outpatient records into coded data. The supply of coding professionals in the United States was limited after the Inpatient Prospective Payment System (IPPS) became legally required in 1982. After IPPS was introduced, payment for inpatient stays had to be reported to payers using ICD codes, so most hospitals focused their more experienced coding resources on inpatient cases. In contrast, outpatient coding professionals tended to have less coding experience than those who worked with inpatient documentation. However, with the increase in regulations for claims submissions and the complexity of outpatient care and treatment, outpatient coding professionals are now required to have a higher-level skill set than in the past.

Well-trained and skilled coders are required in the outpatient setting to handle the increasing volume of services provided as well as the variety of outpatient payment methodologies. Additionally, when facilities use a one-patient-one-coder workflow in the outpatient setting, the outpatient coding professional codes both the facility claim and the physician practice claim. This workflow makes sense because insurance payers monitor both claims for code consistency. The clinical diagnostic and treatment information documented in the outpatient and professional practice clinical records should be consistent. For example, the association between diabetes and related peripheral vascular disease should be documented by the providers in both settings so that the ICD-10-CM code for diabetes with this complication is submitted on both claims.

The outpatient CDS's knowledge base should include the items shown in figure 2.5. Each of the classification and reimbursement systems are discussed in further detail in chapter 3.

Because the skills required of CDSs in the outpatient setting are related to clinical documentation requirements in the ambulatory setting and professional practices, as well as the various payment and coding systems in those settings, the outpatient CDS should have both a CDI credential, such as the **clinical documentation improvement practitioner (CDIP)**, and a coding credential specific to the outpatient setting, such as the **certified coding associate (CCA), certified coding specialist (CCS), certified coding specialist–physician-based (CCS-P)**, or other specific outpatient coding credential (AHIMA 2017). These certifications are further defined as:

- **CDIP** is an AHIMA credential awarded to individuals who have achieved specialized skills in clinical documentation improvement.
- **CCA** is an AHIMA credential awarded to entry-level coding professionals who have demonstrated skill in classifying medical data by passing a certification exam.
- **CCS** is an AHIMA credential awarded to individuals who have demonstrated skill in classifying medical data from patient records, generally in the hospital setting, by passing a certification examination.
- **CCS–P** is an AHIMA credential awarded to individuals who have demonstrated coding expertise in physician-based settings, such as group practices, by passing a certification examination.

Establishing the Medical Necessity of Brief Encounters

The brevity of the typical outpatient encounter presents a specific clinical documentation challenge for providers because the documentation for each encounter must support its medical necessity and ensure that accurate claims are submitted in a timely manner. Clinical records from each outpatient facility record must support the clinical documentation in the physician practice record for the same illness or treatment provided, and the documentation must also

Figure 2.5. Recommended knowledge base for the outpatient clinical documentation specialist

- ✔ Ambulatory and physician practice clinical record standards
- ✔ ICD-10-CM diagnostic coding
- ✔ CPT and HCPCS procedural coding
- ✔ Charge description master guidelines
- ✔ OPPS and APC payment systems
- ✔ Physician fee schedule payment systems
- ✔ Risk-adjustment payment systems
- ✔ Value-based payment systems
- ✔ Healthcare quality measurement programs

show that medical necessity is supported based on the local coverage determinations (LCDs) and national coverage determinations (NCDs) established as guidelines by payers such as CMS. These coverage determination guidelines list specific diagnosis codes that establish the medical necessity for particular treatments. When a provider gives a patient treatment but does not document a corresponding diagnosis code listed in the NCD or LCD, the payer will deny the claim for that treatment. Documentation of chronic illnesses is essential for accurate payment in the physician practice setting for HCC risk-based payment. These many requirements are a challenge for the outpatient CDS to monitor during a brief visit. To ensure that the clinical record is specific enough to support medical necessity and accurate payment, the clinical documentation workflow may likely need to be redesigned so that case review can be performed both prior to and after the visit. Refer to chapters 5, 8, and 10 for more information on CDI workflow redesign.

Chapter 2 Review Exercises

1. The use of EHRs was mandated by which of the following?
    a. ONC
    b. HITECH Act of 2009
    c. HIPAA Privacy Rule
    d. HL7 Standard of 2002

2. The types of information contained within the patient's health record are divided into two classifications. The type of health information documenting the patient's diagnoses and treatment provided is referred to as:
    a. Hybrid information
    b. Clinical information
    c. Standard information
    d. Administrative information

3. Which of the following requirements for an EHR System and its use are included in the final rule for Stage 1 Meaningful Use?
   a. The use of templates to gather additional details for clinical indicators
   b. Interoperability of the EHR between inpatient and rehabilitation settings
   c. Establishment of security requirements that prevent the patient from receiving copies of their treatment records
   d. Generation of lists of patients by specific conditions for quality improvement, reduction of disparities, research, and outreach

4. During the patient encounter, a provider documents all medications currently being administered. The CDS may use this list when evaluating the diagnoses documented and potentially generate a physician query if the _____ indicates a medication was provided but does not have a corresponding diagnosis documented in the record.
   a. Medicare access request
   b. Medical admission registration
   c. Moderate asthma rehabilitation
   d. Medication administration record

5. When a patient's EHR is composed of scanned documents and various electronic records, what is it called?
   a. Multimedia record
   b. Legal health record
   c. Hybrid health record
   d. Designated record set

6. Similar to the information found in a discharge summary in the inpatient setting, a(n) _____ includes information related to the diagnosis, treatment, prognosis, and instructions for follow-up care for an outpatient visit.
   a. Patient history and physician examination
   b. Encounter summary
   c. Progress note
   d. Consultation report

7. If different physicians are treating a patient and their documentation is inconsistent, which physician is queried by the coding professional to provide the final documented response?
   a. Emergency department physician
   b. Surgeon
   c. Attending physician
   d. Consultant physician

8. Which of the following is an example of a "hands-on" or treating provider whose clinical documentation may be used for coding purposes?
   a. Diagnostic radiologist
   b. Pathologist
   c. Diagnostic cardiologist
   d. Anesthesiologist

9. The _____ of the decubitus ulcer documented in the bedside nurse's, wound care nurse's, or physical therapist's note would be useful for final coding purposes.
   a. Size
   b. Stage
   c. Prognosis
   d. Symptoms

10. _____ is a set of standards for the exchange, integration sharing, and retrieval of electronic health information.
    a. HL7
    b. CPT
    c. HITCS
    d. HCPCS

References

42 CFR 412.46: Medical review requirements: Physician acknowledgment. 2002 (October). https://www.gpo.gov/fdsys/pkg/CFR-2002-title42-vol2/pdf/CFR-2002-title42-vol2-sec412-46.pdf.

Acker, B., J. Bronnert, T. Brown, et al. 2011. Problem list guidance in the EHR. *Journal of AHIMA* 82(9):52–58. http://library.ahima.org/doc?oid=104997#.WacbI8h97b0.

American Health Information Management Association (AHIMA). 2017. Certification. http://www.ahima.org/certification.

American Health Information Management Association (AHIMA). 2011. Practice Brief: Fundamentals of the legal health record and designated record set. *Journal of AHIMA* 82(2). http://library.ahima.org/doc?oid=104008#.WsuvaIjwbcs

American Hospital Association (AHA). 2000, 2004, 2005. *Coding Clinic*. Chicago: AHA.

American Medical Association (AMA). 2017. Medicare physician payment schedules. https://www.ama-assn.org/practice-management/medicare-physician-payment-schedules.

American Recovery and Reinvestment Act (ARRA) of 2009. Public Law 111-5.

Centers for Medicare and Medicaid Services (CMS) and National Center for Health Statistics (NCHS). 2018. ICD-10-CM Official Guidelines for Coding and Reporting. https://www.cdc.gov/nchs/data/icd/10cmguidelines_fy2018_final.pdf.

Centers for Medicare and Medicaid Services (CMS). 2017a. Medicare Program Integrity Manual. Chapter 3: Verifying potential errors and taking corrective actions. Section 3.3.24: Signature requirements. https://www.cms.gov/Regulations-and-Guidance/Guidance/Manuals/downloads/pim83c03.pdf.

Centers for Medicare and Medicaid Services (CMS). 2017b (March 10). CMS Transmittal 234, Change Request 9979. Clarification of admission order and medical review requirements. https://www.cms.gov/Regulations-and-Guidance/Guidance/Transmittals/2017Downloads/R234BP.pdf.

Centers for Medicare and Medicaid Services (CMS). 2017c. Risk adjustment. https://www.cms.gov/Medicare/Health-Plans/MedicareAdvtgSpecRateStats/Risk-Adjustors.html.

Centers for Medicare and Medicaid Services (CMS) Glossary. 2017d. https://www.cms.gov/apps/glossary/default.asp?Letter=ALL.

Centers for Medicare and Medicaid Services (CMS). 2017e. Hospital Outpatient Prospective Payment System. APCs. https://www.cms.gov/Medicare/Medicare-Fee-for-Service-Payment/HospitalOutpatientPPS/index.html.

Charles, D., M. Gabriel, and T. Searcy. 2015. Adoption of electronic health record systems among U.S. non-federal acute care hospitals: 2008–2014. ONC Data Brief No. 23. https://www.healthit.gov/sites/default/files/data-brief/2014HospitalAdoptionDataBrief.pdf.

Ericson, C. 2014. Successful documentation of wound care. *Wound Care Advisor* 3(3). http://woundcareadvisor.com/successful-documentation-of-wound-care-vol3-no3.

Glasgow Coma Scale. 2014. http://www.glasgowcomascale.org.

Health IT Standards Committee (HITSC). 2017. https://www.healthit.gov/facas/health-it-standards-committee.

Health Level 7 International (HL7). 2017. Introduction to HL7 standards. http://www.hl7.org/implement/standards.

Hess, P. 2015. *Clinical Documentation Improvement, Principles and Practice.* Chicago: AHIMA.

The Joint Commission. 2017. The Joint Commission's Electronic Accreditation and Certification Manuals. https://www.jointcommission.org/standards_information/edition.aspx.

Medicare Access and CHIP Reauthorization Act of 2015. Public Law 114–10.

Office of Civil Rights (OCR), US Department of Health and Human Services. 2015. Guidance regarding methods for de-identification of protected health information in accordance with the Health Insurance Portability and Accountability Act (HIPAA) Privacy Rule. https://www.hhs.gov/hipaa/for-professionals/privacy/special-topics/de-identification/index.html#protected https://www.hipaa.com/hipaa-protected-health-information-what-does-phi-include.

Office of Inspector General (OIG), US Department of Health and Human Services. 2017 (January). Vidant Medical Center incorrectly billed Medicare inpatient claims with severe malnutrition. https://oig.hhs.gov/oas/reports/region3/31500011.asp.

Office of the National Coordinator for Health Information Technology (ONC). 2017. ONC Tech Lab standards coordination. https://oncprojecttracking.healthit.gov/wiki/display/TechLabSC/ONC+Tech+Lab+Standards+Coordination+Home.

Sayles, N. 2014. *Health Information Management Technology: An Applied Approach.* 4th ed. Chicago: AHIMA.

US Department of Health and Human Services (HHS). 2017. The Health Information Portability and Accessibility Act: The Security Rule. https://www.hhs.gov/hipaa/for-professionals/security/index.html.

The Translation of Clinical Documentation into Coded Data

3

Learning Objectives

- Describe classification systems specific to the outpatient setting that are used for coding diagnoses, treatments, procedures, and services, as well as the process of converting clinical information to coded data.
- Discuss the challenges of interoperability in the facility and professional practice setting.
- Explain the relationship between clinical documentation and coding in the clinical documentation improvement workflow.
- Differentiate between classification systems used in the outpatient facility and those used in the professional practice setting.
- Explain reimbursement systems for the outpatient facility and physician practice.
- Describe the purpose and functionality of the hospital chargemaster and physician fee schedule.
- Identify methodologies for assigning the level of evaluation and management services in the emergency department.

Key Terms

837i
837p
Ambulatory payment classification (APC) weight
Chargemaster
CMS 1450
CMS 1500
Comprehensive APC (C-APC)
Diagnosis-related groups (DRGs)
Foundational interoperability
Geographic practice cost index (GPCI)
Hierarchical Condition Category (HCC) codes
International Classification of Diseases, Tenth Revision, Clinical Modification (ICD-10-CM)
International Classification of Diseases, Tenth Revision, Procedure Coding System (ICD-10-PCS)

Interoperability
Medicare Advantage
Monitor, evaluate, assess/address, or treat (MEAT)
National Uniform Billing Committee (NUBC)
National Uniform Claim Committee (NUCC)
Risk Adjustment Data Validation (RADV)
Risk Adjustment Factor (RAF) score
Semantic interoperability
Shared Nationwide Interoperability Roadmap
Structural interoperability
UB-04 Uniform Bill format
World Health Organization (WHO)

The use of disease and treatment classification systems to code clinical information supports many priorities of the healthcare industry, such as reimbursement, epidemiology, medical research, strategic planning of healthcare delivery, and quality of care monitoring. Various disease and procedure classification systems are used for coding clinical information in the outpatient setting. This chapter discusses the *International Classification of Diseases, Tenth Revision, Clinical Modification (ICD-10-CM)*, Current Procedural Terminology (CPT), Healthcare Common Procedure Coding System (HCPCS), and related reimbursement systems in the outpatient setting, including the Outpatient Prospective Payment System (OPPS), relative value units (RVUs), and Hierarchical Condition Categories (HCCs).

The Coding Process

As noted in chapter 2, coding of clinical information in the outpatient setting requires multiple classifications and reimbursement systems. **ICD-10-CM** is used to classify diagnoses, signs, and symptoms. In the inpatient setting, *International Classification of Diseases, Tenth Revision, Procedure Coding System (ICD-10-PCS)* is used to classify procedures and treatments provided to the patient. ICD-10-PCS is not used in the outpatient setting. Instead, CPT and HCPCS are used to code procedures, treatment, supplies, and medications. When coders submit a final claim for outpatient services, they are responsible for using the ICD-10-CM and CPT/HCPCS systems to classify diagnoses and treatments. ICD-10-CM codes are selected from an ICD-10-CM codebook or encoder. CPT procedures codes are selected from the American Medical Association (AMA) CPT codebook or encoder (AMA 2017). An *encoder* is a software tool that assists the coder or CDS in code selection.

The appropriate form to submit claims for reimbursement depends on the setting. In the physician practice setting, an industry-standard form called the **837p** is used for electronic billing to payers. The **CMS 1500** form is the standard paper claim form used to bill Medicare Fee for Service claims; it is the counterpart of the 837p used for electronic billing (CMS 2016a). The form includes demographic and patient payer–specific information as well as the

ICD-10-CM and CPT/HCPCS codes corresponding to the patient's diagnosis and treatment. Changes to the CMS 1500 form are approved by the **National Uniform Claim Committee (NUCC)** (NUCC 2013). The NUCC is a national group that replaced the Uniform Claim Form Task Force in 1995 and developed a standard data set to be used in the transmission of noninstitutional provider claims to and from third-party payers (NUCC 2017). The AMA is the Secretariat of the NUCC. After changes to the CMS 1500 form are approved by the NUCC, they are submitted to the Centers for Medicare and Medicaid Services (CMS) for approval.

In the outpatient setting, facilities submit claims in either the paper **UB-04 Uniform Bill** format or the electronic format known as the **837i** (CMS 2014). Uniform Bill-04 (UB-04), also called form **CMS 1450**, is a uniform, institutional provider hard-copy claim form suitable for use in billing multiple third-party payers. The UB-04 is the only hard-copy claim form that CMS accepts from institutional providers (CMS 2017a). The UB-04 is used to submit claims for both inpatient and outpatient facility services. The **National Uniform Billing Committee (NUBC)**, a national group responsible for identifying data elements and designing the UB-92, publishes the Official UB-04 Data Specifications Manual and is the official source for UB-04 billing information (NUBC 2017).

Outpatient clinical documentation specialists (CDSs) must be highly skilled in the use of ICD-10-CM, CPT, and HCPCS code sets. Inaccurate codes submitted on claims forms often result in denials of payment or inaccurate payments. Inaccurate coding also contributes to the miscalculation of risk-adjusted scores, which are used for negotiating contracts with payers and calculating shared-risk bonus payments.

Official guidelines and detailed specifications for the use of the ICD-10-CM, CPT, and HCPCS classification systems are found in the following publications:

- ICD-10-CM Official Guidelines for Coding and Reporting (CDC 2017)
- Current Procedural Terminology, Professional Edition 2018 (AMA 2017)
- HCPCS 2017 Alpha-Numeric HCPCS Code List (CMS 2017b)

These guidelines should be readily available to the CDS during the case review and data analytics process.

Most outpatient facilities and physician practices have functional electronic health record (EHR) systems that provide an electronic view of the clinical record. However, CDSs must be aware of exceptions in which hard-copy documentation augments or replaces the EHR. All available information should be used during the coding and CDS case review process to ensure high-quality coding and clinical documentation.

Some common EHR systems are EPIC, Meditech, Cerner, and McKesson. Each EHR system has its own look and feel. Some hospitals use a single system for outpatient and inpatient clinical documentation. A physician practice setting may use the same EHR as the hospital, but, in many cases, physician practices have a separate system for clinical documentation. Some examples of these systems are NextGen, Greenway, and Allscripts.

Interoperability

Providers in hospitals and physician practices often document in multiple systems. When clinical information about a patient is not shared between systems, the clinical information may be inconsistent and conflicting. Thus, when multiple documentation systems are used, their interoperability may be an issue for providers and CDSs. **Interoperability** refers to the ability of systems to exchange information and, ideally, use or interpret each other's data. The definition of interoperability offered by the Healthcare Information and Management Systems Society includes three levels (HIMSS 2013):

- **Foundational interoperability** allows data exchange from one information technology (IT) system to be received by another and does not require the ability for the receiving IT system to interpret the data.

- **Structural interoperability** is an intermediate level that defines the structure or format of data exchange (that is, the message format standards) where there is uniform movement of healthcare data from one system to another such that the clinical or operational purpose and meaning of the data are preserved and unaltered.

- **Semantic interoperability** provides interoperability at the highest level, which is the ability of two or more systems or elements to exchange information and use the information that has been exchanged (HIMSS 2013).

Lack of interoperability in the outpatient setting is a substantial barrier to the outpatient clinical documentation improvement (CDI) program because data from many systems are needed to conduct a case review for a single patient encounter.

Case Example

To identify all diagnoses eligible for HCC assignment in a physician practice encounter, the CDS must review the patient's inpatient and outpatient clinic records. However, the physician practice clinical record resides in its own EHR system, which is not interoperable with the hospital EHR. Therefore, the CDS needs to separately access both the hospital EHR and physician practice EHR to identify all allowable diagnoses for HCC assignment. Because the systems are not interoperable, the review process takes more time and may increase the likelihood of coding errors.

Figure 3.1 lists the set of guiding principles for nationwide interoperability established by the Office of the National Coordinator for Health Information Technology (ONC) (ONC 2015). These principles reflect stakeholder feedback and are part of a 10-year vision to create a health IT infrastructure that guides the development of strategy to improve future interoperability and focus efforts for progress and future innovation (ONC 2015). The American Health Information Management Association (AHIMA) is a proponent of operational

Figure 3.1. Guiding principles for nationwide interoperability

- ✔ Focus on value.
- ✔ Be person-centered.
- ✔ Protect privacy and security in all aspects of interoperability and respect individual preferences.
- ✔ Build a culture of electronic access and use.
- ✔ Encourage innovation and competition.
- ✔ Build upon the existing health IT infrastructure.
- ✔ One size does not fit all.
- ✔ Simplify.
- ✔ Maintain modularity.
- ✔ Consider current environment and support multiple levels of advancement.

Source: Adapted from ONC 2015

interoperability initiatives and supports the ONC Interoperability Standards Advisory (Butler 2016).

The ONC has also created the **Shared Nationwide Interoperability Roadmap** that outlines the strategy and direction to be taken to improve the exchange of health information between systems across the nation (ONC 2015). The roadmap's high-level goals are shown in figure 3.2.

Figure 3.2. Three high-level goals for nationwide health IT interoperability

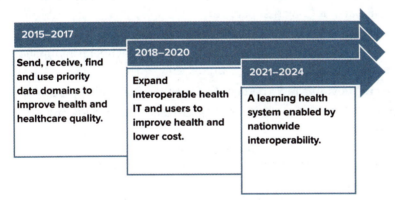

Source: Adapted from ONC 2015

When beginning work at an outpatient facility or physician practice, outpatient CDSs should conduct a review of its EHR systems and hard-copy record storage sites. Each system and site should be studied to determine the types of clinical information available and the most efficient methods to navigate the EHR and storage areas to review essential information needed for CDS case review as well as for internal and external payer audits. During the EHR assessment, the CDS should identify interoperability challenges and develop solutions so that a comprehensive clinical record is available to support high-quality clinical documentation and accurate reimbursement.

Relationship between Clinical Documentation and Coding

Coding professionals and CDSs play essential roles in the process of ensuring high-quality clinical documentation, coding, and claims submission. The clinical record must be complete before it is coded to ensure that all essential aspects of the patient's diagnosis and treatment are reflected on the claim. Also, to support the medical necessity of the treatment provided, the clinical record must include specific documentation supporting the diagnosis and procedure codes submitted on the claim form. CDSs should work to strengthen communication between providers and coders. The goal is to have accurate and complete clinical documentation throughout the health record prior to coding.

The job descriptions shown in figures 3.3 and 3.4 can be used to customize facility-specific coding specialist and CDS position descriptions. Each description includes the title, supervisor, list of responsibilities, and qualifications. The list of responsibilities may be modified to reflect the workflow for a specific facility.

Figure 3.3. Sample job description for a clinical coding specialist

Position Title: Clinical Coding Specialist

Immediate Supervisor: Director of Health Information Management, Manager of Clinical Data, or Coding Supervisor

Position Purpose: The purpose of this position is to apply the appropriate diagnostic and procedural codes to individual patient health information for data retrieval, analysis, and claims processing.

Responsibilities: Abstracts pertinent information from patient records.

- Assigns ICD-10-CM or HCPCS codes, creating APC or DRG group assignments.
- Queries physicians when code assignments are not straightforward or documentation in the record is inadequate, ambiguous, or unclear for coding purposes.
- Keeps abreast of coding guidelines and reimbursement reporting requirements. Brings identified concerns to supervisor or department manager for resolution.
- Abides by the Standards of Ethical Coding as set forth by the American Health Information Management Association and adheres to official coding guidelines.

Position Qualifications: Minimum of successful completion of a coding certificate program in a program with AHIMA approval status. RHIA, RHIT, CCS, CCS-P, and CCA certification status preferred. Coding certification preferred by the American Health Information Management Association. Prefer someone with work experience as a coder or strong training background in coding and reimbursement.

Source: AHIMA 2016

Figure 3.4. Sample job description for an outpatient clinical documentation specialist

Position Title: Outpatient Clinical Documentation Specialist

Immediate Supervisor: Director of Health Information Management, Manager of Clinical Documentation Improvement

Position Purpose: The purpose of this position is to assess requirements for high-quality clinical documentation improvement and educate providers about those requirements to support provider collaboration, quality of patient care, healthcare reimbursement, and other healthcare-related business requirements.

Responsibilities: Review of all hard-copy and electronic portions of the clinical record for documentation gaps.

- This process may be conducted as part of an audit to identify trends and develop redesigned workflow and documentation practices.
- Alternatively, this process may be conducted just prior to or after the patient encounter to further clarify missing documentation to support more specific or missing codes.

Conduct workflow and documentation redesign to streamline the physician clarification process so that the process is more timely and efficient for the provider.

Conduct educational sessions with the providers and coders to improve clinical documentation and code accuracy.

Identify denials and documentation gap trends and develop solutions by leading a collaborative team of providers, coders, and clinical documentation specialists.

Review the chargemaster and fee schedules for missing CPT/HCPCS codes and for unusually high or low volumes of codes that might point to a clinical documentation or coding issue.

Monitor progress of documentation improvement activities and present metrics to support the CDI program and confirm sustainability.

Establish a methodology for clarifying return on investment of the program.

Present program metrics to medical staff leaders, the clinical documentation improvement taskforce, and executive sponsors.

Position Qualifications: Minimum successful completion of a CAHIIM-approved RHIA or RHIT program or has a registered nurse license and CCS or CCS-P certification. Coding certification from the American Health Information Management Association is preferred. A CCDS (Certified Clinical Documentation Specialist) or CDIP (Clinical Documentation Improvement Professional) certification is preferred but not required. Prefer someone with work experience as a clinical documentation specialist or coder or a strong training background in coding, clinical documentation guidelines, and outpatient reimbursement systems.

Basic Coding Guidelines

The following sections review classification and reimbursement systems used for coding diagnoses and procedures in the outpatient setting. However, the coding guidelines are complex, and a full explanation is beyond the scope of this textbook.

ICD-10-CM

ICD-10-CM is based on the *International Classification of Diseases, 10th Revision* (ICD-10) statistical classification of disease published by the **World Health Organization (WHO)**. As the United Nations specialized agency created to ensure the attainment by all peoples of the highest possible levels of health, WHO is responsible for a number of international classifications, including ICD-10 and *International Classification of Functioning, Disability and Health* (ICF) (WHO 2017). ICD-10-CM classifies morbidity data from inpatient and outpatient records and physician office documentation. CMS and the National Center for Health Statistics (NCHS), two departments within the US Department of Health and Human Services (HHS), copublish *ICD-10-CM Official Guidelines for Coding and Reporting* (CDC 2017). The Official Guidelines, which are approved by the Cooperating Parties (four organizations that govern the rules and guidelines for the use of ICD-10-CM), include rules for using the ICD-10-CM Tabular List and Alphabetic Index. In the Tabular List, the ICD-10-CM codes are listed in alphanumeric order and organized into 21 chapters, which tend to group diagnoses by either body system or disease etiology. The Alphabetic Index is an index of diseases and the corresponding ICD-10-CM codes. To code a sign, symptom, or diagnosis, coders first look in the Alphabetic Index for the diagnosis name and then check the corresponding code in the Tabular List, where additional instructions are noted.

Coding professionals should always review the entire record for the encounter to identify all reportable codes. Where signs, symptoms, and abnormal diagnostic results are identified without a definitive diagnosis, the CDS should query the provider for greater specificity in the documentation. The *ICD-10-CM Official Guidelines for Coding and Reporting* Section IV, Diagnostic Coding and Reporting Guidelines for Outpatient Services, explains how to code symptoms, conditions, problems, complaints, or other reason(s) for the outpatient encounter as well as how to sequence ICD-10-CM codes on an outpatient claim. The coding conventions of ICD-10-CM and the general and disease-specific guidelines should be used to determine the first condition that is listed on the outpatient claim. The Official Guidelines instruct coders to "list first the ICD-10-CM code for the diagnosis, condition, problem, or other reason for encounter/visit shown in the medical record to be chiefly responsible for the services provided" (CDC 2017). If the case is a surgical encounter, the reason for the surgery is the first-listed ICD-10-CM code, even if the surgery is not performed. For patients admitted to the observation area for a medical condition, the reason for the admission to the observation area is the first-listed ICD-10-CM code. If a patient develops a complication from an outpatient surgical procedure, the code for the reason for the surgery is listed first, followed by the surgical complication code. The rule-out and suspected diagnosis guidelines followed when coding diagnoses in the inpatient setting do not apply in the outpatient setting. Instead, in outpatient records, the most definitive sign, symptom, or diagnosis is coded. Chronic illnesses may be coded when treatment or care is provided for the condition. History of codes in categories Z80–Z87 should be used to report conditions that no longer exist (CDC 2017).

The outpatient CDS should become proficient in the use of Section IV of the *ICD-10-CM Official Guidelines for Coding and Reporting* during case review. The application and interpretation of the guidelines are critical to high-quality outpatient clinical documentation, accurate reimbursement, and prevention of payer denials.

CPT and HCPCS

As noted earlier, Current Procedural Terminology (CPT) and HCPCS are used for reporting procedures in the outpatient setting. CPT is a comprehensive, descriptive list of terms and associated numeric and alphanumeric codes used for reporting diagnostic and therapeutic procedures and other medical services performed by physicians (AMA 2017). The AMA maintains an editorial panel of physicians that ensures the currency of the CPT classification system by periodically revising, deleting, and adding new procedure codes. The following are the eight code sections of CPT:

99201–99499 Evaluation and Management
00100–01999 Anesthesia
10021–69990 Surgery
70010–79999 Radiology
80047–89356 Pathology and Laboratory
90281–99607 Medicine
Category II 0001F–9007F
Category III 0042T–0463T

The CPT classification also has appendices that include modifiers; a summary of additions, deletions, and revision; clinical examples; and other classification system guidance (AMA 2017).

The Category II codes are "supplemental tracking codes that can be used for performance measurement" (AMA 2017). Category III codes are temporary codes used to classify emerging technology, services, and procedures. Codes are organized in the CPT code book alphabetically, using the following four categories:

- Procedure or service
- Organ or anatomic site
- Condition
- Synonym, eponym, or abbreviation

Healthcare Common Procedure Coding System (HCPCS) is published by CMS for reporting outpatient and physician services. The classification system is a "collection of codes and descriptors used to represent healthcare procedures, supplies, products, and services" (Sayles 2014). It has two levels: HCPCS Level I and HCPCS Level II. Level I refers to the AMA's CPT codebook, and the codes are used primarily for procedures and treatments. Level II is maintained by CMS. Most of these codes are used to identify medical products, supplies, and services not included in the CPT code set jurisdiction, such as medications, some types of medical equipment, and ambulance services. Level II codes also include G codes, which are "used to identify professional health care procedures and services that would otherwise be coded in CPT-4 [Current Procedural Terminology, fourth edition] but for which there are no CPT-4 codes" (CMS 2015). The Level II codes are updated annually and are effective January 1. Each year, there are multiple changes to the Level II codes.

Certain procedures and treatments have both Level I and Level II code options. An example of this is the coding for colonoscopies. CPT codes for this procedure are found in the range 45378 through 45393. However, CMS has created the following Level II HCPCS codes to be used when coding Medicare claims for colonoscopies to screen for cancer:

> Colorectal cancer screening; colonoscopy on individual not meeting criteria for high risk: G0121
> Colorectal cancer screening; colonoscopy on individual at high risk: G0105

In this example, CMS created HCPCS Level II codes to differentiate between colonoscopy performed on patients at high risk of colorectal cancer and the same procedure performed on patients not at high risk. Chapter 18: Preventive Screening Services, section 60.3, Determining High Risk for Developing Colorectal Cancer, of the Medicare Claims Processing Manual provides the characteristics of the high-risk individual (CMS 2017a). An individual at high risk for developing colorectal cancer has one or more of the following:

> A close relative (sibling, parent, or child) who has had colorectal cancer or an adenomatous polyp;
> A family history of familial adenomatous polyposis;
> A family history of hereditary nonpolyposis colorectal cancer;
> A personal history of adenomatous polyps;
> A personal history of colorectal cancer; or
> Inflammatory bowel disease, including Crohn's disease, and ulcerative colitis (CMS 2017a).

Medicare's calculation of reimbursement varies depending on which code is appropriate, and claims that report an incorrect code may be denied. Section 60.3.C of the Medicare Claims Processing Manual provides a partial list of ICD-10-CM codes indicating a high risk for colorectal cancer. If the CDS identifies a trend of claims for screening colonoscopy coded with G0105 being denied, he or she should review a sample of cases for clinical documentation gaps based on this list of ICD-10-CM codes (see table 3.1 for examples of such codes). Separate HCPCS codes for screening colonoscopy have been established by CMS to differentiate between screening and diagnostic colonoscopies.

Other examples where multiple CPT and HCPCS codes describe the same procedure or treatment include the following:

> 99183, Physician attendance and supervision of hyperbaric oxygen therapy, per session (CPT), versus G0277, Hyperbaric oxygen under pressure, full body chamber, per 30-minute interval (HCPCS)
> 27096, Sacroiliac joint injection without fluoroscopic guidance (CPT), versus G0259/G0260, Injection procedure for sacroiliac joint; arthrography (HCPCS)
> 97014, Electrical stimulation (unattended) (CPT), versus G0281/G0283, Electrical stimulation (unattended), one or more areas (HCPCS)

Table 3.1. Examples of ICD-10-CM codes that support the medical necessity of colonoscopy to screen patients at high risk for colorectal cancer

ICD-10-CM Code	Diagnosis
K51.90	Ulcerative colitis, unspecified, without complications
K51.911	Ulcerative colitis, unspecified with rectal bleeding
K51.912	Ulcerative colitis, unspecified with intestinal obstruction
K51.913	Ulcerative colitis, unspecified with fistula
K51.914	Ulcerative colitis, unspecified with abscess
K51.918	Ulcerative colitis, unspecified with other complication
K51.919	Ulcerative colitis, unspecified with unspecified complications
K52.1	Toxic gastroenteritis and colitis
K52.89	Other specified noninfective gastroenteritis and colitis
K52.9	Noninfective gastroenteritis and colitis, unspecified
Z12.12	Encounter for screening for malignant neoplasm of rectum
Z15.09	Genetic susceptibility to other malignant neoplasm
Z80.0	Family history of malignant neoplasm of digestive organs
Z83.71	Family history of colonic polyps
Z85.038	Personal history of other malignant neoplasm of large intestine
Z85.048	Personal history of other malignant neoplasm of rectum, rectosigmoid junction, and anus

Source: CMS 2017b

The practice of using multiple codes to bill for the various individual steps in a single procedure rather than using a single code that includes all of the steps of the comprehensive procedure is known as *unbundling*, whereas *bundling* refers to the process used by insurance companies to incorporate several CPT codes into one payment. CMS has established the National Correct Coding Initiative (NCCI) guidelines to assist in correct coding assignment when more than one CPT or HCPCS code could be used to report a given procedure. CMS guidance explains that NCCI edits do not include all possible combinations of CPT and HCPCS codes. Providers must use the CMS and CPT guidelines to validate accurate submission of CPT and HCPS codes (CMS 2016b; AMA 2017).

Table 3.2 presents CPT codes for nail plate procedures. In this example, CPT code 11730, Removal of the nail plate, is assigned a payment rate of $153.12. The add-on code for removal of additional nail plates, CPT code 11732, is assigned a status indicator (SI) of N, which indicates that the removal of additional nail plates during the same episode of care is not reimbursed separately. Instead, the payment for code 11732 is bundled into the payment for the first removal procedure, coded as CPT 11730. (*Bundled* means that the primary code in a code group is payable and the secondary codes are included.)

Table 3.2. Examples of CPT nail plate procedures

HCPCS Code	Short Descriptor	SI	APC	Relative Weight	Payment Rate
11730	Removal of nail plate	Q1	5051	2.0416	$153.12
11732	Removal of nail plate add-on	N			

Source: CMS 2017c

SIs are codes used under the OPPS to indicate whether the services are separately payable or packaged as part of another service. The Medicare OPPS is used for hospital-based outpatient services and procedures and is predicated on the assignment of **ambulatory payment classifications (APCs)**. SI codes are updated by CMS annually in Addendum D1 of the OPPS Final Rule (CMS 2018). The complete list of SI codes for calendar year 2018 is presented below:

ADDENDUM D1—OPPS PAYMENT STATUS INDICATORS FOR CY 2018

Status Indicator	Item/Code/Service	OPPS Payment Status
A	Services furnished to a hospital outpatient that are paid under a fee schedule or payment system other than OPPS,* for example:	Not paid under OPPS. Paid by MACs under a fee schedule or payment system other than OPPS.
		Services are subject to deductible or coinsurance unless indicated otherwise.
	• Ambulance Services	
	• Separately Payable Clinical Diagnostic Laboratory Services	Not subject to deductible or coinsurance.
	• Separately Payable Non-Implantable Prosthetics and Orthotics	
	• Physical, Occupational, and Speech Therapy	
	• Diagnostic Mammography	
	• Screening Mammography	Not subject to deductible or coinsurance.
B	Codes that are not recognized by OPPS when submitted on an outpatient hospital Part B bill type (12x and 13x).	Not paid under OPPS.
		• May be paid by MACs when submitted on a different bill type, for example, 75x (CORF), but not paid under OPPS.
		• An alternate code that is recognized by OPPS when submitted on an outpatient hospital Part B bill type (12x and 13x) may be available.
C	Inpatient Procedures	Not paid under OPPS. Admit patient. Bill as inpatient.
D	Discontinued Codes	Not paid under OPPS or any other Medicare payment system.
E1	Items and Services:	Not paid by Medicare when submitted on outpatient claims (any outpatient bill type).
	• Not covered by any Medicare outpatient benefit category	
	• Statutorily excluded by Medicare	
	• Not reasonable and necessary	

Continued

ADDENDUM D1—OPPS PAYMENT STATUS INDICATORS FOR CY 2018 (Continued)

Status Indicator	Item/Code/Service	OPPS Payment Status
E2	Items and Services:	Not paid by Medicare when submitted on outpatient claims (any outpatient bill type).
	for which pricing information and claims data are not available	
F	Corneal Tissue Acquisition; Certain CRNA Services and Hepatitis B Vaccines	Not paid under OPPS. Paid at a reasonable cost.
G	Pass-Through Drugs and Biologicals	Paid under OPPS; separate APC payment.
H	Pass-Through Device Categories	Separate cost-based pass-through payment; not subject to copayment.
J1	Hospital Part B Services Paid Through a Comprehensive Apc	Paid under OPPS; all covered Part B services on the claim are packaged with the primary "J1" service for the claim, except services with OPPS SI = F, G, H, L, and U; ambulance services; diagnostic and screening mammography; all preventive services; and certain Part B inpatient services.
J2	Hospital Part B Services That May Be Paid Through a Comprehensive APC	Paid under OPPS; Addendum B displays APC assignments when services are separately payable.
		(1) Comprehensive APC payment based on OPPS comprehensive-specific payment criteria. Payment for all covered Part B services on the claim is packaged into a single payment for specific combinations of services, except services with OPPS SI = F, G, H, L, and U; ambulance services; diagnostic and screening mammography; all preventive services; and certain Part B inpatient services.
		(2) Packaged APC payment if billed on the same claim as an HCPCS code assigned status indicator "J1."
		(3) In other circumstances, payment is made through a separate APC payment or packaged into payment for other services.
K	Nonpass-Through Drugs and Nonimplantable Biologicals, Including Therapeutic Radiopharmaceuticals	Paid under OPPS; separate APC payment.
L	Influenza Vaccine; Pneumococcal Pneumonia Vaccine	Not paid under OPPS. Paid at reasonable cost; not subject to deductible or coinsurance.
M	Items and Services Not Billable to the MAC	Not paid under OPPS.
N	Items and Services Packaged into APC Rates	Paid under OPPS; payment is packaged into payment for other services. Therefore, there is no separate APC payment.
P	Partial Hospitalization	Paid under OPPS; per diem APC payment.

Continued

ADDENDUM D1—OPPS PAYMENT STATUS INDICATORS FOR CY 2018 (Continued)

Status Indicator	Item/Code/Service	OPPS Payment Status
Q1	STV-Packaged Codes	Paid under OPPS; Addendum B displays APC assignments when services are separately payable.
		(1) Packaged APC payment if billed on the same claim as an HCPCS code assigned status indicator "S," "T," or "V."
		(2) Composite APC payment if billed with specific combinations of services based on OPPS composite-specific payment criteria. Payment is packaged into a single payment for specific combinations of services.
		(3) In other circumstances, payment is made through a separate APC payment.
Q2	T-Packaged Codes	Paid under OPPS; Addendum B displays APC assignments when services are separately payable.
		(1) Packaged APC payment if billed on the same claim as an HCPCS code assigned status indicator "T."
		(2) In other circumstances, payment is made through a separate APC payment.
Q3	Codes That May Be Paid Through a Composite APC	Paid under OPPS; Addendum B displays APC assignments when services are separately payable.
		Addendum M displays composite APC assignments when codes are paid through a composite APC.
		(1) Composite APC payment based on OPPS composite-specific payment criteria. Payment is packaged into a single payment for specific combinations of services.
		(2) In other circumstances, payment is made through a separate APC payment or packaged into payment for other services.
Q4	Conditionally Packaged Laboratory Tests	Paid under OPPS or CLFS.
		(1) Packaged APC payment if billed on the same claim as an HCPCS code assigned published status indicator "J1," "J2," "S," "T," "V," "Q1," "Q2," or "Q3."
		(2) In other circumstances, laboratory tests should have an SI=A, and payment is made under the CLFS.
R	Blood and Blood Products	Paid under OPPS; separate APC payment.
S	Procedure or Service, Not Discounted When Multiple	Paid under OPPS; separate APC payment.
T	Procedure or Service, Multiple Procedure Reduction Applies	Paid under OPPS; separate APC payment.
U	Brachytherapy Sources	Paid under OPPS; separate APC payment.
V	Clinic or Emergency Department Visit	Paid under OPPS; separate APC payment.
Y	Non-Implantable Durable Medical Equipment	Not paid under OPPS. All institutional providers other than home health agencies bill to a DME MAC.

Note: Payments "under a fee schedule or payment system other than OPPS" may be contractor-priced (CMS 2018).

Coding in the Physician Practice

Coding in the physician practice uses ICD-10-CM diagnosis codes, evaluation and management (E/M) codes (included in the CPT manual), other CPT codes, and HCPCS and HCC codes.

E/M Coding

E/M codes are used in the physician practice setting as well as in the ambulatory facility setting (as shown in table 3.3). These codes are used to report a patient encounter on the claim form and represent the history, examination, and medical decision-making components of the patient visit. Procedures codes (CPT and HCPCS) are also reported for procedures and treatments that are performed during the visit. These procedure codes may be reimbursed in addition to the E/M unless they are considered a bundled service within the E/M code. An example of a bundled service is an additional skin tag removal coded at 11201. Only the first skin tag removal is 11200. Removal of impacted cerumen, CPT 69210, is bundled into the E/M code when performed during the same encounter.

The CPT codebook (AMA 2017) describes the methodology for selecting E/M codes. Additionally, the Medicare Learning Network has published a complete guide to the use of these codes (CMS 2017c). CDSs should familiarize themselves with this guide, which can be used during the case review and physician education process.

Table 3.3. Settings in which evaluation and management codes are used to report patient encounters

Setting	Example of Patient Encounter	CPT Code
Office or other outpatient setting	New patient visit	90201
Inpatient	Initial hospital care	99221
Emergency department	Emergency department visit	99281
Nursing facility	Initial nursing facility care	99304

CMS has published the following two sets of guidelines, which are used by all payers to determine the E/M level for physician or professional practice:

1995 Documentation Guidelines for Evaluation and Management Services
1997 Documentation Guidelines for Evaluation and Management Services

When billing Medicare, physician practices may use either the 1997 or the 1995 documentation guidelines for evaluation and management services, and not a combination of both (CMS 2017c).

The CPT codebook explains that the selection of E/M codes uses the three key components—history, examination, and medical decision making:

> The code sets to bill for E/M services are organized into various categories and levels. In general, the more complex the visit, the higher the level of code you may bill within the appropriate category. To bill any code, the services furnished must meet the definition of the code. You must ensure that the codes selected reflect the services furnished. The three key components when selecting the appropriate level of E/M services provided are *history, examination, and medical decision making*. Visits that consist predominantly of counseling and/or coordination of care are an exception to this rule. For these visits, time is the key or controlling factor to qualify for a particular level of E/M services. (AMA 2017)

Criteria for selecting the level for each key component are listed in both the 1995 and 1997 guidelines. The options for assigning the E/M level based on the complexity of the key components are shown in table 3.4.

Table 3.4. Key components used for selecting the E/M service level (ranked from least to greatest complexity)

	History	Physical Examination	Medical Decision Making
Criteria	• Problem-focused • Expanded problem-focused • Detailed • Comprehensive	• Problem-focused • Expanded problem-focused • Detailed • Comprehensive	• Straightforward • Low complexity • Moderate complexity • High complexity

Once the level of complexity for each key component has been determined, the coding professional or CDS uses the narrative from the codes corresponding to the site of service to determine the correct E/M level. For example, five E/M codes are available to code E/M services for an established patient in the office or other outpatient setting: 99211, 99212, 99213, 99214, and 99215. Code 99213 includes the following levels of complexity for the three key components:

- Expanded problem-focused history
- Expanded problem-focused physical examination
- Medical decision making of low complexity

The percentage utilization of E/M codes in a specific setting is a metric that can be used to compare particular providers with their peers or with national utilization data, which are available from CMS (CMS 2017d). This exercise in comparative analysis can be useful if a payer raises a red flag about the potential overuse of upper-level codes. It can also help identify circumstances in which higher-level E/M codes are underused, which could lead to potential revenue loss. For example, table 3.5 presents national Medicare Part B data about E/M code use in the General Practice specialty category. A CDS could compare the E/M code use of specific general practice providers to these national percentages to assess whether the selected providers were assigning too many or too few high-level codes relative to their peers.

The outpatient CDS can compare the facility's physicians individually against the metrics provided by CMS. If there is a significant discrepancy between the peer group and specific physicians, an audit of 25 records should be performed

Table 3.5. National percentage utilization of E/M codes data for general practice providers

Code	E/M Volume	% Utilization
99201	1,518	1.07%
99202	16,843	11.85%
99203	63,872	44.93%
99204	48,342	34.00%
99205	11,598	8.16%
Total	**142,173**	**100.00%**

Source: CMS 2017d

to determine whether clinical documentation supports the level of assigned codes and to validate the clinical documentation quality if it is questioned in a payer audit.

RVUs and the Physician Fee Schedule

The Medicare Physician Fee schedule (MPFS) is a list of CPT and HCPCS codes with corresponding reimbursement amounts. The MPFS is used by provider practices to determine the accurate Medicare payment (CMS 2017e). The RVU is a unit of measure used to determine Medicare and other payer reimbursement in the physician practice setting. Each CPT code has an RVU assigned to it.

Reimbursement is calculated by multiplying the RVU weight by a conversion factor and a **geographic practice cost index (GPCI)**. GPCI is an index used to adjust the RVUs, which are national averages, to reflect local costs. It was developed by the Centers for Medicare and Medicaid Services to measure the differences in resource costs among fee schedule areas compared to the national average in the three components of the relative value unit (RVU): physician work, practice expenses, and malpractice coverage; separate GPCIs exist for each element of the RVU.

The following is an example of the calculation used to determine the payment for a specific CPT code using the variables RVU Weight, GPCI, Work, Practice Expense, Malpractice Expense, and Conversion Factor (CMS 2016c):

Payment = [(RVU Work × GPCI Work) + (RVU Practice Expense × GPCI Practice Expense) + (RVU Malpractice Expense × GPCI Malpractice Expense)] × (Conversion Factor)

When calculating an RVU payment, the conversion factor for the current year must be used in the formula. The conversion factor for 2017 was $35.8887 for all services except anesthesia, which had its own conversion factor (CMS 2017e).

Each year, CMS publishes the final rule for Medicare Program; Revisions to Payment Policies under the Physician Fee Schedule (PFS) and Other Revisions to Part B (CMS 2017e). The final rule explains in detail the methodology for creation of each component of the RVU calculation in the PFS. CMS continues to study the work, practice expense, and malpractice expense factors that comprise the RVUs to determine weights that reflect the costs of real-world medical practice. The weights are updated annually as part of the proposed final rule process, and stakeholders have an opportunity to comment on the proposed recommendations

Table 3.6. Selected work RVUs used in radiation oncology, 2016–2017

CPT Code		2016 Work RVU	2017 Work RVU
19298	Placement of radiotherapy after loading brachytherapy catheters (multiple tube and button type) into the breast for interstitial radioelement application following (at the time of or subsequent to) partial mastectomy, includes imaging guidance.	6.00	5.75
49411	Placement of interstitial device(s) for radiation therapy guidance (e.g., fiducial markers, dosimeter), percutaneous, intra-abdominal, intra-pelvic (except prostate), and/or retroperitoneum, single or multiple.	3.82	3.57
57155	Insertion of uterine tandem or vaginal ovoids for clinical brachytherapy.	5.40	5.15
77600	Hyperthermia, external, superficial (i.e., heating to a depth of 4 cm or less).	1.56	1.31
77605	Hyperthermia, external, deep (i.e., heating to a depth of greater than 4 cm).	2.09	1.84
77610	Hyperthermia, interstitial probe(s), 5 or fewer interstitial applicators.	1.56	1.31
77615	Hyperthermia, interstitial probe(s), more than 5 interstitial applicators.	2.09	1.84

Source: CMS 2017e

before they are finalized. In 2017, CMS reduced the work RVUs for a number of CPT codes that use moderate sedation within the radiation oncology specialty (CMS 2016c). Table 3.6 shows the reduction in the work RVU for these services.

The outpatient CDS should be aware of changes in RVU payments that affect clinical documentation requirements so that education can be granted to providers and practice managers on new clinical data to support specific CPT codes. CMS also provides a tool to search the PFS where the CDS can enter a code number and see the corresponding prices for specific locations (CMS 2017f). Figure 3.5 is a screenshot of results for a search using CPT code 99213 for Madera, CA. The search results show the nonfacility payment of $76.68 and the facility payment of $52.67. CMS provides further details on the PFS payment methodology and RVUs on its website (CMS 2017e).

The MPFS methodology developed as part of the sustainable growth rate (SGR) program for determining annual updates to physician Medicare payments. The Medicare Access and CHIP Reauthorization Act of 2015 (MACRA) repealed and replaced the SGR program. This law set in place several goals and objectives for future physician practice Medicare payments:

- Positive or flat fee updates that occur annually for a 10-year period and a two-tracked fee update after the 10-year period ends.
- The Merit-Based Incentive Payment System (MIPS) to consolidate Medicare physician fee-for-service incentives.
- A physician pathway to alternative payment models, such as the patient-centered medical home.
- Other changes to physician payment statutes for the Medicare program (AAFP 2017).

Figure 3.5. Example of results from the Medicare Physician Fee Schedule search tool

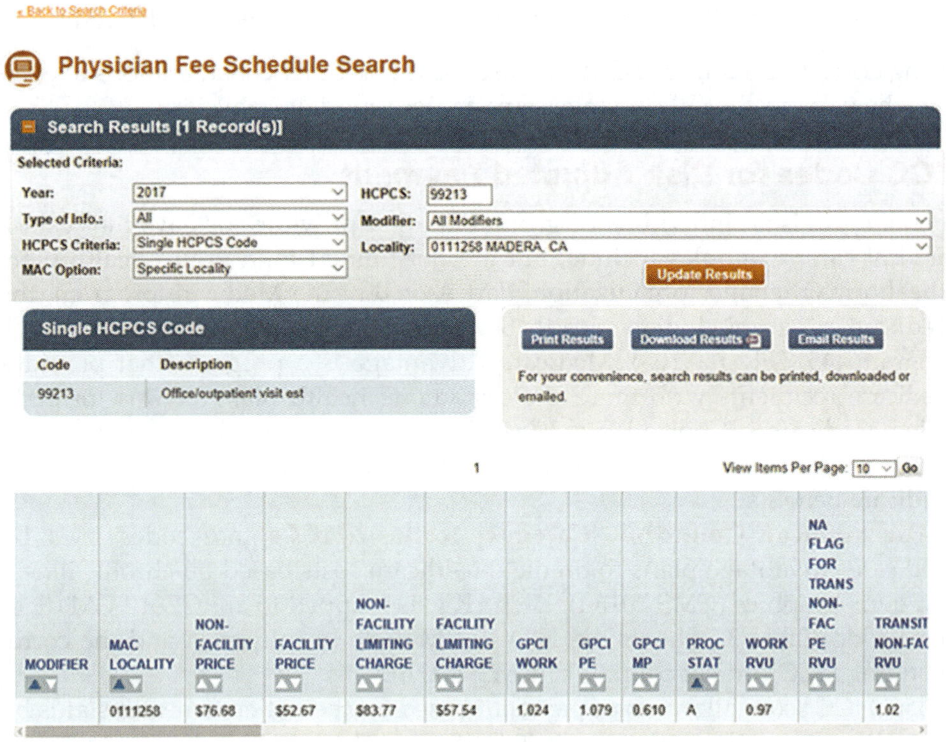

MODIFIER	MAC LOCALITY	NON-FACILITY PRICE	FACILITY PRICE	NON-FACILITY LIMITING CHARGE	FACILITY LIMITING CHARGE	GPCI WORK	GPCI PE	GPCI MP	PROC STAT	WORK RVU	NA FLAG FOR TRANS NON-FAC PE RVU	TRANSIT NON-FAC RVU
	0111258	$76.68	$52.67	$83.77	$57.54	1.024	1.079	0.610	A	0.97		1.02

Source: CMS 2017f

The CMS final rule released on October 14, 2016, provided details of the new MACRA program and the repeal of SGR. This program offers bonuses to physicians based on quality scores monitored through the MIPS and advanced alternative payment models (AMA 2016). MACRA and MIPS are discussed in further detail in chapter 4 of this text.

The outpatient CDS can analyze the average RVUs for individual practitioners in a given specialty for comparison purposes and to evaluate the potential for clinical documentation and reimbursement gaps. For example, within the specialty of interventional cardiology, if the average RVU weight for Dr. A is significantly lower than that for Dr. B, the variation in RVU averages could be related to problems such as incomplete details in documentation or inaccurate coding. Therefore, the following issues should be considered:

- How many intervention procedures and lower-weighted office visits does each physician perform?
- If the ratio of intervention procedures is comparable, is Dr. A's clinical documentation for the interventional procedures complete and detailed enough for accurate coding?
- Do both physicians have the same coders or are their claims assigned to different coders? Has the accuracy of each coder's work been validated?

- Does the charge capture process result in a complete claim with all required CPT codes submitted? Where there are gaps or inaccuracies in charge entry screens, encounter forms, or fee schedule/chargemaster line items, the result may be the omission of a multi-procedure CPT code.

Using critical thinking, the CDS can use these and other considerations to evaluate the variance in RVU averages among peer specialty physicians.

HCC Codes for Risk-Adjusted Payment

A *health plan* is an individual or group plan that provides, or pays the cost of, medical care. Examples include, but are not limited to, a group health plan, a health maintenance organization, Part A or B of the Medicare program, the Medicaid program, Indian Health Services, and the **Medicare Advantage** program (45 CFR 160.103). Medicare Advantage is a program that provides Medicare recipients with more choices among health plans; it was formerly called Medicare + Choice Plans (CMS 2017g). Medicare Advantage, which is also called *Part C Medicare*, is provided by private insurance companies to cover Medicare benefits.

Hierarchical Condition Category codes (HCCs) are codes used by Medicare Advantage plans to predict healthcare costs based on chronic illness and demographics (CMS 2016d). Each HCC is mapped to an ICD-10-CM diagnosis code. Table 3.7 shows the ICD-10-CM code in column A and the corresponding HCC code in column D (CMS 2017h).

The HCC score allows for a payment based on the patient's health status by capturing chronic illness coded in ICD-10-CM. The HCC score is also referred to as a **Risk Adjustment Factor (RAF) score**. The RAF score is the sum of the HCC weights (tied to ICD-10-CM diagnosis codes) for a specific patient over a

Table 3.7. Example of ICD-10-CM/HCC crosswalk

A	B	C	D	E	F	G	H
ICD-10-CM Codes, CMS-HCC and RxHCC Models Includes FY2017 ICD-10 codes							
Diagnosis Code	Description	CMS-HCC PACE/ ESRD Model Category V21	CMS-HCC Model Category V22	RxHCC Model Category V05	CMS-HCC PACE/ESRD Model for 2017 Payment Year	CMS-HCC Model for 2017 Payment Year	RxHCC Model for 2017 Payment Year
A0103	Typhoid pneumonia	115	115		Yes	Yes	No
A0104	Typhoid arthritis	39	39		Yes	Yes	No
A0105	Typhoid osteomyelitis	39	39		Yes	Yes	No
A021	Salmonella sepsis	2	2		Yes	Yes	No
A0222	Salmonella pneumonia	115	115		Yes	Yes	No
A0223	Salmonella arthritis	39	39		Yes	Yes	No
A0224	Salmonella osteomyelitis	39	39		Yes	Yes	No
A065	Amebic lung abscess	115	115		Yes	Yes	No
A072	Cryptosporidiosis	6	6	5	Yes	Yes	Yes

Source: Reprinted from CMS 2017g

12-month period (CMS 2016d). The HCC-related diagnoses are based on clinical information found in the clinical record for any of these settings: physician offices, hospital inpatient, and outpatient facility (CMS 2017h).

The Medicare Advantage per-patient-per-month (PPPM) contract rate is used to calculate the estimated payment *to the Medicare Advantage plan* from implementing an outpatient CDI program. The PPPM rate is published by the Medicare Advantage Plan and is based on the locality of the provider practice (CMS 2017i).

To determine the annual payment for a patient to the Medicare Advantage plan:

1. Identify weights (RAF score) for all unique HCCs during the year. The HCC weights may be downloaded from the 2018 Model Software/ICD-10 Mappings table on the CMS website (CMS 2017h). In the example below, the weight for each HCC corresponding to a diagnosis for a patient is listed to the right of the diagnosis. For example, the HCC weight for diabetes with complications is 0.318. The weights for all HCCs identified for the patient during the year are added together. In this example, the total weight is 1.221. To estimate the total return on investment, add the total weights together for the new HCCs identified by the CDS case review and calculate the total annual payment to the Medicare Advantage plan by adding the payments together.

HCC	Weight
Diabetes with complications	0.318
Vascular disease	0.400
CHF [congestive heart failure]	0.323
Disease interaction (DM [diabetes mellitus] + CHF)	0.180
Total	1.221

2. Identify Medicare Advantage PPPM contract rate.

3. Calculate annual payment to the Medicare Advantage plan using this formula: 1.221 (total weight) × $897.90 (PPPM rate) × 12 (months) = $13,156 (total Medicare Advantage plan payment).

The return on investment to the facility or provider practice is based on the total Medicare Advantage plan dollar improvement from CDI activities adjusted to reflect the Medicare Advantage plan shared bonus agreement. For example, the Medicare Advantage plan could agree to pay the facility or provider practice a percentage of the annual HCC payment. To determine the direct return on investment to the facility, each specific payer contract must be reviewed to calculate the shared dollar amounts agreed upon in the contract for risk adjustment bonus payments. The facility can estimate the increased HCC payments to the Medicare Advantage plan from CDI program activity by first adding the HCC weights together for those patients with provider queries and subsequent addition of unique HCCs and then calculating the corresponding dollar impact for the year estimated using the formula above.

The outpatient CDS provides a valuable service to providers by monitoring the accuracy of HCC assignment through case review, provider clarification, and provider and coder education. The HCC review, clarification, and provider and coder education process is further discussed in chapter 6 of this textbook.

CMS performs a **risk adjustment data validation (RADV)** audit to verify that the clinical documentation is present to support each HCC submitted for payment on the claim. The following list outlines risk-adjustment coding errors often found during CMS RADV audits:

- Illegible signature with credentials.
- Documentation was unauthenticated in the EHR.
- Diagnosis documentation did not include the highest level of specificity for ICD code assignment.
- Clinical record description of the diagnosis did not support the submitted diagnosis code.
- Clinical record did not support the **monitor, evaluate, assess/address, or treat (MEAT)** requirements for each billed diagnosis (Olson 2013):
    - *Monitor:* The clinical record documents that the provider monitored signs, symptoms, and disease progress or regression.
    - *Evaluate:* The clinical record documents that the provider evaluated the test results, effectiveness of medication, and treatment response.
    - *Assess/address:* The clinical record documents that the provider assessed or addressed the clinical indicators by ordering tests, further reviewing records, or counseling the patient.
    - *Treat:* The clinical record indicates that the provider treated the patient using medications, therapies, or other treatment modalities (Premera Blue Cross 2017).

  Note: MEAT criteria are an industry-accepted standard for clinical documentation to support HCC assignment. However, to ensure that documentation meets CMS standards, CDI and coding professionals should also use the *ICD-10-CM Official Guidelines for Coding and Reporting* and *Coding Clinic for ICD-10-CM* to support coding of chronic conditions for HCC assignment.
- Clinical documentation was not specific to indicate a history of or current treatment status of cancer.
- Chronic conditions were not consistently documented as chronic.
- Chronic conditions reported on the claims were not documented annually in the clinical record.
- Manifestation codes for diseases such as diabetes were not consistently reported (Olson 2013).

The outpatient CDI should use this list to perform clinical documentation quality and coding audits in the outpatient setting as they relate to risk-adjusted methodology.

The RAF score is used to calculate the final annual payment to the Medicare Advantage plan. The RAF score calculation includes age, disability status, and chronic illnesses classified using ICD-10-CM and crosswalked to a corresponding HCC. Table 3.8 provides an example of this calculation. The allocation for the patient's age and disability marker is $3,409. The money allocated for the chronic diseases are listed in the next rows, with a total risk factor score of 1.583 and total annual dollar allocation for the patient of $11,810 (Pope et al. 2011).

Table 3.8. Hypothetical example of CMS-HCC (version 12) expenditure predictions and risk score for a community-residing, 76-year-old woman with acute myocardial infarction, angina pectoris, chronic obstructive pulmonary disease, renal failure, chest pain, and ankle sprain

Risk marker	Incremental prediction	Relative risk factor
Female, age 75–79	$3,409	0.457
Acute myocardial infarction (HCC 81)	$2,681	0.359
Angina pectoris (HCC 83)[1]	$0	—
Chronic obstructive pulmonary disease (HCC 108)	$2,975	0.399
Renal failure (HCC 131)	$2,745	0.368
Chest pain (HCC 166)[2]	$0	—
Ankle sprain (HCC 162)[2]	$0	—
Total	**$11,810**	**1,583**

Notes:
[1] HCC 83 Angina Pectoris has an incremental prediction, but the amount is not added because HCC 81 Acute Myocardial Infarction is within the same hierarchy and is the more severe manifestation of cardiovascular disease.
[2] Chest pain (symptom associated with a variety of medical conditions from minor to serious) and ankle sprain (typically transitory) are excluded from the payment model.
Source: Pope et al. 2011

The outpatient CDS can help the physician practice how to identify chronic illnesses through a thorough case review of patients scheduled for upcoming visits. This review should include each patient's clinical record from all sites of service, including inpatient, outpatient, and physician practice. Chronic illnesses that are treated or managed by the provider and documented during the encounter may be reported on the claim, and the corresponding HCC payment will be considered as part of the annual Medicare Advantage payment. The outpatient CDS can also use a database of previously identified HCCs from the last two to three years to clarify previously reported chronic illnesses. A more detailed description of this process is included in chapter 6 of this textbook.

Coding in the Facility Ambulatory Care Setting

As noted, multiple coding and reimbursement systems in the outpatient facility setting are used to determine the final codes for outpatient claims. Coders follow Medicare's OPPS guidelines when coding treatments and services provided to the ambulatory patient in the outpatient facility setting for Medicare claims. The OPPS guidelines provide APC codes to determine Medicare reimbursement. These guidelines are often also used by commercial payers.

To validate supporting clinical documentation for CPT and HCPCS code assignment, the CDS or coding professional must understand OPPS and APC assignment and the relevant CMS regulations. The CDS must also understand CMS regulations related to OPPS and APC assignments, such as OPPS Addendum B, APC weights, comprehensive APCs (C-APCs), and status indicators. The **APC weight** is a number assigned to each APC that, when multiplied by an annually designated conversion factor, identifies the payment by CMS for the specified APC. A **comprehensive APC (C-APC)** is an APC that has a primary service with a high cost, whereby that cost is a large portion of the cost of the patient encounter. A C-APC is similar to a diagnosis-related group (DRG) in that there is an all-inclusive rate for a group of related services. DRGs are explained later in this chapter.

According to CMS's most recent official definition, "a C-APC is defined as a classification for the provision of a primary service and all adjunctive services provided to support the delivery of the primary service" (CMS 2016e).

> When such a primary service is reported on a hospital outpatient claim, taking into consideration [a] few exceptions . . . we make payment for all other items and services reported on the hospital outpatient claim as being integral, ancillary, supportive, dependent, and adjunctive to the primary service (hereinafter collectively referred to as "adjunctive services") and representing components of a complete comprehensive service (78 FR 74865 and 79 FR 66799). Payments for adjunctive services are packaged into the payments for the primary services. This results in a single prospective payment for each of the primary, comprehensive services based on the costs of all reported services at the claim level. (CMS 2016e)

CMS instructs hospitals to report facility resources emergency department (ED) hospital visits using the CPT E/M codes found in the CPT manual (AMA 2017). Facilities should also develop internal hospital guidelines to code appropriate ED E/M visit level. CMS has not developed a national set of hospital-specific codes and guidance, advising hospitals instead to develop their own internal guidelines for assigning the ED E/M levels. The guidelines must take into consideration the intensity of hospital resources at the different E/M levels.

CMS has created alphanumeric HCPCS code G0463 (Hospital outpatient clinic visit for assessment and management of a patient) to be used by hospitals to report clinic visits on OPPS. G0463 is assigned to APC 0634 (Hospital clinic visits) (CMS 2018).

OPPS and APCs

Guidance on the coding and billing of claims in the outpatient facility setting is found on the CMS website (CMS 2017j). CMS uses **diagnosis-related groups (DRGs)** to classify inpatient care for reimbursement. A DRG may refer to (1) a unit of case-mix classification adopted by the federal government and some other payers as a prospective payment mechanism for hospital inpatients in which diseases are placed into groups because related diseases and treatments tend to consume similar amounts of healthcare resources and incur similar amounts of cost; in the Medicare and Medicaid programs, DRGs comprise more than 500 diagnostic classifications in which cases demonstrate similar resource consumption and length-of-stay patterns; or (2) a classification system that groups patients according to diagnosis, type of treatment, age, and other relevant criteria. Under the Prospective Payment System (PPS), hospitals are paid a set fee for treating patients in a single DRG category, regardless of the actual cost of care for the individual (CMS 2017g).

OPPS uses the APC to classify CPT and HCPCS codes. Like DRGs, APCs are assigned an annually updated weight by CMS that corresponds to a payment amount. Each year, CMS publishes "Addendum B. Final OPPS payment by HCPCS code" for use in determining the corresponding payments. In table 3.9, the HCPCS code in column A has a corresponding relative weight in column E. The corresponding payment rate is found in column F (CMS 2017j). Unlike DRGs, payments may be made for multiple APCs for the same encounter.

Table 3.9. Examples of OPPS payment by HCPCS code for calendar year 2017

A	B	C	D	E	F	G	H
	Addendum B.-Final OPPS Payment by HCPCS Code for CY 2017						
	CPT codes and descriptions only are copyright 2016 American Medical Association. All Rights Reserved. Applicable FARS/DFARS Apply. Dental codes (D codes) are copyright 2016 American Dental Association. All Rights Reserved.						
HCPCS Code	**Short Descriptor**	**SI**	**APC**	**Relative Weight**	**Payment Rate**	**National Unadjusted Copayment**	**Minimum Unadjusted Copayment**
25443	Reconstruct wrist joint	J1	5114	69.6200	$5,221.57	.	$1,044.32
25444	Reconstruct wrist joint	J1	5115	127.4814	$9,561.23	.	$1,912.25
25445	Reconstruct wrist joint	J1	5114	69.6200	$5,221.57	.	$1,044.32
25446	Wrist replacement	J1	5116	196.0524	$14,704.13	.	$2,940.83
25447	Repair wrist joints	J1	5113	32.5107	$2,438.34	.	$487.67
25449	Remove wrist joint implant	J1	5114	69.6200	$5,221.57	.	$1,044.32

Source: CMS 2017j

OPPS guidelines use several methodologies for determining payment for services in specific APCs:

- Each APC payment includes ancillary supportive and adjunctive items and services (packaging). There is no additional reimbursement for these packaged services as they are considered to be a part of another service (CMS 2016f, 6).
- Increased payment adjustments are made for rural and certain cancer hospitals (CMS 2016f, 7). APC payments are made for HCPCS codes that are similar clinically. Codes are given a relative weight and are multiplied by a conversion factor to determine payment (CMS 2016f, 7).
- Outlier payments are made when costs are more than the payment rates for a specific APC group.
- Pass-through items such as expensive drugs, devices, and biological as well as new technology items are reimbursed separately (CMS 2016f, 4–6).

The Hospital Chargemaster

Each facility maintains a **chargemaster**, also called a charge description master (CDM), which is a list of descriptions of procedures, services, and supplies with a corresponding department, CDM item code, revenue code, and price. The chargemaster file typically includes more than 10,000 line items, and the accuracy and comprehensiveness of its codes can be a concern for the CDI program. The revenue integrity department (or a related department) is responsible for maintaining the CDM and should conduct an annual evaluation of the file. This assessment should include the following:

- Identification of new supplies, procedures, and services to add to the list
- Annual review of charges for market and cost adjustment
- Monitoring of charge level for the hospital operating room
- Review of E/M levels for the ED
- Addition, deletion, and revision of CPT and HCPCS codes that have changed
- Evaluation of the accuracy of CDM mapping to other systems, such as the pharmacy or laboratory system
- Monitoring of CDM item volumes to screen for issues related to the charge capture process
- Identification and correction of misleading or unclear CDM descriptions that result in an incorrect selection of items from charge capture menus or encounter forms

The outpatient CDS should become familiar with the CDM and be able to identify missing revenue related to CDM code gaps. For example, if a new service or procedure is offered, the outpatient CDS should ensure that the clinical documentation is sufficient to support the new CDM code with regard to accurate coding as well as medical necessity. The CDS will require an understanding of the coding guidelines for the new service or procedure and must research medical necessity requirements so that the coders and providers may be educated in the approved diagnoses listed in the national or local coverage determination (see chapter 2 for discussion of coverage determinations). Where additional detail or specificity is required in the clinical documentation, coders may then query so that clinical documentation supports the more specific diagnosis code. Outpatient CDS staff should be invited to all meetings involving discussion of new procedures and CDM changes.

Coding in the ED

Coding in the ED may be performed by staff in health information management or the ED. The code sets for ED coding include ICD-10-CM, CPT, and HCPCS. In addition to codes for procedures performed in the ED, such as injection, infusion, fracture care, laceration repair, and critical care services, the CPT manual has a limited set of E/M codes (99281–99285) that are used in Type A EDs. A Type A

> provider-based emergency department must meet at least one of the following requirements: (1) It is licensed by the State in which it is located under applicable State law as an emergency room or emergency department and be open 24 hours a

day, 7 days a week; or (2) it is held out to the public (by name, posted signs, advertising, or other means) as a place that provides care for emergency medical conditions on an urgent basis without requiring a previously scheduled appointment and be open 24 hours a day, 7 days a week. (CMS 2017k)

Type B emergency departments use HCPCS codes G0380 through G0384. A Type B

provider-based emergency department must meet at least one of the following requirements: (1) It is licensed by the State in which it is located under applicable State law as an emergency room or emergency department, and open less than 24 hours a day, 7 days a week; or (2) it is held out to the public (by name, posted signs, advertising, or other means) as a place that provides care for emergency medical conditions on an urgent basis without requiring a previously scheduled appointment, and open less than 24 hours a day, 7 days a week; or (3) during the calendar year immediately preceding the calendar year in which a determination under 42 CFR 489.24 is being made, based on a representative sample of patient visits that occurred during that calendar year, it provides at least one-third of all of its outpatient visits for the treatment of emergency medical conditions on an urgent basis without requiring a previously scheduled appointment, regardless of its hours of operation. (CMS 2017k)

There is no national standard for hospital assignment of E/M code levels in the ED. Facilities have the option of using the definitions in the CPT book for these codes, or they can develop a system using facility-specific criteria to identify the level of service. Most of the systems that are criteria-based use ancillary and nursing care services and corresponding points to assign the level code. The American College of Emergency Physicians (ACEP) has reinforced the need for facility billing guidelines to be resource-based and to correspond with the ED CPT code levels reported on the patient claim:

> Facility billing guidelines should be designed to reasonably relate the intensity of hospital services to the different levels of effort represented by the codes. Coding guidelines should be based on facility resources, should be clear to facilitate accurate payments, should only require documentation that is clinically necessary for patient care, and should not facilitate upcoding or gaming. (ACEP 2011)

In this context, *resource-based* refers to criteria and guidelines that consider the extent of staff and other resources used when providing the service.

Professional organizations such as ACEP recommend methodologies for assigning E/M levels in the ED (ACEP 2011). Assigning the wrong level of care when coding claims can result in decreased or inaccurate reimbursement in the ED. The outpatient CDS can assist in ensuring the accuracy of E/M levels by mapping the charge codes to the criteria for assigning the levels. When a certain intervention is charged, the intervention is used to autocalculate the E/M level within the EHR system. For example, when the ACEP facility coding model is used for E/M level code 99284, the clinical documentation must meet the criteria for clinical interventions listed in table 3.10.

Each intervention can be mapped within the EHR to a template or software tool that autocalculates the ED E/M level. This can be done either through the assignment of a CPT/HCPCS code, a check-off box, or a free-format text box in a template (for example, discussion of discharge instructions). These mappings should be validated by the CDI manager for accuracy so that the corresponding E/M level assignment is correct.

Table 3.10. Required clinical interventions for E/M level code 99284 when the ACEP facility coding model is used

	Facility Charge Assignment	
Level	Possible Interventions	Potential Symptoms or Examples which support the interventions
IV CPT 99284 Type A: APC 615 Type B: APC 629 HCPCS: G0383	Could include interventions from previous levels, plus any of: • Preparation for two diagnostics tests: (Labs, EKG, X-ray) • Preparation for plain X-ray (multiple body areas: C-spine & foot, shoulder & pelvis) • Preparation for special imaging study (CT, MRI, Ultrasound, VQ scans) • Cardiac monitoring (2) nebulizer treatments • Port-a-Cath venous access • Administration and monitoring of infusions or parenteral medications (IV, IM, IO, SC) NG/PEG • Tube placement or replacement • Multiple reassessments • Prep or assist with procedures such as: Eye irrigation with Morgan lens, bladder irrigation with 3-way Foley, pelvic exam, etc. • Sexual Assault Exam without specimen collection • Psychotic patient; not suicidal • Discussion of Discharge Instructions (Complex)	• Blunt/penetrating trauma with limited diagnostic testing • Headache with nausea or vomiting • Dehydration requiring treatment • Dyspnea requiring oxygen • Respiratory illness relieved with (2) nebulizer treatments • Chest pain—with limited diagnostic testing • Abdominal pain—with limited diagnostic testing • Non-menstrual vaginal bleeding • Neurological symptoms—with limited diagnostic testing

Source: ACEP 2011

Chapter 3 Review Exercises

1. Three levels of interoperability have been suggested by the HIMSS (HIMSS 2013). Which of these is considered the highest level of interoperability, in which two or more systems or elements are able to exchange information and subsequently use the information that has been exchanged?
   a. Semantic
   b. Structural
   c. Nationwide
   d. Foundational

2. Which of the following is one of the four categories under which codes are organized alphabetically in the CPT code book?
   a. Complication
   b. Numeric reference
   c. Health and physical
   d. Synonym, eponym, or abbreviation

3. Basic outpatient coding guidelines instruct certain sequencing of ICD-10-CM codes for surgical encounters. If documentation includes a rule-out diagnosis, signs and symptoms, and reason for the surgical encounter, and the patient develops a complication during the surgical visit, what do the guidelines instruct?

a. List rule-out diagnosis first.
   b. List signs and symptoms first.
   c. List complication diagnosis first.
   d. List surgical encounter diagnosis first.

4. When selecting the appropriate level of E/M services provided, what are the three key components?
   a. Age, complications, and condition at admission
   b. History, examination, and medical decision making
   c. History, duration of conditions, and medical necessity
   d. Inpatient, outpatient ambulatory, outpatient status not determined

5. OPPS uses status indicators to identify the reimbursement action of a service, such as if a service is separately payable or packaged. The status indicators generating a "Not paid under OPPS" status are:
   a. L, N, Y
   b. D, E1, F
   c. B, E1, M
   d. A, B, C, D, F, L, M, Y

6. Under the Medicare Physician Fee Schedule (MPFS), CPT and HCPCS codes are reimbursed individually. With this method of reimbursement, which of the following is *not* needed to calculate reimbursement by CPT/HCPCS specific to a provider?
   a. GPCI
   b. RAF score
   c. RVU weight
   d. Conversion factor

7. The revenue integrity (or a related) department is typically responsible for maintaining the charge description master and should evaluate the file annually for all but which of the following purposes?
   a. Reviewing charges for market and cost adjustment
   b. Identifying new supplies, procedures, and services to add to the list
   c. Adding, deleting, and revising CPT and HCPCS codes that have changed
   d. Aligning hospital assignment of E/M codes in the ED with national standards

8. HCCs are codes used by Medicare Advantage plans to more accurately predict health cost expenditures of members by adjusting payments based on demographics as well as _____.
   a. RVUs
   b. APC codes
   c. Site of care
   d. Health status

9. Four organizations approve the guidelines for use in ICD-10-CM. This group is referred to as the _____.
   a. WHO
   b. NUCC
   c. Stakeholders
   d. Cooperating Parties

10. The ONC created the _____, which outlines the strategy and direction for improvement to the exchange of health information between systems through the nation.
   a. NUBC
   b. NUCC
   c. UB-04 form
   d. Shared Nationwide Interoperability Roadmap

References

45 CFR 160.103. Definitions. 2013 (Oct. 1).

American Academy of Family Physicians (AAFP). 2017. Medicare Physician Fee Schedule. http://www.aafp.org/advocacy/informed/payment/medicare/internal/medicare-physician-fee-schedule.html.

American College of Emergency Physicians (ACEP). 2011. ED facility level coding guidelines. https://www.acep.org/content.aspx?id=30428.

American Health Information Management Association (AHIMA). 2016. Clinical documentation improvement toolkit. bok.ahima.org/doc?oid=301829.

American Medical Association (AMA). 2017. *Current Procedural Terminology, Professional Edition 2018*. Chicago: AMA.

American Medical Association (AMA). 2016. Medicare Access and CHIP Reauthorization Act (MACRA) Quality Payment Program final rule: AMA summary. https://www.ama-assn.org/sites/default/files/media-browser/public/physicians/macra/macra-qpp-summary.pdf.

Butler, M. 2016 (March 1). AHIMA pledges support for HHS interoperability plan. *Journal of AHIMA* website. http://journal.ahima.org/2016/03/01/ahima-pledges-support-for-hhs-interoperability-plan.

Centers for Disease Control and Prevention (CDC). 2017. ICD-10-CM Official Guidelines for Coding and Reporting FY 2018. https://www.cdc.gov/nchs/data/icd/10cmguidelines_fy2018_final.pdf.

Centers for Medicare and Medicaid Services (CMS). 2018. Hospital Outpatient Prospective Payment—final rule with comment and final CY2017 payment rates. https://www.cms.gov/Medicare/Medicare-Fee-for-Service-Payment/HospitalOutpatientPPS/Hospital-Outpatient-Regulations-and-Notices-Items/CMS-1678-FC.html.

Centers for Medicare and Medicaid Services (CMS). 2017a. The Medicare Claims Processing Manual. Chapter 18: Preventive and screening services. 60.3: Determining high risk for developing colorectal cancer. https://www.cms.gov/Regulations-and-Guidance/Guidance/Manuals/Downloads/clm104c18.pdf.

Centers for Medicare and Medicaid Services (CMS). 2017b. Alpha-numeric HCPCS. https://www.cms.gov/Medicare/Coding/HCPCSReleaseCodeSets/Alpha-Numeric-HCPCS.html.

Centers for Medicare and Medicaid Services (CMS). 2017c. Medicare Learning Network: Evaluation and management services. https://www.cms.gov/Outreach-and-Education/Medicare-Learning-Network-MLN/MLNProducts/Downloads/eval-mgmt-serv-guide-ICN006764.pdf.

Centers for Medicare and Medicaid Services (CMS). 2017d. Medicare utilization for Part B. https://www.cms.gov/Research-Statistics-Data-and-Systems/Statistics-Trends-and-Reports/MedicareFeeforSvcPartsAB/MedicareUtilizationforPartB.html.

Centers for Medicare and Medicaid Services (CMS). 2017e. Medicare Physician Fee Schedule 2018 final rule. https://www.cms.gov/Medicare/Medicare-Fee-for-Service-Payment/PhysicianFeeSched/index.html.

Centers for Medicare and Medicaid Services (CMS). 2017f. Physician Fee Schedule search. https://www.cms.gov/apps/physician-fee-schedule/search/search-results.aspx?Y=0&T=4&HT=0&CT=2&H1=99213&C=13&M=5.

Centers for Medicare and Medicaid Services (CMS) Glossary. 2017g. Glossary. https://www.cms.gov /apps/glossary/default.asp?Letter=ALL&Language=English.

Centers for Medicare and Medicaid Services (CMS). 2017h. 2017 Model Software /ICD-10 Mapping s. https://www.cms.gov/Medicare/Health-Plans/MedicareAdvtgSpecRateStats/Risk-Adjustors-Items/Risk2017.html?DLPage=1&DLEntries=10&DLSort=0&DLSortDir=descending.

Centers for Medicare and Medicaid Services (CMS). 2017i. 2018 MA rate book. https://www.cms.gov/Medicare/Health-Plans/MedicareAdvtgSpecRateStats/Ratebooks-and-Supporting-Data-Items/2018Rates.html?DLPage=1&DLEntries=10&DLSort=0&DLSortDir=descending.

Centers for Medicare and Medicaid Services (CMS). 2017j. Addendum B. Final OPPS payment by HCPCS code for CY 2017. https://www.cms.gov/apps/ama/license.asp?file=/Medicare/Medicare-Fee-for-Service-Payment/Hospitaloutpatientpps/Downloads/2017-January-Addendum-B.zip.

Centers for Medicare and Medicaid Services (CMS). 2017k. OPPS visit codes frequently asked questions. https://www.cms.gov/medicare/medicare-fee-for-service-payment/hospitaloutpatientpps/downloads/opps_qanda.pdf.

Centers for Medicare and Medicaid Services (CMS). 2016a. Medicare Learning Network: Medicare billing: 837P and form CMS-1500. https://www.cms.gov/Outreach-and-Education/Medicare-Learning-Network-MLN/MLNProducts/MLN-Publications-Items/ICN006976.html.

Centers for Medicare and Medicaid Services (CMS). 2016b. Medicare Learning Network: How to use the Medicare National Correct Coding Initiative (NCCI) tools. https://www.cms.gov/Outreach-and-Education/Medicare-Learning-Network-MLN/MLNProducts/downloads/How-to-Use-NCCI-Tools.pdf.

Centers for Medicare and Medicaid Services (CMS). 2016c. Medicare Program; Revisions to payment policies under the Physician Fee Schedule and other revisions to Part B for CY 2017; Medicare Advantage bid pricing data release; Medicare Advantage and Part D Medical loss ratio data release; Medicare Advantage provider network requirements; expansion of Medicare Diabetes Prevention Program Model; Medicare Shared Savings Program requirements: Final rule. Federal Register 81(220):80170. https://www.gpo.gov/fdsys/pkg/FR-2016-11-15/pdf/2016-26668.pdf.

Centers for Medicare and Medicaid Services (CMS). 2016d. March 31, 2016, HHS-operated risk adjustment methodology meeting discussion paper. https://www.cms.gov/CCIIO/Resources/Forms-Reports-and-Other-Resources/Downloads/RA-March-31-White-Paper-032416.pdf.

Centers for Medicare and Medicaid Services (CMS). 2016e. Medicare Program: Hospital Outpatient Prospective Payment and Ambulatory Surgical Center Payment Systems and Quality Reporting Programs; Organ Procurement Organization Reporting and Communication; Transplant Outcome Measures and Documentation Requirements; Electronic Health Record (EHR) Incentive Programs; Payment to Nonexcepted Off-Campus Provider-Based Department of a Hospital; Hospital Value-Based Purchasing (VBP) Program; Establishment of Payment Rates Under the Medicare Physician Fee Schedule for Nonexcepted

Items and Services Furnished by an Off-Campus Provider-Based Department of a Hospital: Final rule with comment period and interim final rule with comment period. Federal Register 81(219):79580. https://www.gpo.gov/fdsys/pkg/FR-2016-11-14/pdf/2016-26515.pdf.

Centers for Medicare and Medicaid Services (CMS). 2016f. Medicare Learning Network: Hospital Outpatient Prospective Payment System. https://www.cms.gov/Outreach-and-Education/Medicare-Learning-Network-MLN/MLNProducts/downloads/HospitalOutpaysysfctsht.pdf.

Centers for Medicare and Medicaid Services (CMS). 2015. Healthcare Common Procedure Coding System (HCPCS) Level II Coding Procedures. https://www.cms.gov/Medicare/Coding/MedHCPCSGenInfo/Downloads/HCPCSLevelIICodingProcedures7-2011.pdf

Centers for Medicare and Medicaid Services (CMS). 2014. Electronic billing and EDI transactions: Institutional paper claim form (CMS-1450). https://www.cms.gov/Medicare/Billing/ElectronicBillingEDITrans/15_1450.html.

Healthcare Information and Management Systems Society (HIMSS). 2013. What is interoperability? http://www.himss.org/library/interoperability-standards/what-is-interoperability.

National Uniform Claim Committee (NUCC). 2017. http://www.nucc.org.

National Uniform Claim Committee (NUCC). 2013. The 02/12 1500 claim form: Understanding the changes to the form. http://www.nucc.org/images/stories/PDF/understanding_the_changes_to_the_0212_1500_claim_form.pdf.

Olson, Carol. 2013. "Top 10 Medicare Risk Adjustment Coding Errors." *AAPC Knowledge Center* (blog), March 20. https://www.aapc.com/blog/23877-top-10-medicare-risk-adjustment-coding-errors/.

Office of the National Coordinator for Health Information Technology (ONC). 2015. Connecting Health and Care for the Nation: A Shared Nation Interoperability Roadmap. Final version 1.0. https://www.healthit.gov/sites/default/files/hie-interoperability/nationwide-interoperability-roadmap-final-version-1.0.pdf.

Pope, G.C., J. Kautter, M.J. Ingber, S. Freeman, R. Sekar, C. Newhart, and RTI International. 2011. Evaluation of CMS-HCC risk adjustment model. Prepared for Centers for Medicare and Medicaid Services. https://www.cms.gov/Medicare/Health-Plans/MedicareAdvtgSpecRateStats/Downloads/Evaluation_Risk_Adj_Model_2011.pdf.

Premera Blue Cross. 2017. Medicare Advantage ICD-10 and risk adjustment presentation. https://www.premera.com/documents/035236.pdf.

Sayles, N. 2014. *Health Information Management Technology: An Applied Approach*. 4th ed. Chicago: AHIMA.

World Health Organization (WHO). 2017. http://www.who.int/en.

Regulation of Outpatient Healthcare and Compliant CDI Practice

4

Learning Objectives

- Explain which agencies and programs regulate and monitor hospital coding, billing, reimbursement, quality, and safety.
- Describe the quality reporting programs for outpatient facility and physician practices.
- Identify the agencies and organizations that publish public data on facility and provider quality.
- Discuss how quality reporting programs affect clinical documentation.
- Illustrate the components of a compliant outpatient clinical documentation improvement program.

Key Terms

Advanced Alternative Payment Models (Advanced APMs)
Advancing Care Information (ACI)
Agency for Healthcare Research and Quality (AHRQ)
Alternative Payment Models (APMs)
Chief compliance officer
Children's Health Insurance Program (CHIP)
Health Insurance Portability and Accountability Act (HIPAA)
Hospital Outpatient Quality Reporting (OQR) Program
Medicare Administrative Contractors (MACs)
Medicare Provider and Analysis Review (MedPAR)
Office of Inspector General (OIG)
OIG Work Plan
Prospective Payment System (PPS)
Research Data Assistance Center (ResDAC)

The quality and delivery of healthcare are regulated by federal and state agencies that establish standards for the healthcare industry. Regulations cover claims submission, reimbursement systems, healthcare practice and quality outcomes, and shared service arrangements for risk-based payment methodologies. The Centers for Medicare and Medicaid Services (CMS) administer many of these regulations and use government contractors to audit claims to identify potential fraud and abuse. Private sector agencies, such as the Leapfrog Group and Healthgrades, also monitor the quality of healthcare delivery and report on quality measures through the Internet and other publicly accessible forums to help consumers select high-quality facilities and providers. This chapter presents an overview of the agencies that regulate, monitor, and report on the quality of healthcare, their guidelines, and the importance of these guidelines to the practice of clinical documentation improvement (CDI) in the outpatient setting. This chapter also presents billing and compliance guidance from the US Department of Health and Human Services (HHS) Office of Inspector General (OIG), CMS, ICD-10-CM Official Guidelines for Coding and Reporting (CDC 2017), US Department of Justice (DOJ), and American Health Information Management Association (AHIMA).

Ambulatory CDI Compliance

Generally, the word *compliance* refers to the act of adhering to official requirements. In the healthcare industry, compliance depends on an organizational culture that promotes the prevention, detection, and resolution of instances of conduct that do not conform to federal, state, or private payer healthcare program requirements or the healthcare organization's ethical and business policies. In CDI and coding, compliance activities involve the process of managing a CDI, coding, or billing department according to the laws, regulations, and guidelines that govern its actors and actions.

Healthcare facilities normally have a **chief compliance officer** who is designated to monitor the compliance process and create a compliance plan. The compliance plan is a process that helps an organization, such as a hospital, accomplish its goal of providing high-quality medical care and efficiently operating a business within the requirements set out in various laws and regulations. These laws and regulations may be referred to as *compliance program guidance*. For example, the OIG of HHS provides compliance program guidance to help healthcare organizations develop internal controls that promote adherence to applicable federal and state guidelines. Appendix 4A of this textbook includes the OIG Compliance Program Guidance for Hospitals (OIG 1998a). Appendix 4B includes the OIG Supplemental Compliance Program Guidance for Hospitals (OIG 2005).

The CDI manager should either maintain a departmental compliance plan or include the CDI program compliance plan guidelines in the overall health information management (HIM) compliance plan. The CDI/HIM program should model the aspects of the OIG Program Guidance for Hospitals and the OIG Supplemental Compliance Program Guidance for Hospitals that focus on the unique regulations and guidelines with which coding and CDI professionals must comply.

Federal Compliance Guidance for CDI Programs

Federal guidance on compliance related to high-quality clinical documentation, coding, and billing practices is published by the OIG, CMS, and DOJ.

OIG Guidance

The **Office of Inspector General (OIG)** is tasked with "detecting and preventing fraud, waste, and abuse; identifying opportunities to improve program economy, efficiency and effectiveness; and holding accountable those who do not meet program requirements or who violate federal health care laws" (OIG 2017). To help with this mission, the OIG has developed a series of guidance documents for voluntary compliance programs in hospitals (OIG 1998a; OIG 2005), small group physician practices (OIG 2000), and third-party medical billing companies (OIG 1998b). This guidance recommends that organizations self-audit claims to ensure that the following standards are met:

- Bills are accurately coded and accurately reflect the services provided (as documented in the medical records).
- Documentation is being completed correctly.
- Services or items provided are reasonable and necessary.
- There are no incentives for unnecessary services.

In an ideal CDI program, the CDI manager and outpatient clinical documentation specialist (CDS) staff work collaboratively with the medical and coding staff to ensure complete and accurate documentation and submission of an accurate claim. CDI managers and CDS staff are encouraged to review the OIG program guidance published in the *Federal Register* to understand the compliance requirements. The CDI manager and the chief compliance officer should meet routinely, and they should on an annual basis review together the most recent **OIG Work Plan**, which outlines the focus for reviews and investigations in various healthcare settings (OIG 2018). The OIG Work Plan is explained in greater detail later in this chapter.

OIG Guidance for Hospitals

The initial OIG guidance for hospitals was published in the *Federal Register* in 1998 (OIG 1998a), with supplemental guidance issued in the *Federal Register* in 2005 (OIG 2005). The supplemental guidance "contains new compliance recommendations and an expanded discussion of risk areas, taking into account recent changes to hospital payment systems and regulations, evolving industry practices, current enforcement priorities, and lessons learned in the area of corporate compliance" (OIG 2005). The CDI manager and ambulatory CDS will be most interested in the guidance on "submission of accurate claims and information" (OIG 2005). OIG has identified the following risks in this area (OIG 2005):

- Inaccurate or incorrect coding.
- Upcoding (the practice of assigning diagnostic or procedural codes that represent higher payment rates than the codes that actually reflect the

services provided to patients). Closely related to upcoding is overcoding, which is the practice of assigning more codes than needed to describe a patient's condition. Some instances of overcoding may be contrary to the guidance provided in the ICD-10-CM Official Guidelines for Coding and Reporting (CDC 2017).

- Unbundling of services (the practice of using multiple codes to bill for the various individual steps in a single procedure, rather than using a single code that includes all steps of the comprehensive procedure).
- Billing for medically unnecessary services or other services not covered by the relevant healthcare program.
- Billing for services not provided.
- Duplicate billing.
- Insufficient documentation.

The OIG notes that, "because incorrect procedure coding may lead to overpayments and subject a hospital to liability for the submission of false claims, hospitals need to pay close attention to coder training and qualifications" (OIG 2005). Furthermore, "hospitals should also review their outpatient documentation practices to ensure that claims are based on complete medical records and that the medical records support the levels of service claimed" (OIG 2005). In some circumstances, the outpatient CDS may be the first team member to identify an incorrect code assignment. For example, on a claim for a Medicare Advantage patient, the outpatient CDS might notice a potential coding problem when the provider selects the *International Classification of Diseases, Tenth Revision, Clinical Modification* (ICD-10-CM) code for diabetic peripheral vascular disease even though the patient record reflects only diabetes and peripheral vascular disease was documented during the previous year. Incorrect use of the ICD-10-CM code for diabetic peripheral vascular disease would result in a higher-level Hierarchical Condition Category (HCC) submission on the claim than is warranted based on the clinical documentation. In this example, if the CDS performs the case review immediately after the visit and requests an addendum to the progress note from the provider, the documentation can be corrected, and the filing of a noncompliant claim can be averted. See chapter 3 for a discussion of HCC code assignment.

OIG Guidance for Individual and Small Group Practices

The OIG guidance for individual and small group practices contains the following seven components for creating a voluntary compliance program (OIG 2000):

- Conducting internal monitoring and external auditing
- Implementing compliance and practice standards
- Designating a compliance officer or contact
- Conducting appropriate training and education
- Responding appropriately to detected offenses and developing corrective action
- Developing open lines of communication
- Enforcing disciplinary standards through well-publicized guidelines

In its guidance, the OIG has made allowances for the smaller practices, giving consideration to their limited financial and staffing resources to implement a full-scale compliance program. However, regardless of the size of the organization, "all health care providers have a duty to reasonably ensure that the claims submitted to Medicare and other federal health care programs are true and accurate" (OIG 2000). Furthermore, the OIG suggests that "the increased accuracy of documentation that may result from a compliance program will actually assist in enhancing patient care," while lowering the risk for federal audits and legal problems and improving billing and reimbursement (OIG 2000). Whether a billing error is an honest mistake or negligence, the physician practice must return any funds that it erroneously claims. If the billing error is not a violation of civil, criminal, or administrative law, only the return of funds is required (OIG 2000).

OIG Guidance for Third-Party Medical Billing Companies

Numerous hospital and physician practices use third-party medical billing companies to assist in claims processing. Some companies simply process the claims, whereas others also code records prior to claims processing. Additionally, providers may ask billing companies to provide timely and accurate advice related to reimbursement. In 1998, the OIG published guidance to assist third-party medical billing companies in developing effective internal controls that promote adherence to applicable federal and state laws and program requirements for federal, state, and private health plans (OIG 1998b). At a minimum, the OIG requires that the third-party company's compliance program include the following seven elements:

(1) The development and distribution of written standards of conduct, as well as written policies and procedures that promote the billing company's commitment to compliance (e.g., by including adherence to the compliance program as an element in evaluating managers and employees) and that address specific areas of potential fraud, such as the claims submission process, code gaming and financial relationships with its providers;

(2) The designation of a chief compliance officer and other appropriate bodies, e.g., a corporate compliance committee, charged with the responsibility of operating and monitoring the compliance program and who report directly to the CEO [chief executive officer] and the governing body;

(3) The development and implementation of regular, effective education and training programs for all affected employees;

(4) The creation and maintenance of a process, such as a hotline, to receive complaints and the adoption of procedures to protect the anonymity of complainants and to protect callers from retaliation;

(5) The development of a system to respond to allegations of improper/illegal activities and the enforcement of appropriate disciplinary action against employees who have violated internal compliance policies, applicable statutes, regulations or federal, state or private payor health care program requirements;

(6) The use of audits and/or other risk evaluation techniques to monitor compliance and assist in the reduction of identified problem areas;

(7) The investigation and correction of identified systemic problems and the development of policies addressing the non-employment of sanctioned individuals. (OIG 1998b)

The OIG has identified the following high-risk areas for medical billing, all of which should be familiar to the CDI manager and ambulatory CDS:

- Billing for items or services not actually documented;
- Unbundling;
- Upcoding [...]
- Lack of integrity in computer systems [system integrity refers to data that is accurate and secure from unauthorized access];
- Computer software programs that encourage billing personnel to enter data in fields indicating services were rendered though not actually performed or documented;
- Failure to maintain the confidentiality of information/records;
- Knowing misuse of provider identification numbers, which results in improper billing; [...]
- Duplicate billing in an attempt to gain duplicate payment;
- Failure to properly use modifiers. (OIG 1998b)

It is important to include these areas in the policies and procedures of both the CDI and HIM coding departments. The CDI program workplan should require a collaborative process with the HIM coding department to ensure that these practices do not occur. For example, the workplan could indicate that the ambulatory CDS will notify the coding department about all compliance concerns and provide physician education on issues related to charging trends for specific procedures that are not properly documented. See chapter 10 for additional information on the CDI workplan.

OIG Work Plan

The OIG's plans for ongoing investigations of fraud and abuse in healthcare are found on the OIG Work Plan website (OIG 2018). The OIG Work Plan is updated monthly, and new Work Plan items are added at that time. The OIG Work Plan covers the following areas:

- Mandatory requirements for OIG reviews, as set forth in laws, regulations, or other directives;
- Requests made or concerns raised by Congress, HHS management, or the Office of Management and Budget;
- Top management and performance challenges facing HHS;
- Work performed by other oversight organizations (e.g., GAO [Government Accountability Office]);
- Management's actions to implement OIG recommendations from previous reviews; and
- Potential for positive impact. (OIG 2018)

The OIG Work Plan also includes the following issues related to legal and OIG investigations:

- Investigating fraud, waste and abuse
- Facilitating compliance in the health care industry
- Excluding bad actors from participation in federal health care programs (OIG 2018)

When new initiatives are added to the OIG Work Plan, they are posted on the OIG website (OIG 2018) and in the annual plan (appendix 4C). For example, the 2017 OIG Work Plan included the following initiatives related to outpatient CDI:

- Monitoring payments for clinical diagnostic laboratory tests
- Medicare payments for transitional care management
- Medicare payments for chronic care management
- Drug waste of single-use vial drugs
- Management review: CMS's implementation of the Quality Payment Program (OIG 2017)

CDI managers should work with the hospital compliance department to develop a workplan that includes areas under review by the OIG and other government agencies. Then, the outpatient CDS can work collaboratively with providers to improve clinical documentation related to issues such as transitional care management, chronic care management, and HCC code assignment. For example, the OIG aims to stop overpayments to Medicare Advantage plans for HCCs that were not properly documented in the clinical record. Therefore, the outpatient CDS should ensure that the previsit and concurrent visit or postvisit case reviews include assessment of complete clinical documentation for each ICD-10-CM code that crosswalks to an HCC code.

Guidance from CMS

CMS regulations and guidance are among the primary standards used by facilities and providers for compliant coding and billing practices. CMS publishes its claims submission requirements in a series of online manuals. When coding, billing, and clinical documentation questions arise, the outpatient CDS should use these detailed manuals, such as the Medicare Claims Processing Manual (CMS 2017a), as a key reference. The claims processing requirements for each state Medicaid program may be found in the Medicaid Provider Manual for each state (for example, RI EOHHS 2018). Each CMS manual is updated annually to correspond with changes to the ICD-10-CM and *International Classification of Diseases, Tenth Revision, Procedure Coding System* (ICD-10-PCS) and Current Procedural Terminology/Healthcare Common Procedure Coding System (CPT/HCPCS) for that year. It is important for each CDS to keep abreast of these annual changes because they affect the claims submission process and prevent denials. Further details about the claims submission process are discussed in chapters 6 and 7 of this text.

DOJ Compliance Memorandum

In 2017, the Fraud Section of the DOJ published a memorandum that addresses the following 11 important compliance-related topics (DOJ 2017):

- Analysis and remediation of underlying misconduct
- Senior and middle management
- Autonomy and resources
- Policies and procedures

- Operational integration
- Risk assessment
- Training and communications
- Confidential reporting and investigation
- Incentives and disciplinary measures
- Continuous improvement, periodic testing, and review
- Third-party management
- Mergers and acquisitions

For each topic, the memo lists pertinent questions asked by the DOJ to assess the quality of a corporate compliance program. However, the DOJ notes that the document is not meant to be used as a checklist or formula for healthcare compliance, and not all points are relevant to every compliance program (DOJ 2017).

Several of the topics and questions from the DOJ memo that apply to the development of an outpatient CDI program are reviewed here. The outpatient CDI program manager and CDS staff should review the DOJ memo in its entirety.

Analysis and Remediation of Underlying Misconduct

Under this topic, the DOJ memo lists questions about root cause analysis, prior indications, and remediation.

Root Cause Analysis – What is the company's root cause analysis of the misconduct at issue? What systemic issues were identified? Who in the company was involved in making the analysis? (DOJ 2017)

The root cause analysis topic points to the value of root cause identification when staff report billing compliance issues or such issues are being monitored as part of the CDI program. Root cause analysis is an important part of the CDI implementation plan and is conducted after data analysis and audit identify areas of focus around claims submission, such as coding errors due to clinical documentation gaps or inaccurate code assignment. Additional information on root cause analysis may be found in chapter 5.

Prior Indications – Were there prior opportunities to detect the misconduct in question, such as audit reports identifying relevant control failures or allegations, complaints, or investigations involving similar issues? What is the company's analysis of why such opportunities were missed? (DOJ 2017)

DOJ guidance recommends that hospitals monitor issues such as claims submission compliance to self-identify issues and determine the reasons that they occurred. Outpatient facilities should also analyze trend reports about claims submission errors. If trends are identified, the CDI program can perform root cause analysis and help correct the problem through process redesign, education, and monitoring.

Remediation – What specific changes has the company made to reduce the risk that the same or similar issues will not occur in the future? What specific remediation has addressed the issues identified in the root cause and missed opportunity analysis? (DOJ 2017)

Hospitals should monitor claims submission issues and put in place measures to prevent similar issues from occurring in the future. These measures should be included in the CDI workflow.

Senior and Middle Management

In this part of the memo, the DOJ asks questions about conduct at the top of the organization and the commitment of leaders and managers to compliance efforts (DOJ 2017).

Conduct at the Top – How have senior leaders, through their words and actions, encouraged or discouraged the type of misconduct in question? What concrete actions have they taken to demonstrate leadership in the company's compliance and remediation efforts? How does the company monitor its senior leadership's behavior? How has senior leadership modelled proper behavior to subordinates? (DOJ 2017)

Leaders of the CDI program (such as the steering committee and taskforce members) should be ready to provide documented steps reflecting the compliance monitoring process and remediation efforts that are conducted on an ongoing basis (see chapters 5 through 9 for further information on the CDI steering committee and taskforce). Evidence of appropriate compliance-related communication to staff, such as sign-in logs, signed policy and procedure documents, e-mail instructions, and training session minutes should be available upon request.

Shared Commitment – What specific actions have senior leaders and other stakeholders (e.g., business and operational managers, finance, procurement, legal, human resources) taken to demonstrate their commitment to compliance, including their remediation efforts? How is information shared among different components of the company? (DOJ 2017)

Members of the CDI steering committee and taskforce and other stakeholders in CDI must document their personal involvement in the monitoring and remediation efforts for clinical documentation compliance. Minutes of meetings and sign-in logs are important to demonstrate the shared commitment of the executive and middle-management-level staff to compliance.

Compliance Role – Was compliance involved in training and decisions relevant to the misconduct? Did the compliance or relevant control functions (e.g., legal, finance, or audit) ever raise a concern in the area where the misconduct occurred? (DOJ 2017)

Autonomy and Resources

The chief compliance officer and appropriate compliance leadership should be included in the discussions of risk mitigation when issues are identified. Involvement by the compliance team is also critical during the training and decision-making process around prevention of future incidents.

The chief compliance officer should be included as a speaker during CDI program training for the CDS and coding team members. The chief compliance officer should address the importance of high-quality documentation and accurate ICD-10-CM, CPT, and HCPCS code assignments. Executive leadership from the legal, finance, and audit departments are also essential in the discussion, decision-making, and education process to reflect high-level executive support of the risk mitigation process.

Policies and Procedures

Under this topic, the DOJ memo lists questions about compliance policies and procedures.

> **Designing Compliance Policies and Procedures** – What has been the company's process for designing and implementing new policies and procedures? Who has been involved in the design of policies and procedures? Have business units/divisions been consulted prior to rolling them out? (DOJ 2017)

The CDI program manager is responsible for creating and maintaining the department policies and procedures that include the industry guidance from DOJ, OIG, and the Cooperating Parties (the four organizations that oversee ICD-10-CM/PCS). The introduction to the policies and procedures should establish a process for maintenance and updates; participation and approval from executive and middle management leadership should be required as part of this process.

> **Applicable Policies and Procedures** – Has the company had policies and procedures that prohibited the misconduct? How has the company assessed whether these policies and procedures have been effectively implemented? How have the functions that had ownership of these policies and procedures been held accountable for supervisory oversight? (DOJ 2017)

The CDI program policies and procedures should specify prohibited misconduct related to claims submission, clinical documentation, and compliant query practice. They should also document the staff training process to ensure compliance and explain the accountability of not only the executive and middle management staff but also the supervisory staff. Chapter 15 of this text provides additional guidance on compliant query process.

> **Accessibility** – How has the company communicated the policies and procedures relevant to the misconduct to relevant employees and third parties? How has the company evaluated the usefulness of these policies and procedures? (DOJ 2017)

The CDI manager should document communications related to misconduct and be able to produce the information upon request. If the communication was a spoken exchange, the record can be a memo or other written document that summarizes the content of the conversation. The CDI manager should monitor compliance practices, report noncompliant incidents, and be able to produce minutes of meetings reflecting the effective use of these policies and procedures to handle noncompliance.

Operational Integration

Responsibility for Integration – Who has been responsible for integrating policies and procedures? With whom have they consulted (e.g., officers, business segments)? How have they been rolled out (e.g., do compliance personnel assess whether employees understand the policies)? (DOJ 2017)

The CDI manager should document the integration process for CDI policies and procedures throughout the organization. This documentation should reflect training programs, sign-in logs, and discussions related to changes in the clinical documentation workflow within specific stakeholder departments. When staff training programs are held, posttraining testing should be conducted to validate the understanding of the participants. These records should be maintained as evidence of the organization's compliance activities. The CDI manager should discuss record maintenance requirements with the chief compliance officer.

Controls – What controls failed or were absent that would have detected or prevented the misconduct? Are they there now? (DOJ 2017)

The CDI manager should document incidents where policies and procedural controls were ineffective in preventing compliance-related incidents. The documentation should include a discussion of policy and procedure revisions, training, and future monitoring for similar incidents.

Training and Communications

This section of the DOJ memo presents questions focused on the training of staff involved in compliance.

Risk-Based Training – What training have employees in relevant control functions received? Has the company provided tailored training for high-risk and control employees that addressed the risks in the area where the misconduct occurred? What analysis has the company undertaken to determine who should be trained and on what subjects? (DOJ 2017)

Where trends of noncompliance are identified, the CDI manager should document specific training for those staff members working in the high-risk areas. The discussion of who should be trained and the decision-making process around training topics should also be included in the documentation.

Confidential Reporting and Investigation

This part of the DOJ memo provides guidance on how compliance-related concerns are reported and investigated.

Effectiveness of the Reporting Mechanism – How has the company collected, analyzed, and used information from its reporting mechanisms? How has the company assessed the seriousness of the allegations it received? Has the compliance function had full access to reporting and investigative information? (DOJ 2017)

When there is a noncompliance issue, the CDI manager should document how the data related to that issue are collected and how the information is shared.

The subsequent process of how the issue is addressed, including persons notified, information shared, corrective action plan, and monitoring activities, should also be documented by the CDI manager. The documentation should support a confidential reporting mechanism to protect the person reporting the incident from retaliation. The CDI manager should discuss the facility policy and procedures on compliance reporting with the chief compliance officer to determine the proper method of maintaining confidentiality during the reporting process.

Continuous Improvement, Periodic Testing, and Review

In this section of the memo, the DOJ poses questions about internal audits and other assessment of compliance within the organization.

> **Internal Audit** – What types of audits would have identified issues relevant to the misconduct? Did those audits occur and what were the findings? What types of relevant audit findings and remediation progress have been reported to management and the board on a regular basis? How have management and the board followed up? How often has internal audit generally conducted assessments in high-risk areas? (DOJ 2017)

The CDI manager should document in detail the type of monitoring assessments that will be conducted if a noncompliance issue arises. For example, the CDI policy could state that if the CDS observes that patients are admitted to the observation area before a provider order is given, or without a provider order, the CDS should review a focused sample of concurrent cases to determine whether education and training for the nursing staff and providers on documentation requirements for observation were effective. The policy could also require that monitoring results are documented in detail and in an executive summary format, with the results presented to the CDI taskforce and steering committee and the results and corresponding discussion documented in the committee minutes.

AHIMA Standards of Ethical Coding and Coding Compliance

AHIMA offers Standards of Ethical Coding as guidance for ethical diagnostic and procedure coding. These standards, which are published on the AHIMA website, are intended to assist coding professionals and managers in decision-making processes and actions, outline expectations for making ethical decisions in the workplace, and demonstrate coding professionals' commitment to integrity during the coding process, regardless of the purpose for which the codes are being reported. The standards are relevant to all coding professionals and those who manage the coding function, regardless of the healthcare setting in which they work or whether they are AHIMA members or nonmembers. Every CDS who collaborates on and recommends code assignment in the ambulatory setting should follow them (AHIMA 2016).

Since 2016, AHIMA's ethical standards have included the principle, "Refuse to participate in the development of coding and coding-related technology that is not designed in accordance with requirements" (AHIMA 2016). This requirement was added to address the increase in coding-related technology, including the electronic health record (EHR). This standard emphasizes that HIM professionals, including CDSs and coders, cannot ethically participate in the development of technology solutions that do not comply with ethical coding practices as specified in the AHIMA Standards of Ethical Coding. For example, it would be unethical for the CDS to support the use of an EHR template that encourages the provider to merely check the smoking cessation counseling box to indicate that the counseling service was provided to the patient—in this case, the clinical record must clearly define the counseling session (that is, what was discussed and with whom); a checked box alone is not adequate documentation to support this service.

Operationalizing Program Compliance

In general, the steps to resolve a compliance issue are identification of the issue; understanding the cause; creation of a solution; and validation of the solution. To identify and resolve the issue, the CDI manager may incorporate the following steps into the CDI program policies and procedures. These steps reflect a high-level view of the process:

- *Step 1: Monitor and trend data:* At the start of the new CDI program, data analytics will be used to monitor the key metrics important to program success. Information found in compliance reports, coding audits, chargemaster revenue and usage reports, claims editors, denials reports, and HCC capture reports will be used for this purpose to identify possible clinical documentation, coding, reimbursement, and billing compliance issues.
- *Step 2: Identify focus areas:* From the information gathered in the analytics review, the CDI manager will select the issues to be included as part of the CDI process. The focused issue list will be presented to the CDI taskforce for implementation discussions.
- *Step 3: Address governance structure accountability:* The CDI manager will provide an overview of the responsibilities and accountability of the executive steering committee members and CDI taskforce members with regard to compliance issues. The executive steering committee should include the chief compliance officer as an ad hoc member to be present during compliance-related discussions. The roles, responsibilities, and accountability should be included in the committee minutes as well as the CDI policies and procedures.
- *Step 4: Perform case audit:* Once the focused issue list has been established, the CDI taskforce will determine the staffing requirements and implementation process. Based on the type of focused item, the sample selection and case review methodology will be determined. Sample selection may be random or subjective. Case review may be previsit, concurrent, postvisit, or retrospective.
- *Step 5: Conduct root cause analysis:* After the audit is complete, the CDI manager in conjunction with the CDS case reviewer or HIM code auditor will discuss the possible root causes of the focused issues. Where needed, specialty providers and outpatient clinic or physician practice staff may be asked to join the discussion.

- *Step 6: Create corrective action plan:* An essential part of the compliance program is the corrective action plan. The plan will outline the details of the issue(s), how issues were identified, the root cause(s), and a detailed description of the recommended process redesign, accountability for the new process, and the monitoring process to validate the solution.
- *Step 7: Revise CDI policies and procedures:* Once the corrective action plan is in place and the solution has been validated, the corresponding policy and procedures must be updated and shared with stakeholders.
- *Step 8: Redesign CDS query integration:* When the root cause, corrective action plan, and policy and procedures are in place, the redesigned process can be implemented. Implementation will likely involve the intervention of the CDS in the previsit, concurrent, and postvisit case review and corresponding query process.
- *Step 9: Educate providers and coding staff:* After the CDS has piloted the redesign process, provider and coding staff education will be conducted. In cases where a specialty-specific provider is included in root cause and workflow redesign discussions, the appropriate education can be provided at that time.
- *Step 10: Monitor the new process:* Steps 1 and 2 will be repeated after the new workflow process is implemented. The data will be analyzed to determine whether the process has resolved the focused issue, without creating new issues to address. An audit (Step 4) will also be conducted to validate correction of the focused issue.

Government Agencies Regulating Healthcare

HHS is the primary federal department that regulates US healthcare. The chief policy officer and general manager of HHS is the Secretary of Health and Human Services, and the Office of the Secretary is responsible for overseeing the department's programs and activities (HHS 2015). Within HHS, there are three human services divisions and eight US Public Health Service agencies (see figure 4.1) (HHS 2017a). Among the agencies that are most familiar to the CDI specialists are the following (HHS 2015):

- *CMS*, which oversees Medicare; federal aspects of Medicaid and the Children's Health Insurance Program (CHIP), which are jointly sponsored and funded by the federal and state governments; the Health Insurance Marketplace; and quality assurance activities associated with the following programs:
  - *Medicare Part A:* Part A insurance helps cover the cost of inpatient care in hospitals, including critical access hospitals, and skilled nursing facilities (not custodial or long-term care) for Medicare beneficiaries. Part A also assists in covering hospice care and some home healthcare. Beneficiaries must meet certain conditions to get these benefits.
  - *Medicare Part B:* Part B is an optional and supplemental portion of Medicare into which beneficiaries pay a monthly premium. It helps cover doctors' services and outpatient care. It also covers some other

Figure 4.1. Organization chart for the US Department of Health and Human Services

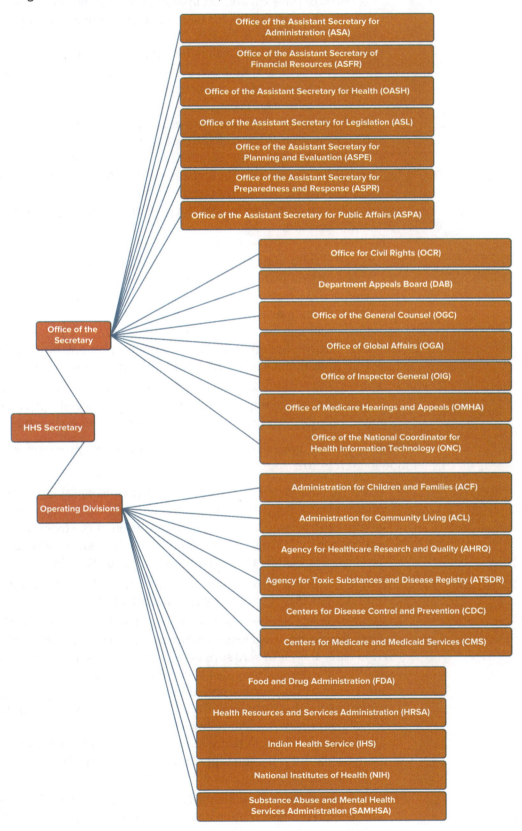

Source: Adapted from HHS 2017a

medical services that Part A does not cover, such as some of the services of physical and occupational therapists, and some home healthcare. Part B pays for these covered services and supplies when they are medically necessary.
- *Medicare Part C:* Part C offers health insurance through private companies, such as health maintenance organizations and preferred provider organizations, to Medicare beneficiaries. These plans are also called *Medicare Advantage plans.*
- *Medicare Part D:* Part D covers prescription drugs and assists Medicare beneficiaries by lowering the cost of drugs.
- *Medicaid:* Medicaid is a joint federal and state program that helps pay the medical costs for some people with low incomes and limited resources. Medicaid programs vary from state to state, but most healthcare costs are covered if a patient qualifies for both Medicare and Medicaid.
- The **Children's Health Insurance Program (CHIP)**: As mentioned, CHIP is funded through states as well as the federal government. It offers health insurance to eligible uninsured children (up to age 19 years) and pregnant women; eligibility is determined by the states and is based on financial need (CSM 2017b).
- *Centers for Disease Control and Prevention (CDC):* CDC oversees efforts to control and prevent diseases and other preventable conditions, as well as initiatives to address public health emergencies.
- **Agency for Healthcare Research and Quality (AHRQ)**: AHRQ aims to find evidence to improve the safety, quality, accessibility, equitability, and affordability of healthcare and promote the use of such evidence.

HHS administers more than 100 programs, including programs related to the following (HHS 2015):

- *The privacy and security of protected health information (PHI):* The **Health Insurance Portability and Accountability Act of 1996 (HIPAA)** is the law that enforces and mandates the adoption of the federal privacy protections for individual patient information, including national standards for electronic healthcare transactions and security (HHS 2017b).
- Health insurance provided through the Patient Protection and Affordable Care Act (ACA), Medicare, Medicaid, and CHIP.
- *Social services:* For example, the Office of Family Assistance (OFA) supports Temporary Assistance for Needy Families (TANF), Head Start, child care, and child care support to help families and communities. The TANF program provides a way for needy families to achieve self-sufficiency through state-funded block grants that design and operate programs for this purpose (OFA 2017a). Other OFA programs include Tribal Temporary Assistance for Needy Families (Tribal TANF), Native Employment Works, Healthy Marriage and Responsible Fatherhood grants, Health Profession Opportunity Grants, and Tribal TANF-Child Welfare Coordination grants (OFA 2017b).
- *Disease prevention and wellness:* Multiple agencies have programs that offer resources to encourage healthy lifestyles and provide routine health screenings and vaccinations.

- *Public health and safety:* Multiple agencies are involved in protecting public health and safety as related to food, drugs, medical devices, and violence prevention.
- *Education and training:* HHS offers opportunities, including loans, scholarships, and training programs, for health professionals and students to advance in their careers and improve their expertise.
- *Research:* HHS supports research that expands scientific understanding of healthcare, public health, human services, biomedical research, and food safety.

CMS is the agency with the greatest impact on clinical documentation requirements. It establishes guidelines for health claims submission, coding, and reimbursement methodologies. Most commercial insurance companies follow CMS guidelines for claims submission and coding.

Medicare Administrative Contractors (MACs), which were established by CMS to administer the Medicare program, and other contractors help CMS monitor and enforce its regulations. A MAC is a private healthcare insurance company that has jurisdiction for Medicare Part A and Part B claims as well as for durable medical equipment (DME) and Fee-for-Service (FFS) claims for Medicare beneficiaries in a specific geographic region. In each region, the MAC is "the primary operational contact between the Medicare FFS program and the health care providers enrolled in the program" (CMS 2017c).

CMS has established multiple reimbursement methodologies and corresponding guidelines to facilitate the payment of healthcare claims for the various settings in the continuum of care:

- *Fee schedule–based payments:* "A fee schedule is a complete listing of fees used by Medicare to pay doctors or other providers/suppliers. This comprehensive listing of fee maximums is used to reimburse a physician and/or other providers on a fee-for-service basis. CMS develops fee schedules for physicians, ambulance services, clinical laboratory services, and durable medical equipment, prosthetics, orthotics, and supplies" (CMS 2017d).
- **Prospective Payment System (PPS)**: PPS is a reimbursement methodology for Medicare payment that is based on a predetermined and fixed amount. Payments for services are based on a classification system such as diagnosis-related groups (DRGs) or ambulatory payment classifications (APCs), making it possible for healthcare facilities to predict what the payment will be for a specific encounter. Separate PPSs exist for acute inpatient hospitals, hospital outpatient settings, home health agencies, skilled nursing facilities, long-term care hospitals, inpatient rehabilitation facilities, hospice, and inpatient psychiatric facilities (CMS 2017e).
- *Value-based programs:* These programs reward healthcare providers by giving bonuses for high-quality and more efficient healthcare delivery. CMS initially established the following four value-based programs: Hospital Acquired Conditions program; Hospital Readmission Reduction program; Hospital Value-Based Purchasing program; and Value Modifier (VM) program, which is also called the Physician Value-Based Modifier program. Other programs have been subsequently added (CMS 2017f).

Public Data and Quality Reporting

Public data related to healthcare quality are increasingly available through the Internet and other public forums. The data focus on a wide range of topics, such as patient safety and satisfaction, quality, and reimbursement (Buttner et al. 2016), and are used to report about and compare providers. The increased availability and awareness of public data about healthcare allow health systems and patients alike to assess the quality of care and consider the various options and services available in the marketplace. However, publicly available healthcare data cannot include PHI (see chapter 2). To ensure the privacy and security of PHI, healthcare data reporting requirements have been established through federal regulations associated with HIPAA, the Health Information Technology for Economic and Clinical Health (HITECH) Act (including the EHR incentive program), and the ACA (Buttner et al. 2016).

Publicly available healthcare data, with PHI removed, are typically stored in a database or other electronic storage format. Software tools are required to download and manipulate the data for analysis. For example, the **Research Data Assistance Center (ResDAC)**, a CMS contractor that provides data to healthcare organizations and researchers, offers the **Medicare Provider and Analysis Review (MedPAR)** database, which contains data on 100 percent of Medicare beneficiaries using hospital inpatient services (ResDAC 2017; CMS 2017g).

Outpatient claims data are also available for use by healthcare organizations for statistical analysis. For example, the following limited data set (LDS) files are among those available online from CMS (CMS 2017h):

- Skilled nursing facility MEDPAR LDS
- Long-term care hospital PPS expanded modified MedPAR
- Hospital Outpatient Prospective Payment System (OPPS)
- Ambulatory surgical center (ASC) payment system
- OPPS partial hospitalization program LDS
- Standard analytical files (Medicare claims) LDS

Data are used by agencies to score healthcare providers by benchmarking them against their peers. The following three categories group most of the types of data currently available:

- Quality or performance measure data collected by public and private organizations
- Utilization data
- Clinical condition data

Some federal agencies and other organizations that offer publicly reported data are listed in table 4.1. Several of the quality programs that focus on the outpatient facility and professional practice setting are discussed in the following sections.

Table 4.1. Selected agencies and organizations offering publicly reported data

Organization	Examples of Available Data
Agency for Healthcare Research and Quality (AHRQ)	• Medical Expenditure Panel Survey • Consumer Assessment of Healthcare Providers and Systems • Healthcare Cost and Utilization Project State Ambulatory Surgery Database (34 states) • Healthcare Cost and Utilization Project State Emergency Department Database (32 states) • Healthcare Cost and Utilization Project State Inpatient Database (48 states)
Centers for Disease Control and Prevention (CDC)	• US cancer statistics • National Center for Health Statistics (NCHS) data files • CDC Wide-ranging Online Data for Epidemiologic Research (WONDER) online databases • Behavioral Risk Factor Surveillance System (BRFSS) survey data files
Centers for Medicare and Medicaid Services (CMS)	• Medicaid statistical information files • Medicaid analytic extract files • Hospital Compare • Nursing Home Compare • Home Health Compare • Short-Term Acute Care Program for Evaluating Payment Patterns Electronic Report (PEPPER)
Healthgrades	• Quality ratings per organization's defined methodology
National Committee for Quality Assurance (NCQA)	• Healthcare Effectiveness Data and Information Set (HEDIS) measures allowing for comparisons of healthcare plan performance
Partners in Information Access for the Public Health Workforce	• Links to numerous health data tools and statistics from government and public health sources, behavioral surveys, and organizational initiatives
The Joint Commission	• Quality Check directory of the accreditation and certification status of healthcare entities surveyed by the Joint Commission
The Leapfrog Group	• Data on overall patient safety and selected procedures per organization's defined methodology

Source: Buttner et al. 2016

Hospital Outpatient Quality Reporting Program

CMS implemented the **Hospital Outpatient Quality Reporting (OQR) Program** specifically for outpatient facility services. The Tax Relief Act of 2006 established the program, which requires hospitals to submit data related to the quality of services provided in the outpatient setting. These quality measures can be categorized as follows:

- Process
- Outcome
- Structure
- Efficiency

The program dictates that hospitals that do not meet the OQR requirements will receive a 2 percent decrease in their annual payment update under OPPS. The data collected through the Hospital OQR Program are publicly available on the Hospital Compare website (CMS 2016a). Hospital Compare was organized by Medicare and the Hospital Quality Alliance, public-private collaboration established in 2002. The data on the website are organized in the following categories:

- General information
- Survey of patients' experiences
- Timely and effective care
- Complications
- Readmissions and deaths
- Use of medical imaging
- Payment and value of care

The Hospital OQR Program is voluntary, and the measures "assess processes of care, imaging efficiency patterns, care transitions, emergency department (ED) throughput efficiency, the use of health information technology, care coordination, patient safety, and volume" (QualityNet n.d.). CMS publicly reports the data gathered through this program. Some examples of OQR measures are listed in table 4.2.

The current version of the *Hospital Outpatient Quality Reporting Specifications Manual* is available on the QualityNet website (QualityNet n.d.). The manual provides detail on each OQR measure. For example, OQR measure 1 (OP-1) and OQR measure 2 (OP-2) relate to the timing of fibrinolytic administration after a patient arrives at the facility (see table 4.2). Fibrinolytic therapy is the administration of a pharmacological agent intended to cause lysis of a thrombus (destruction or dissolution of a blood clot). OP-1 measures the median time to fibrinolysis administration. OP-2 measures the number of patients that received fibrinolytics within 30 minutes of arrival to the ED.

The hospital's quality department will monitor these measures from a clinical perspective and conduct or initiate activities related to fibrinolytic administration if a quality issue is identified. One of those initiatives should be the collaboration with a CDS who can further investigate the root cause of the issue. It is possible that the actual fibrinolytic administration time is right on target, but there is a gap between the actual administration time and the time when it is documented. To investigate the issue, the CDS should observe the patient care team as they enter dates and times in the record. If there is a time gap between the time of administration and the time of documentation, the clinician responsible for recording the information should be notified and given tools to resolve the gap. On the other hand, the investigation might find that there is a patient throughput (flow) issue in the ED that is adversely affecting the timeliness of fibrinolytic administration. If that is the case, the CDS can report this finding to the quality department so that further action may be taken to improve the quality of care. At a later point, the CDS can re-evaluate documentation issues related to measures OP-1 and OP-2 with a sample case review of at least 25 records that involve one of these two quality measures.

The *Hospital Outpatient Quality Reporting Specifications Manual* also provides instruction on clinical record data sources, abstracting data, and reporting quality measures (QualityNet n.d.). The outpatient CDS should be familiar with the

Table 4.2. Hospital Outpatient Quality Reporting measures

Quality Measure	Quality Measure Description
OP-1	Median Time to Fibrinolysis
OP-2	Fibrinolytic Therapy Received Within 30 Minutes of ED Arrival
OP-3	Median Time to Transfer to Another Facility for Acute Coronary Intervention
OP-4	Aspirin at Arrival
OP-5	Median Time to ECG
OP-8	MRI Lumbar Spine for Low Back Pain
OP-9	Mammography Follow-up Rates
OP-10	Abdominal CT—Use of Contrast Material
OP-11	Thorax CT—Use of Contrast Material
OP-12	The Ability for Providers with HIT to Receive Laboratory Data Electronically Directly into their ONC-Certified EHR System as Discrete Searchable Data
OP-13	Cardiac Imaging for Preoperative Risk Assessment for Non-Cardiac Low-Risk Surgery
OP-14	Simultaneous Use of Brain Computed Tomography (CT) and Sinus Computed Tomography (CT)
OP-17	Tracking Clinical Results between Visits
OP-18	Median Time from ED Arrival to ED Departure for Discharged ED Patients
OP-20	Door to Diagnostic Evaluation by a Qualified Medical Professional
OP-21	Median Time to Pain Management for Long Bone Fracture
OP-22	Left Without Being Seen
OP-23	Head CT or MRI Scan Results for Acute Ischemic Stroke or Hemorrhagic Stroke Patients Who Received Head CT or MRI Scan Interpretation Within 45 Minutes of ED Arrival
OP-25	Safe Surgery Checklist Use
OP-26	Hospital Outpatient Volume on Selected Outpatient Surgical Procedures (For a complete list of procedure category and corresponding codes affected, refer to the Hospital OQR Program Specifications Manual.)
OP-27	Influenza Vaccination Coverage among Healthcare Personnel (reported on the National Healthcare Safety Network website)
OP-29	Appropriate Follow-Up Interval for Normal Colonoscopy in Average Risk Patients
OP-30	Colonoscopy Interval for Patients with a History of Adenomatous Polyps—Avoidance of Inappropriate Use
OP-31	Cataracts—Improvement in Patient's Visual Function Within 90 Days Following Cataract Surgery*
OP-32	Facility 7-Day Risk-Standardized Hospital Visit Rate after Outpatient Colonoscopy
OP-33	External Beam Radiotherapy for Bone Metastases

*OP-31 is a voluntary measure; any data submitted will be publicly reported.
Source: QualityNet n.d.

overall reporting requirements and monitor quality outliers through ongoing case review and root cause analysis, as discussed earlier in this chapter. The clinical documentation process for collection of OQR measures can be streamlined using EHR enhancements for data collection. This topic is discussed further in chapter 7.

Quality Payment Program

The Quality Payment Program (QPP) was designed to improve Medicare through a focus on the quality of patient care. The program was created by the Medicare Access and CHIP Reauthorization Act of 2015 (MACRA) and replaces the sustainable growth rate (SGR) program for Medicare physician practice reimbursement. MACRA offers a new approach to paying providers who care for patients covered by Medicare by allowing the providers to select one of two tracks (CMS 2017i):

- The Merit-Based Incentive Payment System (MIPS)
- Advanced Alternative Payment Models (APMs)

As part of the Quality Measure Development Plan (MDP) required by MACRA section 102, CMS has established a focused framework to build and improve quality measures. The quality measures created by MDP are used to support both MIPS and APMs options.

The QPP includes professional practice providers who have signed up for an Advanced APM. Professional practice providers are also included if they have submitted annual Part B Medicare claims for an amount greater than $30,000 and have more than 100 Medicare patients each year (CMS 2017j). CDSs and "HIM professionals will play a central role in many organizations as [the organizations] strive to perform at levels that would make them eligible for additional positive payment adjustments, as well as achieve the highest levels of performance under MACRA" (Marron-Stearns 2017).

MIPS

MIPS consolidates reporting under three Medicare programs—Physician Quality Reporting System (PQRS), VM, and Meaningful Use of Certified Electronic Health Record Technology (CEHRT)—with four performance categories.

> *Certified EHR Technology* means:
> (1) For any federal fiscal year (FY) or calendar year (CY) up to and including 2013:
> (i) A complete EHR that meets the requirements included in the definition of a qualified EHR and has been tested and certified in accordance with the certification program established by the national coordinator as having met all applicable certification criteria adopted by the secretary for the 2011 edition EHR certification criteria or the equivalent 2014 edition EHR certification criteria; or
> (ii) A combination of EHR modules in which each constituent EHR module of the combination has been tested and certified in accordance with the certification program established by the national coordinator as having met all applicable certification criteria adopted by the secretary for the 2011 edition EHR certification criteria or the equivalent 2014 edition EHR certification criteria, and the resultant combination also meets the requirements included in the definition of a qualified EHR; or
> (iii) EHR technology that satisfies the definition for FY and CY 2014 and subsequent years specified in paragraph (2);
> (2) For FY and CY 2014 and subsequent years, the following EHR technology certified under the ONC HIT Certification Program to the 2014 edition EHR certification criteria that has:
> (i) The capabilities required to meet the base EHR definition; and

(ii) All other capabilities that are necessary to meet the objectives and associated measures under 42 CFR 495.6 and successfully report the clinical quality measures selected by CMS in the form and manner specified by CMS (or the states, as applicable) for the stage of Meaningful Use that an eligible professional, eligible hospital, or critical access hospital seeks to achieve. (ONC 2012)

The four performance categories under MIPS are as follows:

- Quality (formerly PQRS)
- Resource Use (formerly VM)
- **Advancing Care Information (ACI)** (the performance category previously referred to as *Meaningful Use* under the CEHRT program; it replaces the Medicare EHR incentive program)
- Clinical Practice Improvement Activities (CPIAs; a new performance category)

The types of providers included in MIPS are as follows:

- Physician
- Physician assistant
- Nurse practitioner
- Clinical nurse specialist
- Certified registered nurse anesthetist (CMS 2017k)

Under MIPS, each provider will receive a composite performance score that ranges from 0 to 100 points. Each of the performance categories has a corresponding weight, as shown in figure 4.2.

Figure 4.2. Weight by category of scores used to calculate a composite performance score in MIPS

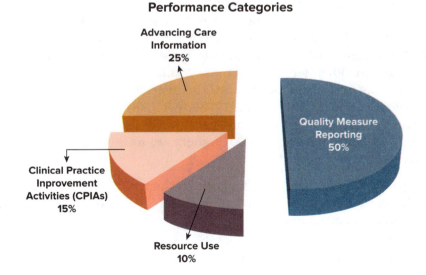

For 2017, first-year Medicare providers were not included in the MIPS track of the QPP. The timeline and process for participation in the QPP are shown in figure 4.3 and further explained below.

Figure 4.3. Timeline and process for participation in the QPP

2017	March 31, 2018	2018	January 1, 2019
Performance: The first performance period opens January 1, 2017 and closes December 31, 2017. During 2017, record quality data and how you used technology to support your practice. If an Advanced APM fits your practice, then you can join and provide care during the year through that model.	**Send in performance data:** To potentially earn a positive payment adjustment under MIPS, send in data about the care you provided and how your practice used technology in 2017 to MIPS by the deadline, March 31, 2018. In order to earn the 5% Incentive payment by significantly participating in an Advanced APM, just send quality data through your Advanced APM.	**Feedback:** Medicare gives you feedback about your performance after you send your data.	**Payment:** you may earn a positive MIPS payment adjustment for 2019 if you submit 2017 data by march 31, 2018. If you participate in an Advanced APM in 2017, then you may earn a 5% Incentive payment in 2019.

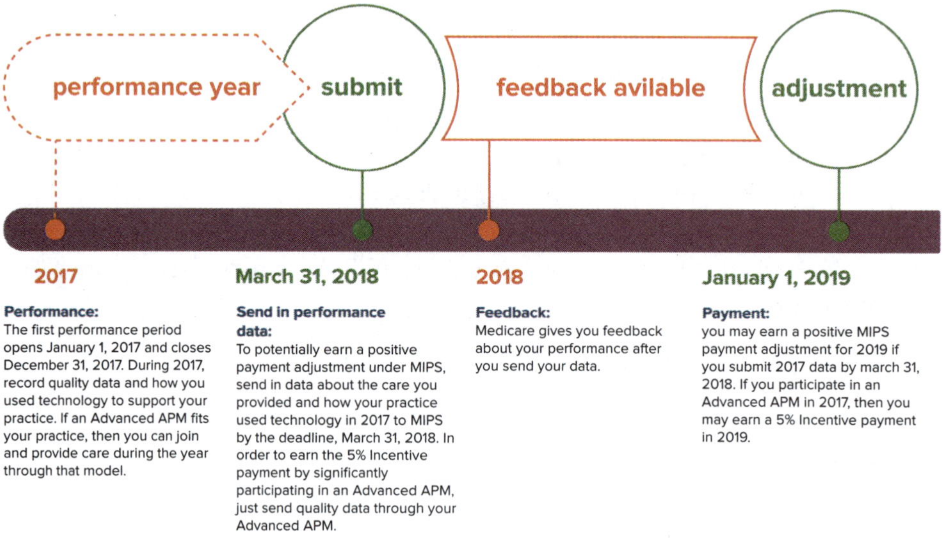

Source: Reprinted from CMS 2017k

During the first year of participation, providers record quality data. The deadline for submitting 2017 data was March 31, 2018. Data collection could begin anytime between January 1, 2017, and October 2, 2017.

After the data are submitted, Medicare provides feedback on the data. Providers are eligible for a positive MIPS payment adjustment in 2019 if the data requirements for 2017 are met. However, CMS may adjust payments up, down, or not at all. The MIPS program is budget neutral, and the total payment adjustments are balanced to equal zero. The program is also based on pay-for-performance. Reporting the MIPS information does not necessarily mean that a bonus will be received. The bonus is based on the scores obtained in each category. The payment is based on a percentage of the Medicare Part B for each provider billing. The available money in the MIPS program will be distributed to those who meet the quality score requirement. In other words, the money collected from all providers in the program as part of the penalty will be distributed as part of the bonus adjustment. Remember, the program is budget neutral. The score thresholds will change each year, and the bonus and penalties will increase over the coming years. For payment year 2019, there are four options for participation (figure 4.4).

- *No participation:* If providers did not participate in in QPP in 2017, they will receive a 4 percent payment reduction (penalty) based on their total Medicare payment amounts.

- *Test:* If providers submitted the minimum payment amount in 2017 (that is, if they submitted one quality measure or one improvement activity), they will receive no bonus and no penalty.

- *Partial:* If providers submitted 90 days' worth of data in 2017, they may receive no penalty or bonus, or they may earn a positive adjustment based on their MIPS scores and available money in the MIPS program.
- *Full data submission:* If providers submitted the full year's worth of data in 2017, they will earn a bonus based on their MIPS scores and available money in the MIPS program (CMS 2017j).

Figure 4.4. 2019 options to participate in Quality Payment Program

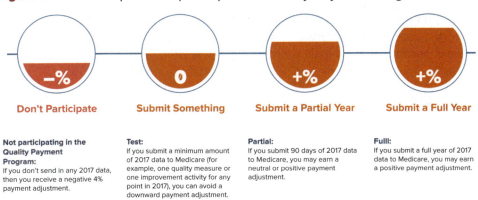

Not participating in the Quality Payment Program: If you don't send in any 2017 data, then you receive a negative 4% payment adjustment.

Test: If you submit a minimum amount of 2017 data to Medicare (for example, one quality measure or one improvement activity for any point in 2017), you can avoid a downward payment adjustment.

Partial: If you submit 90 days of 2017 data to Medicare, you may earn a neutral or positive payment adjustment.

Full: If you submit a full year of 2017 data to Medicare, you may earn a positive payment adjustment.

Source: Reprinted from CMS 2017k

The payment received by providers under the MIPS program depends on the amount of data submitted as well as the performance results (CMS 2017j). CMS estimated that approximately 90 percent of eligible clinicians would be in the MIPS program in 2017 and 10 percent were in an Advanced APM (Marron-Stearns 2016). In 2017, providers could choose "to report for a full 90-day period or, ideally, the full year as to allow them to qualify for up to 4 percent positive payment adjustment and an additional exceptional performance bonus based on the 2017 performance year" (Marron-Stearns 2017).

Advanced APMs

An **Alternative Payment Model (APM)** "is a payment approach, developed in partnership with the clinician community, that provides added incentives to clinicians to provide high-quality and cost-efficient care. APMs can be applied to a specific clinical condition, a care episode, or a population" (CMS 2017j). **Advanced APMs** are a subset of APMs that allow practices to take on risk (receive less payment) or receive bonus payments related to patient outcome (CMS 2017j). APMs are set up to apply to certain clinical conditions or patient populations. Advanced APMs allow providers to earn a 5 percent incentive bonus payment by improving patient care (CMS 2017j).

The final rule with comment period defined the risk requirement for an advanced APM to be in terms of either total Medicare expenditures or participating organizations' Medicare revenue. This new APM option allows for the creation of more advanced APMs tailored to physicians and other clinicians, such as advanced practice nurses, generally, and small practice participation in particular (CMS 2017j).

To qualify for advanced APM status, the APM must meet these criteria:

- The APM must require participants to use CEHRT.
- The APM must provide for payment for covered professional services based on quality measures comparable to those in the quality performance category under MIPS.
- The APM must either require that participating APM entities bear the risk for monetary losses of more than the nominal amount under the APM or be a Medical Home Model under MACRA.

If providers received 25 percent of Medicare payments or saw 20 percent of their Medicare patients through the advanced APM model in 2017, they would earn a 5 percent incentive payment in 2019. The program payment percentages change annually according to the schedule in figure 4.5 (CMS 2017k).

Figure 4.5. Alternative Payment Model (APM) payment percentages over time

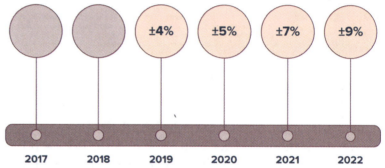

Source: CMS 2017j

The following APMs are available to providers (CMS 2017j):

- *Comprehensive ESRD Care (CEC)—Two-Sided Risk:* This APM allows providers to test, evaluate, and improve patient care for Medicare beneficiaries with end-stage renal disease (ESRD). CMS offers to partner with providers to test new payment and patient-centered delivery models to improve the quality of care.
- *Comprehensive Primary Care Plus (CPC+):* CPC+ is a primary care model that focuses on delivery transformation to home care.
- *Next Generation ACO Model*: This APM offers improvements to care through better care coordination.
- *Shared Savings Program—Track 2:* This APM focuses on population health management and offers shared savings (bonuses) or penalties depending on performance based on Medicare expenditures.
- *Shared Savings Program—Track 3:* This APM offers a higher level of risk than the Shared Savings Program—Track 2 but has a higher bonus potential.
- *Oncology Care Model (OCM)—Two-Sided Risk:* OCM is a payment and delivery model based on treatment efficiencies and effectiveness for cancer patients. The program focuses on the accountability of providers for efficient episodes of care surrounding chemotherapy administration.
- *Comprehensive Care for Joint Replacement (CJR) Payment Model (Track 1—CEHRT):* CJR is a model based on improving care for patients receiving

inpatient hip and knee replacements. The model includes bundled payments and quality measurement to improve the coordination of care during hospitalization and posthospital treatment.

CMS has established the following requirements for advanced APMs:

- Be part of a CMS Innovation Center model, Shared Savings Program track, or certain federal demonstration programs.
- Require participants qualify for the ACI performance category by using CEHRT, meaning that the practice will use the stage 2 or stage 3 CEHRT in 2017 and the 2015 edition CEHRT for a 90-day minimum reporting period in 2018 (Marron-Stearns 2017).
- Base payments for services on quality measures comparable to those in MIPS.
- Be a Medical Home Model expanded under Innovation Center authority or require participants to bear more than nominal financial risk for losses (CMS 2017j).

Advancing Care Information Performance Measure

With the implementation of MACRA, CMS has overhauled Meaningful Use with the implementation of the ACI performance measure. See chapter 2 of this textbook for more information on Meaningful Use. "The proposal for Advancing Care Information is designed to simplify requirements, support patient care, and be flexible to meet the needs of physician practices. The proposal emphasizes measures that support improved patient engagement and connectivity and reduces reporting burden" (CMS 2016b). Table 4.3 compares the Medicare EHR Incentive Program and the ACI performance category.

Table 4.3. Principle changes from the Medicare EHR Incentive Program to Advancing Care Information Performance Category

Meaningful Use	Advancing Care Information
Must report on all objective and measure requirements.	Advancing Care Information streamlines measures and emphasizes interoperability, information exchange, and security measures. Clinical Decision Support and Computerized Provider Order Entry are no longer required.
One-size-fits-all: every measure reported and weighed equally.	Customizable: Physicians or clinicians can choose which best measures fit their practice.
All-or-nothing: EHR measurement and quality reporting.	Flexible: Multiple paths to success.
Misaligned with other Medicare reporting programs.	Aligned with other Medicare reporting programs. No need to report quality measures as part of this category.

Source: Reprinted from CMS 2016b

CMS advises that the ACI score will account for 25 percent of the MIPS score (CMS 2017k). To qualify for this measure, practices must use a certified EHR and report measures reflecting how their practice uses the EHR functionality. The ACI performance category focuses on interoperability and information exchange. The ACI score is made up of a base and a performance score. The base score accounts for 50 points. Table 4.4 lists the six objectives required for reporting the base score.

Table 4.4. Base Advancing Care Information (ACI) score objectives

Base Score	Maximum 50 points
Protect Patient Health Information	Yes, required
Electronic Prescribing	Both must be reported: Numerator (total meeting measure) and denominator (possible meeting measure)
Patient Electronic Access	Both must be reported: Numerator/Denominator
Coordination of Care Through Patient Engagement	Both must be reported: Numerator/Denominator
Health Information Exchange	Both must be reported: Numerator/Denominator
Public Health and Clinical Data Registry Reporting	Yes, required

Source: CMS 2016b

The performance score accounts for up to 80 points in the ACI category. Physicians and other clinicians select the measures emphasizing patient care and information access that best fit their practice. The performance score objectives are as follows:

- Patient electronic access
- Coordination of care through patient engagement
- Health information exchange

The total ACI score is calculated by adding the points for the base score to the performance score. A score of 100 or more points will allow credit for the full 25 points possible in the ACI category contributing to the total MIPS score (CMS 2016b).

The requirements for compliance with MIPS, APMs, and the ACI performance measure are complex. When assisting physician practices in the implementation of data gathering to support a QPP, CDSs should refer to guidelines and implementation information published by CMS (2017g).

Privately Held Hospital Compare Organizations

As discussed in chapter 1, multiple private organizations monitor the quality of healthcare provided to patients across the United States. CDSs should become familiar with organizations such as the Leapfrog Group and Healthgrades so that they can assist facilities and physician practices in effective and accurate data-gathering processes to demonstrate the high quality of care provided.

The Leapfrog Group

The Leapfrog Group was founded in 2000 by large employers and other purchasers of healthcare. It is a national nonprofit organization that monitors quality and safety of US healthcare services. One of Leapfrog's three major initiatives is the Leapfrog Hospital Survey, which collects and reports data on hospital performance. The Leapfrog Group reports on more than 1,800 hospitals, and the organization reports that approximately half of all US hospitals respond to its survey (Leapfrog 2017a). The hospital report is available on the Leapfrog Group website, and a graphical display offers a quick look at how hospitals compare in five categories associated with the quality of care (figure 4.6). The report in figure 4.6 shows that Hospital A did not answer the survey; Hospital B has a lower score than Hospital C in the Never Events Management category, and Hospital C has a lower score in the Specially Trained Doctors Care for ICU [intensive care unit] Patients category (Leapfrog 2017b).

Figure 4.6. Example of hospital comparison from the Leapfrog Group

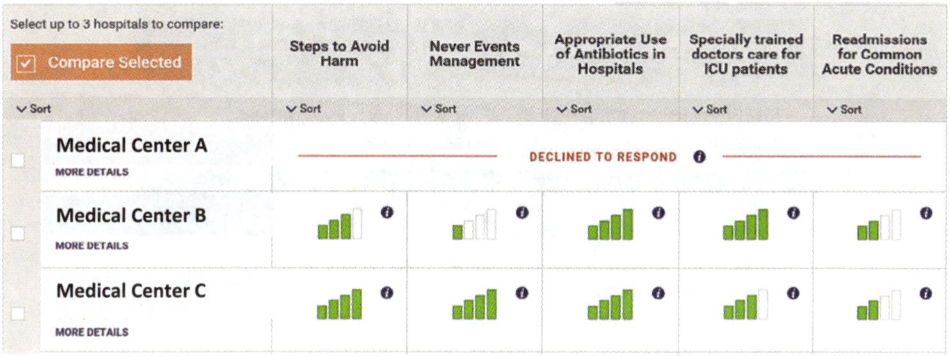

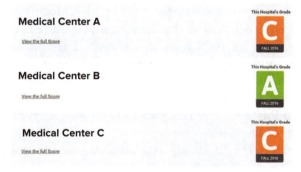

Source: Leapfrog 2017b

A second initiative from the Leapfrog Group is the Leapfrog Hospital Safety Grade (figure 4.7). It assigns letter grades to hospitals based on patient safety criteria related to facility-based errors, injuries, accidents, and infections (Leapfrog 2017c). Grades are given semiannually to more than 2,600 general acute care hospitals and are derived from data from CMS national performance measures, the Leapfrog Group survey, AHRQ, CDC, and the American Hospital Association's annual survey and health information technology supplement (Leapfrog 2017c).

Figure 4.7. Examples of the Leapfrog Group's hospital safety grades

Source: Leapfrog 2017c

In a third major initiative, the Leapfrog Value-Based Purchasing Platform uses the Leapfrog Hospital Survey results to generate an overall value score for each facility that uses the platform. The score is used to rank hospitals and set benchmarks for financial awards or incentives to hospitals in the top decile. Reports are provided twice a year. The overall value score includes weighted scores from five domains, as shown in figure 4.8. The domains, and the measures within them, are weighted based on patient volume, severity of harm, and resource use.

Figure 4.8. Leapfrog overall value score domains, domain weights, and domain measures

Medication Safety (18%)

- Computerized Physician Order Entry (CPOE) and Bar Code Medication Administration (BCMA)

Inpatient Care Management (23%)

- ICU Physician Staffing, NQF Safe Practices, Never Events Policy, Antibiotic Stewardship, and Hospital Readmission

Infections & Injuries (41%)

- Central-Line Associated Blood Stream Infections (ICU only) (CLABSI), Associated Urinary Tract Infections (ICU only) (CAUTI), Facility-wide Inpatient Hospital-onset MRSA, Facility-wide Inpatient Hospital-onset C.Diff., Surgical Site Infection after Colon Surgery (SSI: Colon), Hospital-Acquired Pressure Ulcers, and Hospital-Acquired Injuries

Maternity Care (18%)

- Early Elective Deliveries, NTSV Cesarean Sections, Episiotomies, Newborn Bilirubin Screening, DVT Prophylaxis for Women Undergoing Cesarean Section, and High-Risk Deliveries (i.e. Very Low Birthweight Babies)

Source: Leapfrog 2017a

Healthgrades

Healthgrades is a leading online resource for information about physicians and hospitals. The organization's mission is to make information on physicians and hospitals more transparent so that healthcare consumers can find the right hospitals or physicians for their healthcare needs. The website offers a rating system to locate providers based on patient satisfaction; experience match; and hospital quality. Hospital quality is determined by clinical outcomes. Hospital performance ratings are based on the most common hospital procedures and conditions, with adjustment for risk factors such as age, gender, and medical condition (Healthgrades 2017a).

Healthgrades offers the following reports that provide insight into quality matters:

- America's Best Hospitals
- Annual Report to the Nation
- Hospital Quality and Clinical Excellence
- Outstanding Patient Experience
- Patient Safety in American Hospitals
- Women's Care
- Women's Health

An example of the information available on the Healthgrades website is the infographic in figure 4.9, which highlights the significance of the Distinguished Hospital for Clinical Excellence Award (Healthgrades 2017b).

Figure 4.9. Healthgrades Distinguished Hospital for Clinical Excellence Award infographic

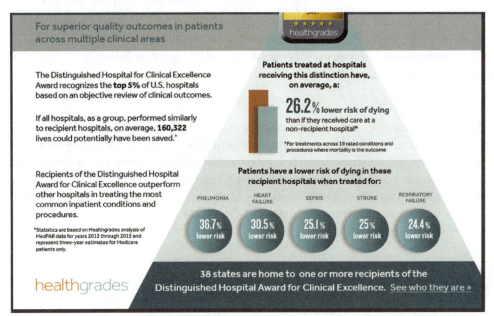

Source: Reprinted from Healthgrades 2017b

Healthgrades also gives out the Distinguished Hospital Award for Clinical Excellence in the following clinical areas, which are of particular importance to a hospital's overall quality rankings:

- Sepsis
- Heart failure
- Pneumonia
- Total knee replacement
- Chronic obstructive pulmonary disease
- Coronary interventional procedures
- Acute myocardial infarction
- Gastrointestinal bleed
- Stroke

In a 2016 report on the treatment of sepsis in facilities that won the clinical excellence award in that area, Healthgrades noted a correlation between improved sepsis risk-adjusted mortality rates and other mortality-based cohorts; on average, a hospital that had a 10 percent reduction in risk-adjusted mortality in sepsis care also reduced risk-adjusted mortality rates in other areas (figure 4.10) (Healthgrades 2016).

CDSs should collaborate with the HIM coding staff and physicians to ensure that severity of illness and risk of mortality (SOI/ROM) scores and related clinical documentation and coding are of high quality. Severity of illness (SOI) refers to a type of supportive documentation reflecting objective clinical indicators of

Figure 4.10. Correlation of the risk-adjusted mortality rate for sepsis and risk-adjusted mortality rates for other conditions in hospitals

On average hospitals that saw a 10% reduction in risk-adjusted mortality in Sepsis care also saw:
A 4.3% reduction in risk-adjusted mortality rates during care for heart failure
A 3.3% reduction in risk-adjusted mortality rates during care for chronic obstructive pulmonary disease
A 3.9% reduction in risk-adjusted mortality rates during care for pneumonia
A 3.2% reduction in risk-adjusted mortality rates during care for stroke
A 4.1% reduction in risk-adjusted mortality rates during care for respiratory failure

Source: Reprinted from Healthgrades 2016

a patient's illness (essentially, the patient is sick enough to qualify for an identified level of care) and referring to the extent of physiological decompensation or organ system loss of function. Risk of mortality (ROM) refers to the likelihood of an inpatient death for a patient. SOI/ROM scores based on ICD-10-CM codes affect each hospital's risk-adjusted mortality rates. Improvements in clinical documentation can dramatically affect SOI/ROM scores and demonstrate the high-quality care provided by the facility.

Chapter 4 Review Exercises

1. Several federal agencies publish guidance on compliance related to high-quality clinical documentation, coding, and billing practices. Which agency provides a document listing pertinent questions to assess the quality of a corporate compliance program?
   a. US Department of Justice (DOJ)
   b. Office of Inspector General (OIG)
   c. National Center for Health Statistics (NCHS)
   d. Centers for Medicare and Medicaid Services (CMS)

2. The OIG has identified several risks associated with submission of accurate claims and information. The area of risk related to a practice of using multiple codes to bill for the various individual steps in a single procedure rather than using a single code that includes all of the steps of the comprehensive procedure is considered:
   a. Upcoding
   b. Unbundling
   c. Duplicate billing
   d. Billing for services not provided

3. The overarching agency that regulates healthcare in the United States is the:
   a. Office of Inspector General (OIG)
   b. National Center for Health Statistics (NCHS)
   c. Centers for Medicare and Medicaid Services (CMS)
   d. US Department of Health and Human Services (HHS)

4. MACRA offers a new approach to paying physicians by allowing them to select one of two tracks:
   a. ACI or MDP
   b. SGR or CHIP
   c. BCMA or CEHRT
   d. MIPS or Advanced APMs

5. The performance category under MIPS that replaces the Medicare EHR incentive program and was previously referred to as Meaningful Use is:
   a. Quality
   b. Resource Use
   c. Advancing Care Information
   d. Clinical Practice Improvement Activities

6. The Leapfrog Group uses survey results to generate an overall value score for each facility that uses its platform. Among the four domains that contribute to this overall value score, the most heavily weighted is:
   a. Maternity Care
   b. Medication Safety
   c. Infections and Injuries
   d. Inpatient Care Management

7. The OIG recommends that voluntarily compliant healthcare organizations self-audit claims to ensure all but which of the following standards are met?
   a. There are no incentives for unnecessary services.
   b. Services or items provided are reasonable and necessary.
   c. Necessary services are provided at a fair and affordable cost.
   d. Bills are accurately coded and accurately reflect the services provided.

8. The steps to resolve a _____ issue include identifying the issue, understanding the cause, creating a solution, and validating the solution.
   a. Compliance
   b. Quality-of-care
   c. Patient satisfaction
   d. Billing and payment

9. The Agency for Healthcare Research and Quality (AHRQ) is an operating division of HHS. The agency aims to find evidence to improve the safety, quality, accessibility, equitability, and _____ of healthcare and promote the use of such evidence.
   a. Proximity
   b. Reliability
   c. Expediency
   d. Affordability

10. In the ACI, _____ MIPS points are allotted for a score of 100 or more points in the ACI.
    a. 10
    b. 15
    c. 20
    d. 25

References

American Health Information Management Association (AHIMA). 2016. American Health Information Management Association Standards of Ethical Coding [2016 version]. http://bok.ahima.org/CodingStandards#.Ws4zN4jwbcs

Buttner, P., S.H. Houser, J. Flanigan, R. Mikaelian, B. Ryznar, and C.P. Smith. 2016. Understanding publicly available healthcare data (2016). American Health Information Management Association Practice Brief. http://bok.ahima.org/doc?oid=301870#.WdTqsGhSw2w.

Centers for Disease Control and Prevention (CDC). 2017. ICD-10-CM Official Guidelines for Coding and Reporting FY 2018. https://www.cdc.gov/nchs/data/icd/10cmguidelines_fy2018_final.pdf.

Centers for Medicare and Medicaid Services (CMS). 2017a. Medicare Claims Processing Manual. Chapter 32: Billing requirements for special services. https://www.cms.gov/Regulations-and-Guidance/Guidance/Manuals/downloads/clm104c32.pdf.

Centers for Medicare and Medicaid Services (CMS). 2017b. Children's Health Insurance Program. https://www.medicaid.gov/affordable-care-act/chip/index.html.

Centers for Medicare and Medicaid Services (CMS). 2017c. Medicare Administrative Contractors: What is a MAC. https://www.cms.gov/Medicare/Medicare-Contracting/Medicare-Administrative-Contractors/What-is-a-MAC.html.

Centers for Medicare and Medicaid Services (CMS). 2017d. Fee schedules—general information. https://www.cms.gov/Medicare/Medicare-Fee-for-Service-Payment/FeeScheduleGenInfo/index.html.

Centers for Medicare and Medicaid Services (CMS). 2017e. Prospective Payment Systems—general information. https://www.cms.gov/Medicare/Medicare-Fee-for-Service-Payment/ProspMedicareFeeSvcPmtGen/index.html.

Centers for Medicare and Medicaid Services (CMS). 2017f. Value-based programs. https://www.cms.gov/Medicare/Quality-Initiatives-Patient-Assessment-Instruments/Value-Based-Programs/Value-Based-Programs.html.

Centers for Medicare and Medicaid Cervices (CMS). 2017g. MEDPAR. https://www.cms.gov/Research-Statistics-Data-and-Systems/Statistics-Trends-and-Reports/MedicareFeeforSvcPartsAB/MEDPAR.html.

Centers for Medicare and Medicaid Services (CMS). 2017h. Limited data set (LDS) files. https://www.cms.gov/Research-Statistics-Data-and-Systems/Files-for-Order/LimitedDataSets/index.html.

Centers for Medicare and Medicaid Services (CMS). 2017i. Quality Payment Program: What's the Quality Payment Program? https://www.cms.gov/Medicare/Quality-Payment-Program/Quality-Payment-Program.html.

Centers for Medicare and Medicaid Services (CMS). 2017j. Quality Payment Program. https://qpp.cms.gov.

Centers for Medicare and Medicaid Services (CMS). 2017k. MIPS: Advancing Care Information deep dive. https://www.cms.gov/Medicare/Quality-Initiatives-Patient-Assessment-Instruments/Value-Based-Programs/MACRA-MIPS-and-APMs/MIPS-ACI-Deep-Dive-Webinar-Slides.pdf

Centers for Medicare and Medicaid Services (CMS). 2016a. Hospital Compare. https://www.cms.gov/Medicare/Quality-Initiatives-Patient-Assessment-Instruments/HospitalQualityInits/HospitalCompare.html.

Centers for Medicare and Medicaid Services (CMS). 2016b. Merit-Based Incentive Payment System: Advancing Care Information. https://www.cms.gov/Medicare/Quality-Initiatives-Patient-Assessment-Instruments/Value-Based-Programs/MACRA-MIPS-and-APMs/Advancing-Care-Information-Fact-Sheet.pdf.

Healthgrades. 2016. Major differences in improvement in treating sepsis for Distinguished Hospital Recipients. Healthgrades 2016 Distinguished Hospital Award for Clinical Excellence analysis and white paper. https://www.healthgrades.com/quality/2016-healthgrades-hospital-quality-clinical-excellence-report.

Healthgrades. 2017a. About Us. https://www.healthgrades.com/about.

Healthgrades. 2017b. 2017 Distinguished Hospital Award for Clinical Excellence. https://www.healthgrades.com/quality/2017-healthgrades-hospital-quality-clinical-excellence-report.

The Leapfrog Group. 2017a. Leapfrog VBP Compare. http://www.leapfroggroup.org/sites/default/files/Files/2017LVBPP_ScoringMethodology_090117_Final.pdf.

The Leapfrog Group. 2017b. Hospital ratings. http://www.leapfroggroup.org/compare-hospitals.

The Leapfrog Group. 2017c. Leapfrog hospital safety grade. http://www.hospitalsafetygrade.org.

Marron-Stearns, M. 2017. How MACRA changes HIM. *Journal of AHIMA* 88(3):22–25.

Marron-Stearns, M. 2016 (November 7). MACRA strategies for 2017: Advantages and disadvantages of four options. *Journal of AHIMA* website. http://journal.ahima.org/2016/11/07/macra-strategies-for-2017-advantages-and-disadvantages-of-four-options.

Office of Family Assistance (OFA), US Department of Health and Human Services. 2017a.Temporary Assistance for Needy Families (TANF). https://www.acf.hhs.gov/ofa/programs/tanf.

Office of Family Assistance (OFA), US Department of Health and Human Services. 2017b. About OFA. https://www.acf.hhs.gov/ofa/about.

Office of Inspector General (OIG), US Department of Health and Human Services. 2018. OIG Work Plan. https://oig.hhs.gov/reports-and-publications/workplan/index.asp.

Office of Inspector General (OIG), US Department of Health and Human Services. 2017. HHS OIG Work Plan 2017. https://oig.hhs.gov/reports-and-publications/archives/workplan/2017/HHS%20OIG%20Work%20Plan%202017_508.pdf.

Office of Inspector General (OIG), US Department of Health and Human Services. 2005. Supplemental compliance program guidance for hospitals. *Federal Register* 70(19):4858–4876. https://oig.hhs.gov/fraud/docs/complianceguidance/012705HospSupplementalGuidance.pdf.

Office of Inspector General (OIG), US Department of Health and Human Services. 2000. Compliance program guidance for individual and small group physician practices. *Federal Register* 64(194): 59434–59452. https://oig.hhs.gov/authorities/docs/physician.pdf.

Office of Inspector General (OIG), US Department of Health and Human Services. 1998a. OIG compliance program guidance for hospitals. *Federal Register* 63(35):8987–8998. https://oig.hhs.gov/authorities/docs/cpghosp.pdf

Office of Inspector General (OIG), US Department of Health and Human Services. 1998b. Compliance program guidance for third-party medical billing companies. *Federal Register* 63(243):70138–70152. https://oig.hhs.gov/fraud/docs/complianceguidance/thirdparty.pdf.

Office of the National Coordinator for Health Information Technology (ONC), US Department of Health and Human Services. 2012. Standards, implementation specifications, and certification criteria for electronic health record technology, 2014 edition; revisions to the Permanent Certification Program for Health Information Technology. *Federal Register* 77(171):54163–54292. https://www.federalregister.gov/documents/2012/09/04/2012-20982/health-information-technology-standards-implementation-specifications-and-certification-criteria-for.

QualityNet. n.d. Hospital Outpatient Quality Reporting (OQR) Program. https://www.qualitynet.org/dcs/ContentServer?c=Page&pagename=QnetPublic%2FPage%2FQnetTier3&cid=1192804531207.

Research Data Assistance Center (ResDAC). 2017. Find a CMS data file. https://www.resdac.org/cms-data.

Rhode Island Executive Office of Health and Human Resources (RI EOHHS). 2018. Claims processing. http://www.eohhs.ri.gov/ProvidersPartners/BillingampClaims/ClaimsProcessing.aspx.

US Department of Health and Human Services (HHS). 2017a. HHS Organizational Chart. https://www.hhs.gov/about/agencies/orgchart/index.html.

US Department of Health and Human Services (HHS). 2017b. HIPAA for Professionals. https://www.hhs.gov/hipaa/for-professionals/index.html.

US Department of Health and Human Services (HHS). 2015. HHS Agencies and Offices. https://www.hhs.gov/about/agencies/hhs-agencies-and-offices/index.html.

US Department of Justice (DOJ). 2017. Evaluation of corporate compliance programs. https://www.justice.gov/criminal-fraud/page/file/937501/download.

Outpatient CDI Assessment

5

Learning Objectives

- Explain the importance of an initial assessment of outpatient clinical documentation to determine the feasibility of and return on investment for a clinical documentation improvement (CDI) program.
- Describe the steps in an initial outpatient clinical documentation assessment.
- Identify the resources needed to assess outpatient clinical documentation and implement the outpatient CDI process.
- Explain the importance of executive level and key stakeholder buy-in for CDI.
- Recommend solutions to the challenges of high-quality outpatient clinical documentation.
- Illustrate how to present the outpatient CDI program to executive stakeholders.

Key Terms

Ambulatory payment classification (APC)
Key performance indicator (KPI)

Needs assessment

Many hospitals that have implemented clinical documentation improvement (CDI) programs have reduced the volume of claims denials and improved appropriate reimbursement payments and the accuracy of quality scores. For these reasons, CDI programs have become very popular in the inpatient setting and are now beginning to expand into the outpatient setting (Combs 2016). Outpatient facilities and professional practices are now also beginning to realize the benefits of improving clinical documentation in the outpatient continuum of care. Outpatient CDI programs can ensure accurate reimbursement and assist providers in achieving shared bonuses from programs established by payers to encourage high-quality, cost-effective patient care (Arrowood et al. 2015). The process and concepts described in this chapter can be adapted for outpatient CDI programs in any outpatient setting, such as the outpatient facility clinic, emergency department, provider practice, or ambulatory surgical center.

Among the first steps in the CDI program in the outpatient setting is the selection of an outpatient clinic or provider practice to serve as a pilot program. The use of a pilot clinic will allow the CDI manager to develop a preliminary process, observe the process during implementation, and conduct process redesign where needed to streamline the program. The more efficient, streamlined process can then be rolled out to additional facility or professional practice sites. Selection of the pilot clinic should be based on size, complexity, and the presence of physician leadership willing to work through the development of the program in the pilot clinic. A moderate-size family medicine or internal medicine clinic is a good place to start, particularly if it has a physician champion who is recognized and respected in the area of clinical documentation. This champion can encourage other providers at the clinic to participate in CDI. Refer to chapters 8 and 10 for additional information on pilot clinic implementation.

The challenge for the CDI professional is to understand the CDI program requirements in the outpatient setting and implement a comprehensive program throughout the continuum of care that not only incorporates outpatient and professional practice requirements but also uses interoperability and streamlined clinical documentation processes to document pertinent diagnoses identified in the inpatient setting. This premise assumes the skill sets and qualifications of the outpatient clinical documentation specialist (CDS) include knowledge of the vast array of disease and procedure classifications, reimbursement systems, technology solutions, and quality measurement programs in the ambulatory healthcare industry today.

A well-thought-out outpatient CDI program begins with the assessment of the program's feasibility and return on investment (ROI) and the creation of a high-level workplan through strategic collaboration with key leaders and stakeholders from the facility's executive leadership group, medical staff, practice management, and clinic management, as well as the health information management (HIM), CDI, quality, care management, revenue integrity, and revenue cycle departments. This chapter provides a framework that the leadership taskforce can use to assess the outpatient CDI program.

Assessing the Feasibility of CDI

When considering the feasibility of CDI for the outpatient setting, CDI leaders must consider both the benefits of CDI and any potential barriers to the creation of a CDI program (Combs 2016). The process of evaluating the benefits and barriers can be referred to as a **needs assessment**. This type of evaluation is similar to a cost–benefit analysis, where the evaluator reviews the benefits of a project against the cost of the project. However, the needs assessment goes one step further to also assess the political, operational, and resource issues related to the proposed project.

Benefits of Outpatient CDI

The benefits of CDI in the outpatient setting are far-reaching and include the following:

- *Accurate assignment of* International Classification of Diseases, Tenth Revision, Clinical Modification *(ICD-10-CM) code assignment:* "Specificity in diagnoses is just as important in the outpatient world as it is in the inpatient world. Each diagnosis should be documented to the highest level of specificity that is supported by the clinical evidence. This will impact Hierarchical Condition Category (HCC) assignment, which will impact the risk adjustment factor (RAF) to accurately reflect the patient population cared for by a facility" (Combs 2016). Refer to chapter 3 for more information on disease classifications.
- *Accurate Current Procedural Terminology (CPT) and Healthcare Common Procedure Coding System (HCPCS) code assignment:* These codes "capture procedural specificity in the outpatient setting. This is obtained through detailed procedure notes to ensure the correct procedure is reflected" (Combs 2016). Refer to chapter 3 for more information on procedure classifications.
- *Accurate* **ambulatory payment classification (APC)** *assignment:* "APC is the Outpatient Prospective Payment System applicable to hospitals. It is just as important that documentation supports the appropriate APC assignment in the outpatient setting as DRG [diagnosis-related group] assignment is in the inpatient setting" (Combs 2016). Refer to chapter 3 for more information on APC classifications.
- *Appropriate reimbursement:* "High-quality clinical documentation is just as important in the outpatient setting [as in the inpatient setting] to receive appropriate reimbursement for the care provided" (Combs 2016).
- *Accurate quality scores:* "Just as inpatient is measured on various quality scores, so is outpatient. It is important that the documentation in the outpatient setting is of the same excellence to capture the correct quality scores" (Combs 2016). Refer to chapters 2 and 4 for more information on quality measurement.
- *Fewer claims denials:* "Payment denials are seen in the outpatient environment just as they are in the inpatient world. Many times, denials are a result of missing documentation to support medical necessity of the care provided" (Combs 2016). Refer to chapters 2, 6, 7, 10, 12, 14, and 16 for more information on denials management.
- *Fewer days for claims in accounts receivable:* In a CDI program, the outpatient CDS can collaborate with providers to streamline the clinical documentation process so that gaps in documentation are identified at the time and site of service, not weeks or months later. When clinical

documentation queries to providers from coders are monitored on a daily basis, claims are not delayed because coders are waiting for provider responses.

- *High-quality clinical documentation for provider-to-provider collaboration:* CDI can help overcome system interoperability issues and allow providers across the continuum of care (inpatient, outpatient, and professional practice settings) to access critical health information. Provider collaboration relies on accurate documentation throughout the health record, and the CDS must therefore ensure that documentation errors in one setting do not spread to the records of other providers. For example, if a patient never used tobacco but one provider erroneously documents that the patient smokes, the CDS can help prevent a situation in which other providers automatically document the incorrect information. Refer to chapter 3 for more information on interoperability.

Potential Barriers to an Outpatient CDI Program

Possible barriers to a comprehensive outpatient CDI program include CDS staffing issues, the short time frame for bill drop, and issues related to the adoption of the outpatient query process by the medical staff (Combs 2016). In addition, limits to interoperability of systems can pose a roadblock to streamlined case view by the outpatient CDS.

Staffing Issues

Because the outpatient CDI program involves staffing challenges not faced in the inpatient CDI program, productivity standards and the appropriate number of staff need to be identified specifically for the outpatient CDI program. In the outpatient setting, patients are seen more quickly than in the inpatient setting, and outpatient documentation therefore includes fewer notes. The CDI manager should conduct a time study to determine the average number of outpatient case reviews that can be performed in an hour. This hourly case review standard can then be used to establish a productivity rate for the average percentage of time the CDSs spend performing case reviews in a given day, week, or month. In addition to case review, CDS activities may include presentations at educational sessions, provider communication, educational material development, data analytics, healthcare informatics, and subject matter expert support related to technology solutions. Because of the variable number of activities and workflows included as part of the CDS job description, each facility must assess the facility-specific productivity and performance measures for the CDS position. See chapter 3 for a sample job description for the CDS.

Timing of Documentation Review

Inpatient CDI professionals usually have several days to review documentation and query providers during the patient's admission. In the outpatient setting, patients are seen within a much shorter time frame and a concurrent review of outpatient records by the CDI professional may not be possible. Therefore, CDI programs need to establish a process for the review to be performed soon after the visit and before the bill is completed.

Lack of Physician Buy-In

In all settings, the success of a CDI program relies on physician buy-in. The physicians are the ones who document a patient's care and respond to queries about clinical documentation. Without timely responses to queries, the CDI program is at risk for failure. The rationale for developing a CDI program in the outpatient setting must be explained to physicians. For example, CDI can make the clinical documentation process easier for the provider. By performing the following activities, CDSs can assist providers in this process and improve physician adoption of CDI measures:

- Evaluate the clinical documentation workflow and determine where the process can be redesigned.
- Identify technology solutions to improve the electronic health record (EHR) documentation process through the use of templates and dropdowns.
- Improve query workflow with the use of technology solutions and streamlining of the query process.

Lack of EHR Interoperability

A lack of interoperability among multiple EHRs in the outpatient and inpatient settings is a barrier to high-quality outpatient clinical documentation because it fosters gaps in clinical documentation from one site to another. For example, to assess HCC capture throughout the continuum of care, the CDI program must identify HCC-related chronic illness diagnoses in all settings. Where the EHR in the physician practice does not interface with the EHR in the inpatient setting, chronic illnesses identified during an inpatient admission may be missed by the outpatient CDS working in the physician practice setting.

Steps in the Outpatient CDI Assessment Program

After careful consideration of the benefits of and barriers to an outpatient CDI program, the healthcare entity's executives and CDI leaders can decide whether to move forward with the program. An outside consultant may assist with this feasibility assessment. In most cases, the benefits outweigh the barriers because high-quality documentation in the outpatient setting is a significant health system goal. Once the decision is made to move forward with the outpatient CDI program, an assessment of the current state of clinical documentation is required to determine the extent of the program as well as the program priorities. Participants in a CDI program should customize the following assessment steps as needed to reflect variables such as the facility type, service lines, and number of outpatient clinics and professional practices.

Because the outpatient setting is expansive, CDI program leadership must focus efforts toward high-volume, high-risk areas to ensure the ROI for the program costs. After the CDI program manager or project manager is in place, the next steps in this process are gathering data and establishing a CDI taskforce as a resource for information on possible gaps in the clinical documentation process. After data is gathered, the CDI manager analyzes data to identify the initial areas of focus and conducts case reviews to determine root causes and develop the process redesign methodology.

Step 1: Gather Data and Identify Areas of Focus

The outpatient CDI assessment requires the analysis of several types of data. Each data set will be used to further analyze the potential issues related to accurate billing and coding as well as clinical documentation gaps that may be affecting quality scores or claims denials.

When establishing areas of focus, CDI governance committees (the CDI taskforce and CDI steering committee) should consider both quality measurement and case volume, as well as reimbursement risk. As discussed in chapter 4, quality scores are tied to reimbursement in value-based purchasing and risk-sharing payment plans. Some areas of focus will be selected based on cash-flow issues. For example, claims edits hold up the claims submission or delay payment because of back-end denials. Both quality scores and cash-flow issues affect reimbursement and revenue generation for the facility or professional practice. For example, providers in the Merit-based Incentive Payment System who have poor quality scores could incur penalties or not earn bonuses. Poor quality scores can also adversely affect publicly available quality data about the facility or practice and thus decrease its market share (see chapter 4). The following types of data should be included in the analysis.

Claims Data with ICD-10-CM, CPT, HCPCS, and APC Codes

Data analytics software tools are used to evaluate potential coding and billing errors. Where the software tool is not part of the overall EHR system, 837 claims data files may be required to upload the patient data. An 837 file is a file format that is used to submit healthcare claims to the payers electronically. There are a variety of software tools available for analyzing claims data. These tools will be discussed in more detail in chapter 7. See chapter 6 for more information on data analytics using ICD-10-0CM, CPT, HCPCS, and APC codes.

Results of Previous ICD-10-CM, CPT, HCPCS, and APC Code Audits for Coding and Billing Accuracy

Most facilities and physician practices periodically audit the coding accuracy of a random or subjective sample of patient claims. A subjective sample may be used when high error rates have been associated with specific ICD-10-CM, CPT, APC, or HCPCS codes. The past audit results can be used to identify areas of focus for the outpatient CDI program. See chapter 6 for more information on data analytics using ICD-10-0CM, CPT, HCPCS, and APC codes.

Hospital Outpatient Charge Description Master (CDM) and Physician Practice Fee Schedules

Clinical documentation and CDM gaps are often the result of missing procedure or service CPT or HCPCS codes in the hospital CDM or physician fee schedule (see chapter 3). These files should be available to the outpatient CDS during the assessment process to validate the accuracy of descriptions in the CDM or fee schedule and the corresponding description in the charge capture document or screen. Incorrect linking of the CDM or fee schedule with the charge entry document or screen can produce a claims error that recurs every time the item is selected. Reviewing the CDM or fee schedule also allows the outpatient CDS to identify procedures that are not provided as options during the charge capture process. This type of problem can occur when new codes are added to a classification system or new services are provided in the facility or practice without the update of the CDM or fee schedule. The CDS should work closely with the finance or reimbursement staff to fully understand the CDM. Refer to chapters 3 and 6 for more information on the use of the CDM for outpatient CDI activities.

Denials Trend Reports for Facility and Physician Practices

The denials or revenue integrity department may have software that can generate trend information on denials by specialty, physician, coder, or CPT/HCPCS, APC, or ICD-10-CM classification. This information should be used to identify high-volume and high-dollar denials that could become an initial area of focus for the outpatient CDI program. For example, the denials trend reports could identify that claims for a specific procedure are frequently denied, and subsequent investigation could determine that the CPT code for that procedure is tied to a national coverage determination (NCD) or local coverage determination (LCD) but the clinical documentation for the denied claims does not include the specificity required to code the diagnosis to an ICD-10-CM code on the NCD/LCD medically necessary diagnosis list. See chapter 2 for further discussion of NCD and LCD and chapters 2, 6, 7, 12, and 15 for more information on denials management activities.

Claims Edit Trends and Reports

A claims edit or automated claims review is a claims review and determination made using system logic (edits). Automated claims reviews never require the intervention of a human to make a claim determination (CMS 2017a). These automated edits are processed using software called a *claims scrubber* or *clinical editor*. These software tools are integrated into the hospital billing system and review the claims prior to the final bill submission. This review will flag potential coding problems in a claim and allows the billing and coding departments to correct the claim before submission. There are a variety of claims edits such as the Medically Unlikely Edit (MUE), which was developed by the Centers for Medicare and Medicaid Services (CMS) to reduce the incidence of reimbursement for Medicare Part B claims that contain HCPCS/CPT coding errors (CMS 2017b). Claims edits and MUEs are further discussed in chapter 6.

The outpatient CDS should become familiar with claims edits and which edit-related issues are most often delaying the processing of claims. The National Correct Coding Initiative (NCCI) is another CMS program involving claims edits related to HCPCS/CPT coding. Refer to chapter 3 for further discussion of NCCI edits. Such delays can dramatically affect the number of accounts receivable days, which is a measure used by CFOs and other business department leaders as a **key performance indicator (KPI)**. In healthcare, a KPI is a quantifiable measure used over time to determine whether some structure, process, or outcome in the provision of care to a patient supports high-quality performance as measured against best practice criteria. Edit issues related to high-volume, high-dollar claims should be included in the CDI program's initial target list for root cause analysis. The CDS can assist charge auditors in the billing offices to set up computer edits to avoid these types of claims denials.

Step 2: Establish an Outpatient CDI Taskforce

Establishment of the outpatient CDI taskforce is the next step in the assessment process. These key stakeholders are essential to the success of the assessment process because their buy-in will help streamline the process and minimize roadblocks. The following are stakeholders to include on the taskforce:

- Chief financial officer (CFO)
- Revenue integrity leader
- HIM director
- Admitting or central scheduling director
- Care management director
- CDI director and outpatient CDI leader
- Physician leadership
- Denials management leader
- Quality department leader
- Clinic management leaders (Select which clinic manager to invite based on the topic of discussion. For example, when discussing wound care, invite the wound care clinic manager.)
- Physician practice management leaders
- Payer contract leader

Refer to chapters 6, 8, and 9 for more information on how to establish an effective CDI taskforce.

The CFO's support is essential to the successful operation of this taskforce. He or she should encourage each member to participate in monthly taskforce meetings.

The first taskforce meeting should include a discussion of the taskforce's objectives, a presentation on the complete outpatient CDI assessment process, a discussion of the role each of the members will play, and the tentative time frame for the tasks. Steps 2 through 6 in the CDI assessment process should be customized to meet the needs of the health system based on the complexity and number of outpatient clinics and physician practices. Sub-taskforce groups may be needed to monitor the progress of large clinics and practices or work on a specific project. The need for this strategy can be considered at the first taskforce meeting.

Step 3: Conduct Focused Case Review

After the data identified in step 2 have been gathered, the next step is to review a sample of the high-volume, high-dollar issues that were identified. A sample of 10 to 15 cases is a good starting point for each major category.

Additional case reviews may be required when the results of the initial review are unclear.

The focused case review includes five areas of focus that are commonly identified as clinical documentation opportunities in the outpatient setting: CPT, HCPCS, and APC errors; HCC code gaps; medical necessity denials; claims edit issues; and charge capture gaps.

CPT, HCPCS, and APC Errors

If an error trend for a specific CPT, HCPCS, or APC code has been identified during previous audits, a sample case review should be conducted to determine root causes of the errors. The root causes of errors in this category are typically traced to low-quality clinical documentation, inadequate coder skills, or charge capture issues. Refer to chapter 3 for more information on CPT, HCPCS, and APC codes.

Case Example

> A primary care practice manages behavioral health patients. Initial data gathering during the CDI assessment program reveals that this practice used HCPCS code G0502 for the initial 70-minute patient encounter in the first calendar month of behavior healthcare management activities, but an external audit found that the clinical record did not support billing for 70 minutes for assessment of the patient and development of a treatment plan. Upon further investigation by the CDI team, a trend of payer denials was identified for code G0502. This HCPCS code should therefore be included as part of the focused case review activities as part of the outpatient CDI program. This trend reflected denials for inaccurate CPT/HCPCS coding based on the lack of documentation to support the 70 minutes of behavioral healthcare management time required for code G0502.

Gaps in HCC Codes

HCC is a payment model that identifies patients with serious or chronic illness and assigns a risk factor score to each patient based on a combination of the individual's health conditions and demographic details. The individual's health conditions are identified via ICD-10-CM diagnoses that are submitted by providers on incoming claims, and the risk factor score is one variable used to determine the reimbursement amount for Medicare Advantage beneficiaries. If the ICD-10-CM code assignment is incorrect, the HCC assignment could also be incorrect, and reimbursement may be denied or inaccurate. Refer to chapter 3 for more detail on HCCs.

A review of HCC accuracy can be conducted using the following steps:

- Review the HCCs identified in previous years for each patient whose case has been selected for focused review. Compare the HCCs for the previous years to those identified in the current year to establish whether there seem to be gaps. Capture the missing ICD-10-CM-coded HCCs for the current year for an ROI calculation (discussed in the section Step 4: Analyze Results of Case Review, later in this chapter).
- Review the current year's clinical documentation for the physician practice, as well as clinical documentation in the inpatient, emergency department, and other outpatient settings, to identify missing ICD-10-CM-coded HCC diagnoses.

- If clinical indicators of chronic diseases captured in HCCs, medications reflecting treatment of such diseases, or relevant diagnoses from previous encounters or settings are identified, query the physician for possible updates to the clinical record and addition of the missing ICD-10-CM codes.

Figure 5.1 presents an example of a case review spreadsheet. This type of spreadsheet can be used if an HCC software tool is not available. The spreadsheet allows for entry of the patient number, date of service, name, original ICD-10-CM code, auditor ICD-10-CM code, and case comment. The spreadsheet uses a VLOOKUP formula in Microsoft Excel, linked to the CMS HCC payment codes and weight files, to automatically calculate the HCC and HCC weight from the ICD-10-CM code.

Figure 5.1. Sample case review spreadsheet

Review Location:			HCC Internal Medicine Clinic								
Auditor			Jane Smith								
Basic Case Information					Code Data Sets					Clinical Documentation Statisics	
Case #	MR#/ID#/ Encounter#	Date-of-Service	Patient Name	Provider	Original ICD-10	Original HCC Code	Original HCC Wt	Auditor ICD-10	Auditor HCC Code	Auditor HCC Wt	New HCC Each Year	Comments
1	34567	12/08/16	Alberson, E.	Smith, G.				I5030	85	0.323	1	Query for clarification of congestive heart failure and type.
1	34567	12/08/16	Alberson, E.	Smith, G.	C9110	10	0.677	C9110	10	0.677		
1	34567	12/08/16	Alberson, E.	Smith, G.	I4891	96	0.268	I4891	96	0.268		
1	34567	12/08/16	Alberson, E.	Smith, G.	F39	58	0.395	F39	58	0.395		
1	34567	01/10/17	Alberson, E.	Smith, G.	I480	96	0.268	I480	96	0.268		
1	34567	03/14/17	Alberson, E.	Smith, G.				E119	19	0.104	1	Diagnosis found on progress note 3/14/17
1	34567	06/14/17	Alberson, E.	Smith, G.	I5022	85	0.323	I5022	85	0.323		

Source: ©AHIMA

Medical Necessity Denials

Claims denied for missing or incorrect diagnoses codes based on the NCD or LCD should be evaluated to determine the root causes of the denials. The NCD and LCD identify the payable ICD-10-CM codes for specific CPT/HCPCS procedure codes (see chapter 2). The causes of these errors may be a lack of specific clinical documentation, inaccurate coding, or the lack of proper preauthorization screening. For example, the diagnosis on a claim for a positron emission tomography (PET) scan may have been coded as lung cancer, unspecified, but the NCD for PET scans requires a more specific code, such as lung cancer of the upper lobe.

Preauthorization, or prior approval authorization, is the process of obtaining approval for specific healthcare services from a healthcare insurance company before the patient receives those services. Preauthorization is also called precertification. In some circumstances, payers will not reimburse claims for services that are not preauthorized.

Claims Edit Issues

Claims scrubbers and clinical editors provide feedback on many types of claims submission issues that delay the processing of the claim (see chapter 6). The issue can be related to the lack of documentation demonstrating medical necessity for the NCD or LCD, an incorrect or missing CPT/HCPCS modifier, a missing component of CPT/HCPCS code, and other errors in claims data. The cause of these errors can be low-quality clinical documentation, coder error, charge capture issues, or lack of preauthorization screening.

Charge Capture Gaps

Gaps in charge captures can occur for several reasons, including the following:

- CPT/HCPCS options could be missing from a charge entry template or form.
- The link between a charge capture screen and the CDM or fee schedule could be incorrect.
- The descriptions in charge entry screens, the CDM, or the fee schedule could be misleading.
- Charge entry staff could be insufficiently educated about how to capture charges.
- Charge entry screens and forms might not be properly revised when updates are made to code classification systems, such as CPT/HCPCS (updated each January) or ICD-10-CM (updated annually on October 1).

Step 4: Analyze Results of Case Review

Once the case reviews are complete, the findings should be evaluated to determine the priority of each issue identified. This evaluation can be done by analyzing each issue, the corresponding potential volume of cases, and the error rate identified during the case review.

CPT, HCPCS, and APC Codes

For each CPT, HCPCS, or APC code where an error trend is identified, the CDS can assess the total volume of that code within the practice or facility and use the audit error rate to estimate the potential error rate. APC codes are used for facilities only. CPT and HCPCS codes apply to both physician practices and facilities.

HCC Codes

HCC code review should be a priority and area of focus for the outpatient CDI program. If a problem with HCC assignment is found in the initial assessment, further analysis of the findings from missing HCCs in previous years, as well as the current year, will identify providers whose cases may be included in the pilot project based on their total RAF score points missed.

Medical Necessity Denials

Denials trends and corresponding case review results should be used to identify issues related to specific providers, CPT or HCPCS codes, or ICD-10-CM codes. High-volume, high-dollar issues should be included in the initial target list for

CDI. The workplan of the Office of Inspector General of the US Department of Health and Human Services includes a review of outpatient outliers for short-stay claims (OIG 2016), which can help the outpatient CDS work to decrease such outliers. See chapter 4 for additional information on the OIG Work Plan.

Claims Edits

Analysis of claims edit trends can be used to determine items with a high-volume, high-dollar impact. The CDI program may prioritize those items where education and training or a streamlined outpatient clinical documentation query process can quickly resolve the issue. If software is available to track these trends, claims edits can be identified and further assessed based on volume and charge information.

Multiple vendors sell data analytics software to evaluate healthcare claims data. For example, MedeAnalytics is a data analytics firm that sells software tools to hospitals and health systems for use in strategy and operations activities (MedeAnalytics 2017). When a healthcare entity licenses such software, its claims data for a specified period are uploaded into the tool and then the entity can run data analysis reports. Where these tools are available for use in healthcare facilities, CDSs should be given access to use the tools to perform their job functions.

Figure 5.2 is a report from MedeAnalytics that provides a list of top revenue risks grouped into the following seven categories:

- *Unit count:* This category indicates that the expected number of units (procedure codes) for the specific treatment or medication is higher or lower than the typical number of units ordered.
- *Bundled payment:* This category flags codes that were submitted on the claim but should be bundled into another code that is also submitted on the claim. (See chapter 3 for more information on bundled payments.)
- *Procedure-related:* This category includes issues related to procedure code errors. For example, this category notes when a procedure is reported that requires more than one procedure code and the second code is not reported on the claim, or when a CPT add-on code is coded alone.
- *Missing charges:* Some clinical codes require another corresponding code to complete the claims submission. This category identifies claims that lack the corresponding codes. For example, a claim that includes a code for an injected medication without the required medication administration code would be included in the missing charges section of the report.
- *Diagnosis-related:* This category flags reported CPT codes that do not have a corresponding diagnosis to justify the treatment provided, such as a CPT code for a chest x-ray when the documented diagnosis is a urinary tract infection.
- *Noncovered service:* This category includes codes for services or treatments that are not covered by the payer, such as cosmetic surgery.
- *Obstetrical (OB) billing and care:* This category includes OB-related coding and claims issues associated with global OB care.

In figure 5.2, each category includes the volume of claims, the percentage of total claims issues that the category represents, the average charge amount for claims in the category, average payer payments, and the total charge amount for the month to date. This information can be used to determine which areas of focus would result in the greatest ROI for the outpatient CDI program. For example, the total volume of missing charges is 8,449, which represents 13.29% of all revenue risks tallied within the seven reported categories. The average charge in the missing charge category is $5,891. The average payments for claims with missing charges are $154 from Medicare and $1,898 from commercial payers and others. The average combined payment from all payers is $1,372, and the number of claims received for the month to date is 997.

Figure 5.2. Sample report showing data for a specific facility's top revenue risks. The report includes all physicians and all primary payers in these risk categories: Unit Count, Bundled Payments, Procedure Related, Missing Charges, Diagnosis Related, Noncovered Service, and OB Billing and Care, for a specified period

Risk Category	Volume	% of Total	Average Charges	Avg Commercial/Other Pmts	Avg Medicaid Pmts	Avg Medicare Pmts	Average Pmts	Claims MTD	Commercial/Other Pmts	Medicaid Pmts
Unit Count	21,955	34.54%	$10,108	$1,535	$0	$474	$2,010	460	$33,334,705	$0
Bundled Payment	15,042	23.67%	$5,554	$795	$0	$330	$1,125	246	$11,617,159	$0
Proc Related	11,796	18.56%	$9,256	$1,784	$0	$550	$2,334	206	$20,701,925	$0
Missing Charges	8,449	13.29%	$5,891	$1,898	$0	$154	$2,052	86	$15,975,022	$0
Diag Related	6,250	9.83%	$2,752	$706	$0	$96	$802	24	$4,412,339	$0
Noncovered Service	66	0.10%	$4,344	$497	$0	$33	$531	6	$32,833	$0
OB Billing and Care	1	0.00%	$1,047	$181	$0	$0	$181		$181	$0
Total: All	63,559	100.00%	$7,582	$1,372	$0	$374	$1,746	997	$80,288,686	$0

Source: MedeAnalytics 2017. Reprinted with permission. The example screenshots and dashboards for Revenue Integrity were provided by MedeAnalytics, Inc. MedeAnalytics offers a cloud-based analytics platform that aggregates and normalizes data across multiple sources, delivering it in an intuitive format that inspires clear and actionable insights into healthcare organizations' revenue, cost, quality, and risk. MedeAnalytics and Revenue Integrity are registered trademarks of MedeAnalytics, Inc. All rights reserved.

Charge Capture

To resolve denials, incorrect reimbursement, and claims edit issues related to the charge capture process, further analysis of the root cause is required. Initial areas of focus should be those high-volume, high-dollar categories that can be quickly resolved through education or a system update.

Step 5: Estimate the Return on Investment

The ROI for CDI can be estimated by determining the impact of reducing errors in each category identified in the CDI assessment. In particular, three categories should be considered when calculating ROI: HCC RAF scores, CPT/HCPCS code errors, and related charge capture issues and denials.

HCC Codes

If CDI leads to increased reporting of HCC codes for patients enrolled in Medicare Advantage, the amount of Medicare Advantage plan reimbursement should increase. The increased reimbursement to the plan is based on the increase in weight of the RAF scores. To calculate the ROI to the health system, hospital, or physician practice, the CDI manager should further review the Medicare Advantage contracts or discuss the contracts with the health plan contract manager to determine the formula used to share in the risk. For example, the risk share reimbursement may be set as a percentage of reimbursement to the Medicare Advantage plan. Further detail on calculating RAF scores to estimate Medicare Advantage reimbursement can be found in chapter 3 of this text.

Issues Related to CPT/HCPCS Codes, Charge Capture, and Denials

Several steps are required for calculating the impact of a specific CPT/HCPCS or denials issue. The impact (ROI) of CPT/HCPCS capture issues can be estimated by using the following steps:

1. Identify the total volume for the specific CPT/HCPCS service.
2. Determine the reimbursement impact of eliminating the charge capture issue for each unit.
3. Multiply the per-unit reimbursement impact by the total volume and the error rate percentage identified during the assessment of the issue.

Case Example

An audit was conducted of the chemotherapy clinic billing and coding process. The CDS identified a charge capture issue and determined that it was due to the charge entry clerk in the chemotherapy clinic selecting or entering the incorrect CPT code, perhaps because she was given the wrong information or was inadequately trained. CPT code 96409, Chemo IV push, single drug (Medicare reimbursement $191.08), was billed instead of 96413, Chemo IV infusion, 1 hour (Medicare reimbursement $297.54). This error occurred from March 2017 to August 2017. The total number of units billed in error was 3,659. The error rate percentage was 100%.

1. 3,659 unit hours: Chemotherapy infusion, billed as IV push
2. $106.46 reimbursement impact ($297.54 − $191.08)
3. $106.46 (impact) × 3,659 × 1 (100% error rate) = $389,537.14 (ROI)

The estimated impact for denials can be calculated using a similar method as that described for CPT/HCPCS codes.

Case Example

The CDS identified a pattern of medical necessity denials related to the use of an unspecified ICD-10-CM code that was excluded for reimbursement under the payer's LCD for a sinus x-ray. The CDS investigated further and found that the issue could be resolved through a technology solution that includes elimination of the unspecified code from the automated drop-down list of available ICD-10-CM codes. To calculate the ROI, the CDI identified 1,027 occurrences of the error over the past year. The reimbursement for the sinus x-ray by the payer for CPT code 70210, x-ray exam of sinuses, was $62.11.

1. Identify the total volume of like denials (1,027 cases).
2. Identify the reimbursement impact of the denied charge ($62.11 reimbursement).
3. Multiply the total volume by the reimbursement impact (1,027 × $62.11 = $63,786.97).

In the case of denials, the CDI manager can also estimate the cost (staff salary) of correcting a resubmitting a specific denial type. The salary cost can be multiplied by the number of denials to get an estimated salary cost ROI for the denials. Then, the reimbursement impact and the salary cost impact can be added together to calculate the total ROI of the program.

Where the CDI manager has access to denials management software, the denials trends can be reviewed over time for specific denials categories improved through CDI activities. The reimbursement impact of the improvements can be estimated by multiplying the average impact of the category by the denial-type count. Some denials software also provides dollar impact of denials built into the software. In those cases, the ROI for the software can be taken from the denials management software.

Step 6: Create a High-Level Workplan

After steps 1 through 5 of the outpatient CDI assessment program are completed, the CDI manager should draft a focused list of target issues for the initial outpatient CDI program at the pilot clinic, with priority placed on high-volume, high-dollar issues. As stated previously, the pilot clinic is selected based on patient volume, complexity, specialty, and access to a physician champion. The appropriate focused targets will vary based on the services provided and the quality of the existing clinical documentation, coding, and charge capture processes.

Once the targets are identified, the CDI manager and team can develop a high-level workplan for presentation to the executive leadership responsible for program approval. The CDI workplan is an instructional roadmap to CDI program implementation. It can be created using spreadsheets (for example, an Excel workbook) or project management software (such as Microsoft Project). Each step in the workplan includes a task and subtasks. As the implementation process moves along, the original workplan tasks that are presented to the CDI taskforce and steering committee will be further detailed and new subtasks will be defined.

As explained in greater detail in chapter 10, the tasks in the workplan are as follows (*Note:* The workplan is an all-inclusive list of CDI program activities. The plan should include all program activities from inception to completion, including the initial data request and taskforce activities, which may already be complete at the time the workplan is generated.):

- **Task 1—Data analytics request:** Each outpatient CDI project requires an initial data request to stakeholders for claims files, the CDM, professional practice fee schedules, denials reports, claims scrubber reports, coding audit reports, and other information that will help the project team.

- **Task 2—On-site kickoff meeting and interviews:** After the data for analysis have been requested and received, the kickoff meeting and stakeholder interviews will be conducted. A formal presentation will be given during the kickoff meeting. See appendix 5A for a sample presentation in Microsoft Powerpoint format.

- **Task 3—CDI program governance and oversight:** Task 3 includes the development of the executive oversight steering committee and CDI taskforce. There may be more than one taskforce, depending on the size and complexity of the facility or health system.

- **Task 4—Outpatient and professional practice case review:** This task includes the professional practice and outpatient facility case review for clinical documentation and coding issues. The review will include the following:
  - Assessment of the clinical record to determine gaps in high-quality clinical documentation

- Review of coding accuracy (ICD-10-CM, CPT, and HCPCS)
- Review of HCC assignment and related clinical documentation gaps for all sites of services (inpatient, outpatient, and professional fee)

- **Task 5—High-level assessment of technology to support the outpatient CDI program:** This assessment should be conducted by the project manager in conjunction with the information technology (IT) department. The following issues related to facility software applications and technology tools should be included during the assessment process:
  - Denials management
  - EHR interoperability
  - HCC suspecting (*Suspecting* means using natural language processing [NLP] software to identify potential chronic illnesses by scanning diagnostic test results, clinical signs and symptoms, and other clinical information in the EHR. NLP is a technology that converts structured or unstructured human language into data that can be translated then manipulated by computer systems.)
  - Ambulatory coding compliance edits

- **Task 6—Outpatient clinical documentation assessment report:** The CDI manager completes an outpatient assessment report that recommends areas of focus for the new outpatient CDI case review process. The findings will address clinical documentation gaps, coding issues, charge capture issues, and technology requirements.

- **Task 7—Rapid redesign of pilot clinic workflow:** This task includes the steps to visit the clinic and evaluate the clinical documentation workflow and develop an implementation plan for the redesigned workflow. During this redesign process, the clinical documentation workflow will be streamlined and made more efficient.

- **Task 8—Physician collaboration and education:** As noted previously, physician buy-in is essential to the CDI program's success. Educating physicians about clinical documentation in the outpatient and professional fee settings will make the CDI program more efficient by reducing the number of provider queries required to resolve documentation gaps. The educational sessions should be short (no longer than 30 minutes), and the content should be specific to the physicians in the specialty area invited to the meeting.

- **Task 9—Rapid redesign of remaining clinics:** This task continues rollout of the CDI program to the remaining clinics in the project. It includes essentially the same steps as the pilot program implementation outlined in tasks 4 through 8, except the timing will depend on the number of facilities, distance, and available resources.

- **Task 10—Ongoing program monitoring:** This task includes steps to ensure the sustainability of the outpatient CDI program. The project manager or program sponsor should conduct monthly calls with the key stakeholders to ensure that the program is progressing as planned.

The format from the excerpted workplan in figure 5.3 can be used to customize the workplan for the executive presentation. The plan includes the task number, task, subtask, disposition, status notes, consultant responsible party,

Figure 5.3. Selection from an outpatient CDI workplan timeline

Medical Center CDI Workplan

Priority: Pending / Complete

Task #	Task	Subtasks	Status Notes	Disposition	Consultant Responsible Party	Facility Responsible Party	Start Date	Due Date	Dec	Jan	Feb	Mar	Apr	May
1	**Data Analytics**													
1.a		Submit Data Requests for 835/837 files, CDM, fee schedules		Complete	Project Mgr		Dec 1	Dec 5	↑					
1.b		Upon receipt of 835/837 files, submit to IT for the denials and ambulatory claims manager tool update.	835/837 files received. Analytics review is under way.	Complete	Project Mgr		Dec 1	Dec 5	↑					
1.c		Gather additional information as needed from client for project assessment.	Files gathered during on-site review: Charge master, fee schedules and Payor Contract Matrix.	Complete	Project Mgr		Dec 15	Dec 30	↑					
1.d.		Analyze data and identify trends for focused outpatient audits and Physician, CDI, and Coder education. These findings and recommendations will be included in Assessment Report.	Updated projected date of focused targets March 15.	Complete	Project Mgr		Dec 20	Mar 15				↑		

PHASE I: CDI PROGRAM ASSESSMENT

Project Timeline

Source: ©AHIMA

facility responsible party, start date, due date, and graphical timeline. A detailed discussion of workplan development and use during the outpatient CDI project is found in chapter 10 of this text.

Executive and Key Stakeholder Buy-in

After the initial steps in the assessment process are complete and the high-level workplan has been created, the plan for the CDI program is presented to the executive leadership and other key stakeholders. An executive-level steering committee or existing executive or leadership meeting is the best place for this presentation. A meeting of the outpatient CDI taskforce could also be used for this purpose.

The CDI manager or director should be the presenter and keep the presentation short—no longer than 15 minutes. The recommended format for the presentation is a slideshow created with PowerPoint or a similar type of presentation software. The three major sections of the presentation and their subsections are as follows:

- Goals and objectives of the outpatient CDI program
    - Program goals
    - Program objectives
- Results of the CDI assessment
    - Data analytics
    - Case review findings
    - Financial impact
    - Conclusions
    - Recommendations
- Next steps
    - Pilot site selection
    - Communicating the pilot site plan
    - Focused target areas
    - Staffing the project
    - Pilot site implementation schedule
    - Remaining clinic and physician practice rollout plan
    - Ongoing monitoring for sustainability
    - Reporting project ROI

At the conclusion of the meeting, the CDI director or manager should encourage discussion of the program's feasibility, pilot site selection, stakeholder communication, start date, and tasks required for final approval implementation. Refer to chapters 6, 7, 8, and 10 for more information on the steps included here in the outpatient CDI assessment.

Chapter 5 Review Exercises

1. Which of the following best describes the recommended starting point for any outpatient CDI program?
   a. Gaining physician buy-in
   b. Selecting a pilot clinic or provider practice
   c. Assessing the program's feasibility and ROI
   d. Focusing efforts on high-volume, high-risk areas

2. When deciding whether CDI would be beneficial in the outpatient setting, which of the following questions is most important for CDI leaders to consider?
   a. Who will be the cardiology CDS?
   b. Does the healthcare entity already have an inpatient CDI program?
   c. Will the medical staff leader participate in the educational programs for physicians?
   d. What are the potential barriers to developing an outpatient CDI program?

3. Which of the following represent the primary barriers to outpatient CDI?
   a. Staffing, timing, and buy-in
   b. Cost, ROI, and relevant skills
   c. ROI, CDS experience, and IT buy-in
   d. ROI, proficiency in inpatient CDI, and IT support

4. CDI in the outpatient setting provides several benefits. Among these is the ability to identify gaps in documentation at the time and site of service, which may lead to _____.
   a. Shortened time for bill drop
   b. More accurate quality scores
   c. Additional staff recruitment opportunities
   d. Fewer days for claims in accounts receivable

5. The assessment of the current state of the clinical documentation stage involves multiple steps. After data have been gathered and areas of review focus have been identified, the next step is to _____.
   a. Estimate the ROI
   b. Create a detailed workplan
   c. Conduct a focused case review
   d. Establish an outpatient CDI taskforce

6. A stakeholder to include on the CDI taskforce is the _____.
   a. HIM director
   b. Utilization review nurse
   c. Respiratory therapy director
   d. Chief executive officer (CEO)

7. One of the steps in the outpatient CDI assessment program involves identifying its areas of focus. Which of the following is least likely to be considered when determining the areas of focus?
   a. Case volume
   b. Stakeholder buy-in
   c. Reimbursement risk
   d. Quality measurement

8. The _____ process of evaluating benefits and barriers is similar to a cost–benefit analysis but progresses one step further to also analyze the political, operational, and resource issues related to the proposed project.
   a. Audit
   b. Case review
   c. Needs assessment
   d. Root cause analysis

9. Which of the following formulas is used to estimate the impact of CPT/HCPCS capture issues?
   a. Impact × ROI × Total volume
   b. Total volume × Impact × Error rate
   c. Total volume × Reimbursement impact
   d. RVU weight × Conversion factor × GPCI

10. A CDI workplan involves a series of tasks, one of which is to conduct a high-level assessment of technology to support the outpatient CDI program. With whom should the IT department work to facilitate this assessment?
    a. CDS
    b. CFO
    c. HIM director
    d. Project manager

References

Arrowood, D., L.M. Johnson, and M.M. Wieczorek. 2015. Clinical documentation improvement in the outpatient setting. *Journal of AHIMA* 86(7):52–54.

Centers for Medicare and Medicaid Services (CMS). 2017a. Glossary. https://www.cms.gov/apps/glossary/default.asp?Letter=ALL.

Centers for Medicare and Medicaid Services (CMS). 2017b. Medically Unlikely Edits (MUE). https://www.cms.gov/Medicare/Coding/NationalCorrectCodInitEd/MUE.html.

Combs, T. 2016 (May 27). Benefits and barriers for outpatient CDI programs. Documentation Detective blog. *Journal of AHIMA* website. http://journal.ahima.org/2016/05/27/benefits-and-barriers-for-outpatient-cdi-programs.

MedeAnalytics. 2017. http://medeanalytics.com.

Office of Inspector General (OIG), US Department of Health and Human Services. 2016. OIG work plan: Outpatient outlier payments for short-stay claims. https://oig.hhs.gov/reports-and-publications/workplan/summary/wp-summary-0000079.asp.

Analyzing Clinical Documentation Data

6

Learning Objectives

- Identify the types of data sets related to clinical documentation improvement (CDI).
- Describe the types of case review used in CDI and the purpose of each.
- Discuss the steps in the process to prepare for a CDI pilot program.
- Learn how to conduct a focused case review.
- Explain how to develop an effective process for reporting CDI outcomes to stakeholders.

Key Terms

Charge description master (CDM) number
Claims edits
Claims scrubber
Denials trend analysis

Medically Unlikely Edits (MUEs)
Outpatient Prospective Payment System (OPPS)
Research identifiable file (RIF)
Structured query language (SQL)

Assessing clinical documentation in the outpatient setting can be a daunting task. The sheer numbers of specialties, locations, data types, and clinical documentation processes can seem overwhelming or leave one wondering where to start. A focused approach to this quandary is the best practice and essential to the outpatient clinical documentation improvement (CDI) program's success. Because CDI has so many moving parts, the first step is to select and review relevant data that identify the areas of focus, which are chosen based on their high volume and high impact (on revenue or quality). The timing of the case review is important to the development of an effective solution. Case review may be performed prior to, during, or after the patient encounter. The CDI program may need to use a combination of these review times to develop a comprehensive solution. Finally, the program will also need a methodology for reporting the findings; such reports are essential to foster buy-in from CDI stakeholders and the sustainability of the program. This chapter provides a streamlined approach to data analysis and focused review.

Selecting Clinical Documentation Data for Analysis

The first step in assessing clinical documentation is to identify the data sets available for analysis. These data sets may come from a variety of sources, such as the **Outpatient Prospective Payment System (OPPS)** claims data file; facility chargemaster and physician practice fee schedule volumes; claims edit frequency; denials tools; previous coding audit reports; and so on. The Hospital OPPS is the reimbursement system created by the Balanced Budget Act of 1997 for hospital outpatient services rendered to Medicare beneficiaries and maintained by CMS (CMS 2016a). The following sections describe examples of the multiple data sets available for use by the CDI manager to determine areas of focus for case review activity.

Chargemaster

The hospital chargemaster, often referred to as a *charge description master* (CDM), is a master price list that includes the items that are billed by the facility on the UB-04 Uniform Bill claim to the insurance company (the UB-04 form is discussed in greater detail later in this chapter and in chapter 3). The list includes "supplies, devices, medications, services, procedures, and other items for which a distinct charge to the patient exists" (AHIMA 2010). This list is updated annually, usually by a specialist in the revenue integrity or revenue cycle department. The specialist must be familiar with Current Procedural Terminology (CPT) and Healthcare Common Procedure Coding System (HCPCS) codes and guidelines because those codes are assigned to specific items in the CDM. For each entry in the list, the chargemaster typically includes the following: charge description, CPT/HCPCS code, revenue code, charge, department code, charge code, and charge status. Table 6.1 provides a snapshot of an abbreviated CDM. The parts of the chargemaster that are relevant to CDI are discussed in the sections that follow.

Charge Description

The charge description identifies the item. There is no industry standard format for charge descriptions, and charge capture errors may be made by those

Table 6.1. Selection from a chargemaster

Charge Description	CPT/HCPCS Code	Revenue Code	Charge	Department Code	Charge Code	Charge Status
Nasal Bone X-ray	70160	320	$150.00	15	2214111000	12/1/18
Thyroid Sonogram	76536	320	$250.00	15	2110410000	1/1/17
Echo Encephalogram	76506	320	$1,500.00	15	2326222111	7/5/17

Source: AHIMA 2010

entering charges if they misinterpret the descriptions and therefore select an incorrect service item. Also, some CDMs limit the number of characters available for the description, which can lead to additional problems when a complete description is not available (especially when the charge involves variables such as dosage, size, level, or type). Many HCPCS descriptions are very similar except for slight differences at their ends. If HCPCS descriptions are uploaded from CMS or the American Medical Association (AMA) into a system that limits the number of characters in the description field, the important distinguishing piece of a description could be omitted.

The lack of industry standards for descriptions can be the root cause of HCPCS code errors. Most chargemaster items are hard coded, which means that the HCPCS code is assigned automatically when an item is selected from a charge entry screen or another input tool, such as a superbill or charge ticket. A coder may not be involved in the HCPCS code selection process. Depending on the facility and organization policies, other items on the chargemaster may be soft coded, such as surgery, emergency department procedures, or clinic procedures. During the soft-coding process, coders assign the correct CPT or HCPCS code on the claim in the billing system. Areas such as laboratory, radiology, and therapies are almost always hard coded.

The outpatient clinical documentation specialist (CDS) can review the volume for procedures and services to determine whether all codes representing the service offerings are being used and that the volumes seem to be reasonable. Where a possible code utilization issue is identified, the outpatient CDS should compare the chargemaster descriptions with the descriptions on the charge entry screen to evaluate whether inconsistencies between these descriptions could be the root cause of the issue. When the specific issue is identified, the CDS should work with the information technology (IT), health informatics, and clinic managers to update the descriptions in the electronic health record (EHR) and train the staff responsible for the charge entry function.

Case Example

A cardiology practice with five interventional cardiologists had a concern related to revenue. The CDS reviewed the chargemaster volumes for the five cardiologists and noticed that Dr. Audubon's total procedure volume was much lower in the first quarter than the volumes for the other partners in the group, even though she was among the hospital's top admitters. Further investigation revealed that the number of procedures by Dr. Audubon billed for the period in question was incorrect, and the cause of the error was a charge capture issue. The CDS worked with IT and the clinic managers to resolve the problem.

CPT or HCPCS Code

As noted, a corresponding CPT or HCPCS code is linked in the chargemaster to many items, such as minor surgical procedures, supplies, and medications. CMS publishes updates to CPT and HCPCS codes in the Addendum B files for OPPS (CMS 2017a). Data from the addendum can be used to determine whether items are reimbursable under the OPPS. Most payers follow Medicare guidelines to determine payable or packaged CPT/HCPCS codes. (*Packaged* means that the primary code in a code group is payable and the secondary codes are included.) See chapter 3 for further discussion of CPT and HCPCS codes.

Revenue Code

A revenue code is a 4-digit code that indicates the department or type of service for each chargemaster item. The same CPT code may be found in more than one revenue code. The revenue code helps the CDS to understand which departments use particular codes. The list is updated each year by the National Uniform Billing Committee (NUBC) and CMS. The complete list of revenue codes can be purchased from NUBC as part of the Official UB-04 Data Specifications Manual (NUBC 2017). A list of revenue codes is also found on the Research Data Assistance Center (ResDAC) website (ResDAC 2016a). ResDAC is a group of faculty and staff from several US universities that offers CMS data to be used for research. The following list is an example of revenue codes for the pharmacy (ResDAC 2016a; NUBC 2017; Noridian Healthcare Solutions 2017):

Pharmacy 025X

0250 General

0251 Generic drugs

0252 Nongeneric drugs

0253 Take-home drugs

0254 Drugs incident to other diagnostic services

0255 Drugs incident to radiology

0256 Experimental drugs

0257 Nonprescription

0258 IV solutions

0259 Other

Department Code

The department code is used to identify the cost center for accounting purposes. Department codes are assigned by each facility, and there is no industry-standard code set. The department code is important to identify the departments using a specific CPT code. The same CPT codes may be found in multiple departments. The CDS uses the codes to understand which charges are being submitted by specific departments.

Charge Code

The charge code is also called the *charge description number, item code,* or **CDM number** (AHIMA 2010). These codes are selected by the facility, and, unlike revenue codes, do not correspond to an industry-standard numbering system. The CDM number is important when determining the volume for a specific CPT or HCPCS code on the chargemaster.

Charge Status

The charge status field for an item lists a date to indicate whether the item is currently being used or, if it is no longer in use, the effective dates. Charge status is often referred to in terms of "active" versus "inactive" item codes. When doing any type of trending or historical review, it is important to know which item codes were active during the time frame under investigation and review. Items are retired based on changes in CPT or HCPCS codes, service line changes, or coding guideline changes.

Claims Edits

Claims edits are flags or error messages produced by a **claims scrubber** (a type of billing software that reviews the coding of claims) when there seems to be a problem with code assignment in a reimbursement claim. Claims edits require correction before the claim is submitted to avoid the denial or rejection of the claim by the payer. Understanding claims edits is therefore important to the outpatient clinical documentation program because the process of resolving them can hold up claims submission and delay reimbursement to the facility or professional practice. Ultimately, it is the goal of the CDI program to identify why claims edits occur and determine how to prevent their occurrence in the future. Preventing the causes of claims edits can lower the cost of the claims submission process. This decrease in cost may also be seen as a return on investment (ROI) for the outpatient CDI program.

It is important to note that there are differences in professional or physician and hospital OPPS claims scrubbers. The facility claims scrubbers use the industry guidelines for facility billing specified for the CMS-1450 form in chapter 1 of the Medicare Claims Processing Manual (CMS 2017b). The CMS-1450 form (also known as the UB-04 Uniform Bill) is a uniform institutional provider hardcopy claims form suitable for use in billing multiple third-party payers. It is the only hard-copy claims form that CMS accepts from institutional providers (CMS 2017b). The professional practice claims scrubbers use edits related to professional fee claims for the CMS 1500 form specified in chapter 1 of the Medicare Claims Processing Manual (CMS 2017b). The CMS-1500 form is the uniform professional claims form used by provider practices to submit claims to insurance companies.

The types of claims scrubber edits can be categorized as follows (Experian 2016):

- *General industry-standard edits:* Edits related to National Correct Coding Initiative (NCCI) bundling, global period, local coverage determination (LCD) and national coverage determination (NCD), deleted codes, CPT modifier validity, frequency limits (allowed number of units within a given time period), or new versus established patients. Refer to chapter 3 of this text for more information on NCCI edits. The *global period* (also referred to as the *global package*) is a payment policy of bundling payment for the various services associated with a surgery into a single payment covering professional services for preoperative care, the surgery itself, and postoperative care. Other industry-standard edits are established to

guide coders and the healthcare industry in the correct use of codes on the claims form to report the following:
- Bilateral procedures (procedures done on both the right and left side).
- Multiple codes requiring modifiers to further specify the circumstances of a code submission. For example, modifier 25 is appended to the end of a CPT code when an evaluation and management (E/M) code is used in addition to a procedure code. Further discussion on the use of modifiers may be found in the CPT manual published by AMA (2018); E/M codes are discussed in chapter 3 of this textbook.
- Component codes required for documenting a procedure that includes multiple steps. An example of component code use is a gastroenterology intervention, such as an esophagoscopy for removal of foreign body, in which multiple, unbundled procedures may be performed. The primary esophagoscopy procedure would be assigned CPT code 43194, and the secondary removal of polyp performed during the same procedure would be assigned CPT code 43217 (AMA 2018). Additional guidance related to the use of component codes may be found in AMA's CPT manual (AMA 2018).

- *Payer-specific edits:* Edits customized to reflect the requirements of individual payers. These include edits similar to the general, industry-standard edits related to issues such as bundling, noncovered services, medical necessity, exclusion and inclusion criteria related to age or gender, and frequency.
- *Custom edits:* Edits designed by the organization to identify facility-specific claims processing and coding issues.

Most of the health information billing systems available in the marketplace include claims scrubbers. The reports generated by these systems are an excellent resource for the outpatient CDS to use in identifying high-volume, high-impact coding and billing issues related to clinical documentation gaps. For example, payers will check documentation of medical necessity for specific CPT or HCPCS codes against a list of approved *International Classification of Diseases, Tenth Revision, Clinical Modification* (ICD-10-CM) codes. The CDS should audit procedures that have a high edit rate for medical necessity to determine the reason why the appropriate ICD-10-CM diagnosis codes were not submitted. Reasons for this problem can vary by provider, but the root cause is usually that the clinical documentation lacks the specificity required to allow for a correct code assignment. The specific reasons for medical necessity edits include the following:

- Lack of specific documentation supporting allowed diagnoses listed in the LCD or NCD notices
- Lack of patient prescreening for medical necessity prior to the encounter

Solutions for these issues can be established using the pre-encounter, concurrent, or postencounter case review process outlined in the Focused Clinical Record Review Process section later in this chapter.

The claims scrubber may also produce compliance-based edits such as **Medically Unlikely Edits (MUEs)**. CMS developed its MUE program to reduce the paid-claims error rate for Medicare Part B claims. An MUE for a CPT/HCPCS code is the maximum units of service that a provider would report under most circumstances for a single beneficiary on a single date of service. Not all HCPCS/CPT codes have an MUE. MUEs are designed to reduce errors specifically associated with clerical entries and incorrect coding based on criteria such as anatomical considerations, CPT/HCPCS code descriptors, CPT coding instructions, established CMS policies, nature of a service or procedure, nature of an analyte, nature of equipment, prescribing information, and clinical data (CMS 2017c).

The claims scrubber workflow process includes a work queue used to identify claims to be reviewed, corrected, and resubmitted. The process of correcting claims edits is time-consuming and costly for the facility. The outpatient CDS can assist by identifying clinical documentation and coding trends that could result in claims edits and a delay in the billing process. Once the root cause is identified through case review and investigation of the clinical documentation process, a solution such as workflow redesign or provider education can be implemented.

Denials Trends and Reports

Denials trend analysis refers to the process of analyzing denials frequency data by category and determining trends for high-volume denials. This process should also include ongoing analysis for denials categories that are decreasing or increasing in volume. This methodology is an essential part of the outpatient CDI process; by using it, the outpatient CDS can highlight improvements to stakeholders and further investigate and develop solutions for denials categories that are on the rise.

Denials reports may be generated by a stand-alone software tool. Alternatively, denials may be entered into a spreadsheet or database by the denials management department for tracking purposes. This function is normally found in the revenue integrity, revenue cycle, or the denials management department. The outpatient CDS should receive access to the denials reports and participate in taskforce meetings where denials trends are discussed.

Coding Audit Reports

Most health information management (HIM) departments perform internal and external coding audits as part of their quality assurance process. The audit reports can provide valuable information related to clinical documentation gaps. The audits normally include not only coding errors but also cases where a provider query could increase the specificity of documentation for accurate coding and to support medical necessity requirements. The outpatient CDS should have access to the audit reports and be included in group discussions so that provider education and ongoing monitoring of the issues can be part of the CDI solution. Often, a process is in place to educate coders about issues identified during the audit, but less attention is typically paid to the provider education component. The outpatient CDS can include providers in group or one-on-one discussions when denials trends are provider-specific.

HCC Reports and Audits

Medicare Advantage payers are interested in accurate capture of Hierarchical Condition Categories (HCCs) by facilities and professional practices because it ensures that the reimbursement received from CMS is correct. Refer to chapter 3 for more information on the Medicare Advantage program. Upon request, payers will provide reports to facilities and providers that indicate which patients were reimbursed under the Medicare Advantage HCC program. Hospitals with a data analytics department may be able to run a similar report listing the claims number, encounter date, ICD-10-CM code, and corresponding HCC code for the past one- or two-year period. This report can be used to audit all encounters for a specific patient to determine whether the HCCs are captured accurately. Proprietary software tools that will provide this type of monitoring and reporting are also available in the marketplace. This technology will be discussed in more detail in chapter 7 of this text.

Quality Measure Scores

Quality measures have been established by CMS for outpatient facilities under the Hospital Outpatient Quality Reporting (OQR) program and under the Medicare Access and CHIP Reauthorization Act of 2015 (MACRA) and Merit-Based Incentive Payment System (MIPS) for the physician practice (see chapter 4). The quality department in the facility or the practice manager in the professional practice setting can provide trend reports on these measures that will allow the outpatient CDS to determine which are affected by clinical documentation gaps. For example, two MIPS program measures are as follows (CMS 2017):

- Dementia—Caregiver Education and Support: Percentage of patients, regardless of age, with a diagnosis of dementia whose caregiver(s) were provided with education on dementia disease management and health behavior changes and referred to additional resources for support within a 12-month period
- Dementia—Cognitive Assessment: Percentage of patients, regardless of age, with a diagnosis of dementia for whom an assessment of cognition is performed and the results reviewed at least once within a 12-month period

Data capture for both of these measures requires specificity in the clinical documentation about caregiver education and cognitive assessment. An effective data capture process for these two measures can be included in the pre-encounter, concurrent, or postencounter case review process outlined in this chapter.

Outpatient Research Identifiable Files

OPPS claims data are available for purchase from the ResDAC as outpatient **research identifiable files (RIFs)**, which include data elements such as diagnosis codes, HCPCS codes, dates of service, reimbursement amounts, outpatient provider numbers, revenue center codes, and beneficiary demographic information. Patient-identifying information has been removed from the file. The updated RIF is available for purchase twice a year, when the OPPS proposed and final rules are published in the *Federal Register* (ResDAC 2016b). Institutional outpatient providers included in this data are "hospital outpatient departments, rural health clinics, renal dialysis facilities, outpatient rehabilitation facilities, comprehensive outpatient rehabilitation facilities, and community mental health centers" (ResDAC 2016b).

RIFs can be used to compare a healthcare entity's HCPCS code use against that of its peer groups to identify missing charge capture opportunities. For example, if different hospitals within a peer group provide similar services, such as wound debridement, chemotherapy infusion or injections, or laceration repairs, the hospitals' use rates for the corresponding CPT/HCPS codes for these services can be compared to see whether the code frequency in a specific hospital is reasonable for a particular service. Table 6.2 compares one medical center's use of three HCPCS codes for wound debridement (11042, 11043, and 11044) to that of its peers. Each of the codes is payable under OPPS. This table indicates the medical center's use of the lowest-weight code (11042) is much higher than that of the peer group (97 percent versus 82 percent). Therefore, the outpatient CDI team for the medical center should conduct an audit of cases with these procedure codes documented to validate the accuracy of coding and identify any documentation gaps. The audit might find that coders use the lowest-level code because the clinical documentation for debridement is not specific enough to identify the more extensive debridement procedures and a process is lacking for effectively querying providers about the potential clinical documentation gaps.

Table 6.2. Comparison of HCPCS debridement code use in one medical center versus its peers

HCPCS Code	Short Descriptor	SI	APC	Relative Weight	Payment Rate	Medical Center	Medical Center Peer Group
11042	Debridement subq tissue 20 sq cm/<	T	5052	3.9015	$292.62	97.00%	82.00%
11043	Debridement musc/fascia 20 sq cm/<	T	5053	6.0412	$453.10	2.00%	12.00%
11044	Debridement bone 20 sq cm/<	J1	5072	16.4881	$1236.62	1.00%	6.00%

Source: CMS, 2017a

To create a report similar to the one in table 6.2, the outpatient RIF can be uploaded into a database using **structured query language (SQL)**, such as Microsoft Access, and reports can be written using a software application, such as Crystal Reports. SQL is a fourth-generation computer language that is used to create and manipulate relational databases.

RIFs are somewhat difficult to obtain. To gain access, the purchaser or researcher must go through an application process and present a strong case about the use of the data. The outpatient RIF is fairly expensive, and only an SAS programmer can manipulate the data. The limited data sets with the standard analytical files (SAFs) and the OPPS files that are used by CMS for proposed and final rule-making are alternatives to the outpatient RIF. These limited data sets are also available for purchase and can be used for the same purpose as RIF to perform a comparative analysis of peers within CPT/HCPCS code groups (ResDAC 2016c).

Other HCPCS Code Utilization Files

Other files with data on the use of HCPCS codes, such as the top 200 Level I HCPCS/CPT codes and the top 200 Level II HCPCS codes, are available from CMS (2017e). These files have Medicare utilization statistics for Part B physician/

supplier national data and do not apply to hospital/facility utilization. Refer to chapter 3 for information on the distinctions between Level I and Level II HCPCS codes.

Tables 6.3 and 6.4 display excerpts of the rankings of Level I HCPCS/CPT and Level II HCPCS codes, respectively, by total allowed charges from CMS's national top 200 data sets (CMS 2017e). These data sets can be used to compare the national frequency of use of certain HCPCS codes with their usage by a specific clinic, physician group, or individual physician. For example, the codes for office visits for established patients (99211–99215) are in the top 200 Level I data set. If the individual physician's use of these codes does not align with the national trend to use low-level codes for most visits by established patients, the outpatient CDS should investigate this finding to determine the root cause. Similarly, the Level II data set could be used for a comparative analysis of the use of codes for medical supplies or medications in the national top 200. If the assignment of such codes to an individual physician's cases varies notably from the national trend, the outpatient CDS should investigate whether the code assignments for the physician's work are correct or if there is a charge capture issue.

Table 6.3. Excerpt from the data set of top 200 Level I HCPCS/CPT codes used for Medicare Part B by physicians and suppliers, ranked nationally by charges for calendar year 2015

Rank by Charges	HCPCS Code	Allowed Charges, Total Dollars	Total No. of Allowed Services
1	99214	9,891,277,157	95,564,075
2	99213	6,925,839,306	99,683,743
3	99232	3,574,920,688	49,154,526
4	99233	2,339,976,735	22,189,676
5	99223	2,215,682,581	10,832,400
6	66984	2,147,710,586	3,187,012

Source: CMS 2017e. Codes copyrighted by the American Medical Association

Table 6.4. Excerpt from the data set of top 200 Level II HCPCS codes used for Medicare Part B by physicians and suppliers, ranked nationally by charges for calendar year 2015

Rank by Charges	HCPCS Code	Allowed Charges, Total Dollars	Total No. of Allowed Services
1	A0427	2,141,667,946	4,992,480
2	J0178	1,735,051,420	1,773,426
3	A0428	1,270,397,503	5,864,317
4	E1390	1,216,483,501	8,451,818
5	J2778	1,130,335,685	2,872,513
6	A0425	1,116,272,322	141,617,936

Source: CMS 2017e. Codes copyrighted by the American Medical Association

Table 6.5 shows an excerpt from CMS's Evaluation and Management Codes by Specialty file (CMS 2017e). This file displays allowed services, allowed charges, and total payment amount by E/M code and physician specialty. It can be used to compare national data on specialty-specific E/M CPT code frequency with data for a specific clinic, physician group, or individual physician. For example, if the distribution of the individual physician's CPT/HCPCS codes for new patient office visits (codes 99201–99205) does not align with the national trend to assign low-level codes most often, the outpatient CDS should investigate this finding to determine the root cause.

Table 6.5. Excerpt from CMS's Evaluation and Management Codes by Specialty file for calendar year 2015[a]

HCPCS CODE	Specialty	Total No. of Allowed Services	Allowed Charges, Total Dollars	Payment Amount, Dollars
99201	General Practice	1,518	63,496	41,404
	General Surgery	26,446	1,042,372	726,691
	Allergy/Immunology	262	10,363	7,144
	Otolaryngology	8,442	344,109	229,699
	Anesthesiology	3,856	117,492	88,658
	Cardiology	2,349	94,109	64,721

[a]Data have been screened to meet CMS privacy guidelines. Sum of columns may not equal
Source: CMS 2017e. Codes copyrighted by the American Medical Association

Preparing to Implement the Pilot CDI Plan

After the data resources relevant to the CDI project are identified, the process of creating a specific strategy for CDI implementation begins. As discussed in chapter 5 of this text, CDI programs are expanding to the outpatient setting to include a variety of sites such as outpatient facility clinics, emergency departments, provider practices, ambulatory surgical centers, and other short-term outpatient settings. The emergency department (ED) could be the pilot site for a new outpatient CDI program, depending on the focus areas selected. For example, if medical necessity denials are a significant issue in the ED, the ED may be an excellent choice as a pilot site. If HCC capture is an area of focus for the CDI program, a family medicine or internal medicine practice may be a better choice for the pilot site.

The pilot-site outpatient CDI implementation process can be broken down into 10 steps, which are discussed in the sections that follow.

Step 1: Identify the Pilot Sites

By selecting one or two clinics (or other appropriate outpatient sites) to begin the outpatient CDI implementation process, the efficiency of the work steps can be tested. If the focus of the CDI program is HCC capture, clinics that have a high volume of primary care services are appropriate pilot sites. If the CDI focus is related to charge capture, medical necessity, and other denials issues, clinics with high-risk, high-volume diagnoses and procedures are good candidates for the pilot project. When selecting pilot sites, consideration should also be given to the willingness of the clinic manager and medical staff to be among the first to work with a new process while it is being streamlined. Formal and informal leaders on the medical staff can advance the overall program through their participation, buy-in, and positive communications with other colleagues.

Case Example

When considering which sites would be the best for a pilot CDI program, the Community Clinic emerges as the first pick for multiple reasons: It is the largest primary care clinic in the health system. The physician leader of the clinic is also the CDI program's physician advisor and has a personal interest in the success of the project at his clinic. Additionally, he has already identified a short list of denials issues that have significantly reduced the practice's revenue over the past year.

Step 2: Review Data

Once the pilot sites are selected, the outpatient CDS should review the data collected from the clinical editor, denials reports, coding audit reports, and quality measure reports to determine trends that have high-volume and high-risk impacts. In this context, *high risk* means that there is a significant reimbursement or quality score impact per case. Those areas that also have high volume in addition to high risk are good targets for the first areas of focus.

Case Example

The outpatient CDI team discusses the concerns of the CDI program physician advisor about the frequent denials patterns he has already identified at the Community Clinic. The CDS then reviews denials trend and detail reports for the clinic and determines that the denials patterns identified by the physician advisor are in fact an area of concern. The CDS also reviews clinical editor reports, coding audit reports, and quality measure reports from the clinic and sets up a meeting to discuss the findings with the key stakeholders in the corresponding areas (denials management, HIM, revenue integrity).

Step 3: Select Focus Areas

Especially at the beginning of the program, when the outpatient CDI workflow is being established with the clinicians, participants in the CDI project should agree on a short list of focus areas as a starting point for the redesign of the clinical documentation workflow. Beginning with too many review items may cause the medical and office staff to become confused and frustrated. As stated in step 2, the areas of highest impact should be selected so that the CDI manager can prove the ROI for the program in a short time frame.

Case Example

During a CDI taskforce meeting, the outpatient CDI team and the stakeholder group discuss the data analysis done in step 2 of the pilot CDI process. Five areas are identified as a starting point for the workflow redesign in the pilot clinic. The list includes HCC code capture and four procedures that are frequently involved in claims denials because the claims do not support the medical necessity of the procedures. The medical necessity issue is related to the lack of specific clinical information and corresponding ICD-10-CM diagnosis codes on the NCD list for these procedures.

Step 4: Review HCPCS/CPT Frequency Reports

Where high-volume issues are identified, the outpatient CDS can review the chargemaster or physician fee schedule volumes to identify coding gaps. The gaps may be related to the charge capture process, the lack of specific clinical documentation for accurate coding, or the lack of chargemaster and fee schedule updates that reflect new services offered and new CPT/HCPCS codes.

Case Example

One of five cardiologists in a busy practice notices on a newly created relative value unit (RVU) report that her historical volume for echocardiography, one of the practice's frequently performed procedures, was much lower than that of her four peers. This finding is not reasonable because she performed a much higher volume of echocardiograms than the other four physicians. The outpatient CDS is notified of this issue by the physician and investigates it further. The CDS determines that the staff member charging for the procedure in the EHR used the final procedure report as the prompt to enter the charge. However, the procedure reports for this physician were not consistently being routed to the staff member who enters the charges because they were hard-copy reports created at another location. In fact, the reports were being scanned without first being submitted for charge entry. Having identified this manual charge process as the root cause of the inaccurate volume on the RVU reports, the outpatient CDS revises the workflow to ensure that, going forward, the staff assisting the physician during the procedure takes care of the charge entry at the time the procedure is completed.

Step 5: Monitor HCC Capture

If one of the focus areas for the CDI pilot program is HCC capture, relevant data and documentation procedures should be monitored at each pilot clinic.

Case Example

The outpatient CDS is charged with improving HCC capture in the primary care clinics. Analysis of the historical reports from the payer reveals that many of the HCCs identified in the previous two years were not being documented and coded in the current year.

Step 6: Audit a Sample of Cases from Each Group of Diagnoses and Procedures Identified in Steps 2 and 3

In this step, the CDS looks for the root cause of each issue targeted in the CDI plan by studying the audit results and trends identified.

Case Example

> Prior to launching a workflow redesign to mitigate the clinical documentation issue in the cardiology practice discussed in the step 4 case example, the CDS audits a sample of Medicare Advantage cases to validate the root cause of the HCC capture issue. The CDS documents the audit results for future reference and for use during educational sessions on the new workflow. Facility-specific case examples are helpful during staff education processes. When case examples are used, patient and physician identifying information should be removed from the presentation.

Step 7: Conduct Key Stakeholder Interviews

Once the focus areas are identified and the audits have been conducted, interviews with the key stakeholders are held to further assess the root cause of each issue and the optimal approach to correct the problem.

Case Example

> After identifying the root cause of the missing echocardiography procedures presented in the step 4 example, the CDS meets with the cardiologist who identified the issue, the clinic manager, and clinic staff to discuss the details of the audit. During the meeting several participants provide additional information that improves the workflow redesign.

Step 8: Identify the Root Cause

After auditing, stakeholder interviews, and workflow analysis are completed, the root cause should be defined. Keep in mind that there may be several reasons for the breakdown in accurate charge capture, coding, and clinical documentation.

Case Example

> The detailed discussion during the stakeholder meeting sheds new light on the true reasons for the breakdown in the echocardiogram charge captures. In addition to the issue related to the hard-copy cardiology procedure report, the taskforce identifies several other reasons for the low volume of charges.

Step 9: Discuss Findings and Recommendations

Once the root cause is identified, the outpatient CDI and taskforce can discuss a preliminary action plan, which may include workflow redesign, coder or provider education, and possible technology solutions.

Case Example

> Once the taskforce finishes its discussion of root causes of the charge capture issue for echocardiograms, the group discusses what should be done about the issues identified. The group decides that several steps should be taken: redesign of the charge capture workflow, reassignment of the charge capture process to staff earlier in the process (immediately after the procedure is complete), staff education on the new process, and an audit of charge capture accuracy during the first week after the changes are made.

Step 10: Implement the Solution

With the help of the stakeholders, the new workflow redesign, education, or technology solution can be implemented.

Case Example

> The CDI taskforce places the responsibility of implementing the new workflow redesign in the hands of the outpatient CDS. The first step is a meeting with the physicians and staff to outline the findings and recommendations. Next, a schedule of implementation and an implementation workplan are presented to the group for discussion. The implementation is scheduled to begin on a specified future date. Once implemented, a series of periodic reviews are conducted to validate the root cause and workflow redesign solutions. The CDS provides education for the providers on the monitor, evaluate, assess/address, or treat (MEAT) guidelines for documenting secondary conditions in the clinical record and implements a process to notify the provider prior to the patient encounter of chronic conditions that could be applicable for the current visit. This process is further discussed in the Focused Clinical Record Review Process section later in this chapter. See chapter 3 for additional information on MEAT guidelines.

Focused Clinical Record Review Process

As noted previously, once the root causes of a clinical documentation gap are identified, the next step is to implement a solution. Provider and coder education is normally part of the overall solution. However, education alone is rarely a sufficient way to resolve the problem. Usually, additional steps, including case review, query, and re-review, need to be taken. These steps are like those taken in inpatient CDI programs, but the timing of the review process is a distinctive challenge in the outpatient setting because patient encounters may last less than an hour.

Pre-encounter and Concurrent Case Review

If possible, the patient encounters that will be relevant to the area of CDI focus should be identified before the visits happen. For example, when performing HCC case review in the physician practice, the outpatient CDS should identify an efficient method of running a report of all Medicare Advantage patients scheduled for appointments on the following day. EHR software can usually generate such a report, including patients' names, medical record numbers, dates of birth, providers, and times of visit. If the area of CDI focus is a specific diagnosis or procedure, office or clinic staff may identify relevant patient encounters by using the previsit registration diagnosis or procedure schedule.

When performing HCC review, the outpatient CDS should review clinical information for each encounter from the previous year. The payer HCC reports, when available, can be useful to determine which patients had a previous HCC claims submission. However, all encounters should be reviewed in case an HCC was previously documented but not coded. A spreadsheet can be used to capture all HCCs identified in any setting within the health system or Medicare

Advantage group (inpatient, outpatient, and professional fee). A specific HCC need only be submitted once per year for the health system or group to receive the corresponding HCC payment (CMS 2016b). Refer to chapter 3 for additional information on the Medicare Advantage program.

Figure 6.1 shows a spreadsheet for a patient who had five outpatient encounters, two in 2016 and three in 2017. In 2016, the outpatient CDS identified two HCCs (HCC 9 and HCC 23) that could have been used in the Medicare Advantage claim, as reflected in the Auditor HCC Code column. However, the Original HCC Code column shows that only HCC 23 was reported on the claim. Again, in 2017, HCC 9 was not reported during the visit on January 19. On May 5, 2017, after reviewing patient encounters scheduled for the next day, the outpatient CDS submitted an electronic query to the physician asking whether carcinoma of the liver (ICD-10-CM code C22.7) was still a chronic condition in this case. On the date of the visit, the physician reviewed the query and agreed that this condition was a chronic condition in the case. The outpatient CDS documented the 0.97 weight increase in the Medicare Advantage payment associated with HCC 9 as part of the CDI program's ROI. The per-patient-per-month (PPPM) contract rate for the group was $744. Multiplying $744 by 12 months and by the weight increase of 0.97 resulted in an annual increase of $8,660 in the Medicare Advantage payment for this patient. Refer to chapter 3 for additional detail on Medicare Advantage plans.

Figure 6.1. Example of a CDI audit report for HCC review of one patient's encounters, 2016–2017

REVIEW TYPE:		HCC Case Review												
CDS REVIEWER:		Jane Smith												
Basic case Information							Code Data Sets				Comments/Queries/ROI			
Case #	MR#/ID#/ Encounter#	Date of Service	Patient Name	Provider	Claim ICD-10	Original HCC Code	Original HCC Wt	Auditor ICD-10	Auditor HCC Code	Auditor HCC Wt	New HCC Each Year	Comments	HCC Impact	Query Submitted	Query Agreed
Example Case															
1	1234	03/28/16	Jones, Jack	J. Frost	A391	23	0.228	C227	9	0.97	1				
1	1234	10/03/16	Jones, Jack	J. Frost				A391	23	0.228		PMH, Medication Admin Record			
1	1234	01/19/17	Jones, Jack	J. Frost	J441	111	0.328	C227	9	0.97		Progress notes			
1	1234	01/19/17	Jones, Jack	J. Frost	F3342	58	0.395	J441	111	0.328					
1	1234	01/19/17	Jones, Jack	J. Frost				F3342	58	0.395		Progress notes			
1	1234	05/06/17	Jones, Jack	J. Frost				C227	9	0.97	1	Added progress note	$8,660	5/06/2017	5/06/2017

Source: ©AHIMA

The pre-encounter case review can be performed either on site or remotely (if an EHR is in place). The physician, practice manager, and CDS should choose the review methodology together so that a streamlined solution can be implemented without significantly interfering with patient care. Most often, providers request an electronic query similar to those used in the inpatient setting. The query may be monitored by the physician at the time of the encounter, by the physician's nurse just before the encounter, or by the CDS if an onsite concurrent model for case review is in place. Any of the diagnoses and procedure areas of focus, whether identified at the start of the CDI program or added as the program progresses, can be monitoring using this methodology.

In many programs, the greatest challenge to a streamlined workflow is identifying the relevant patients before their visits. When the focus area is a specific procedure, patient identification may require concurrent case review in situations where the procedure is not prescheduled. Also, if the focus area is a quality measure applicable to all patients, a concurrent case review may be required for a specific data point, such as smoking cessation counseling for the MIPS quality measure. A technology solution for identifying this type of data point should be considered, as opposed to a live case review. EHR templates or interactive pop-ups or other in-line methods of communication with the physician may be more effective when gathering data for a large portion of the patient population. Chapter 7 discusses technology solutions in greater detail.

Before the workflow redesign begins, the outpatient CDS should discuss the concurrent case review process with the provider and manager and come to an agreement with them about the process methodology. This discussion is best done in person while the CDS is observing the normal workflow for clinical documentation in the physician practice setting. At that time, the CDS can talk with the provider about the desired method to query the provider. Options are alert messages, EHR tasks, e-mail, text messages, or phone calls. Some providers may benefit from prereview of cases along with a concurrent shadowing process on the day of the visit. The outpatient CDS can then remind the physician about the query item at the time of the patient encounter or just prior to the point of clinical documentation.

Postencounter Case Review

Where concurrent case review is in place, postencounter case review is not required. If the prereview of cases is done remotely, the outpatient CDS should check the record after the visit, preferably on the same day, so that the provider may be notified of clinical documentation gaps. Notification on the day of the encounter allows the provider to complete the required documentation before the bill drops. In organizations that hold the bill for several days before dropping it, providers have more time to update the record within the bill-drop window.

Reporting on Program Data

The CDS should promptly and frequently communicate feedback about the CDI areas of focus to providers, clinic managers, and other stakeholders. This feedback reinforces and shares credit for the program successes. The report can be as simple as a spreadsheet with detailed findings about the captured clinical documentation and an executive summary of the number of focus areas identified and captured, as well as the ROI where applicable. Metrics such as query, response, and agreement rates help point out successes and areas for improvement. The following are recommended metrics:

- Total focus items identified (for example, total number of HCCs identified)
- Total queries submitted by the CDS, with a subcategory for each provider
- Total responses and response rate by provider
- Total agreements and agreement rate by provider
- Total impact per each focus area, where applicable (for example, total increase in HCC weight by CDS or provider)

- Monthly trends for each indicator listed above, including totals and averages for each indicator
- Quarterly totals and averages for each indicator

Figure 6.2 provides an example of how to report CDI program data to the stakeholders. The scorecard includes the key metrics that are needed to evaluate the success of the program, as well as graphs of selected key metrics. The CDS can tailor the graphs and metrics shown to include those that the CDI steering committee would benefit from seeing periodically. The CDI steering committee or taskforce should decide whether provider names are to be included in the report. Alternatively, a provider code number could be assigned so that only the individual providers know which data are theirs in the report.

Figure 6.2. Example of an outpatient clinical documentation improvement scorecard

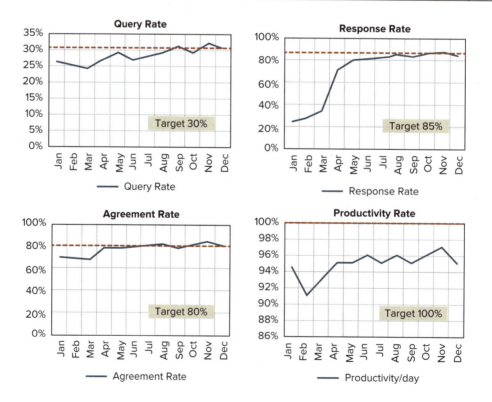

Outpatient CDI Key Performance Indicator Scorecard

Primary Care Clinic
CDS: Rebecca Jones
FY 2017

	Target	Jan	Feb	Mar	Apr	May	Jun	Jul	Aug	Sep	Oct	Nov	Dec	Annual
Pre-encounter Reviews	195	176	171	174	190	194	201	196	199	194	200	203	198	191
Post encounter Reviews	325	315	321	318	330	329	340	335	341	345	340	344	347	333
Total Reviews	520	491	492	492	520	523	541	531	540	539	540	547	545	524
Productivity/day	100%	94%	91%	93%	95%	95%	96%	95%	96%	95%	96%	97%	95%	95%
Query Rate	30%	26%	25%	24%	27%	29%	27%	28%	29%	31%	29%	32%	30%	28%
Response Rate	85%	25%	28%	35%	71%	79%	81%	82%	85%	83%	86%	87%	85%	69%
Agreement Rate	80%	70%	69%	68%	79%	78%	80%	81%	82%	79%	82%	84%	81%	78%

Source: ©AHIMA

Chapter 6 Review Exercises

1. Which of the following is a type of data set that is available to assist in assessing clinical documentation related to clinical documentation gaps and is generally involved in the HIM department's quality assurance process?
   a. Chargemaster
   b. Coding audit reports
   c. Claims edit frequency
   d. Outpatient research identifiable file (RIF)

2. The hospital chargemaster is a master price list that includes the items billed by the facility on a UB-04 claim. The list includes:
   a. Devices and medications
   b. Patient-specific data or start time
   c. DSM codes to support charge capture
   d. Crosswalk of generic and brand name products

3. When reviewing claims edits, the ultimate goal of the CDI program is:
   a. To properly classify edits according to their type
   b. To detect differences in professional/physician and hospital OPPS claims scrubbers
   c. To identify the root cause for an occurrence and determine how to prevent the occurrence in the future
   d. To state a solution for lack of specific documentation supporting allowed diagnoses listed in the LCD or NCD notices

4. The process for implementing an outpatient CDI pilot program can be broken down into 10 steps. Which of the following best describes the reason why the highest-impact review items should be identified at the same time that a focus area is selected?
   a. To test the efficiency of the work steps in real time
   b. To permit monitoring of HCC capture at each pilot clinic
   c. To ensure that a root cause of coding errors can be identified at an early stage
   d. To help the CDI manager prove the ROI for the outpatient program in a short amount of time

5. The department code in the hospital chargemaster is a numeric, alpha, or alphanumeric code used to identify the _____.
   a. Charge status date
   b. Charge description number
   c. Cost center for accounting purposes
   d. General, industry-standard claims edits

6. Claims scrubber edits can be categorized as payer-specific, custom, and _____ edits.
   a. HCC-specific
   b. Denial cause code
   c. Physician-specific
   d. General, industry-standard

7. Denials information is normally found in the revenue integrity, denials management, or _____ department.
   a. CDI
   b. HIM
   c. Revenue cycle
   d. Budget management

8. A _____ code is a 4-digit code indicating the department or type of service for each chargemaster item. The list of these codes is updated annually by the NUBC and CMS.
   a. Item
   b. Charge
   c. Revenue
   d. Department

9. CMS developed the _____ to reduce the paid-claims error rate for Medicare claims related to clerical entries and incorrect coding based on criteria such as anatomical considerations.
   a. MIPS
   b. OPPS
   c. MUE program
   d. Hospital OQR program

10. The _____ is the uniform professional hard-copy claims form used by provider practices to submit claims to insurance companies.
    a. CDM
    b. UB-04
    c. CMS-1450
    d. CMS-1500

References

American Health Information Management Association (AHIMA). 2010 (March). Care and maintenance of chargemasters (2010 update). *Journal of AHIMA*. http://bok.ahima.org/doc?oid=101404#.Wg4c0UqnG70.

American Medical Association (AMA). 2018. *CPT 2018 Professional Edition*. Chicago, IL: AMA.

Centers for Medicare and Medicaid Services (CMS). 2017a. Addendum A and Addendum B Updates. https://www.cms.gov/Medicare/Medicare-Fee-for-Service-Payment/HospitalOutpatientPPS/Addendum-A-and-Addendum-B-Updates.html.

Centers for Medicare and Medicaid Services (CMS). 2017b. Medicare Claims Processing Manual. Chapter 1: General billing requirements. https://www.cms.gov/Regulations-and-Guidance/Guidance/Manuals/downloads/clm104c01.pdf.

Centers for Medicare and Medicaid Services (CMS). 2017c. National Correct Coding Initiative: Medically Unlikely Edits. https://www.cms.gov/Medicare/Coding/NationalCorrectCodInitEd/MUE.html.

Centers for Medicare and Medicaid Services (CMS). 2017d. Quality Payment Program: Quality measures. https://qpp.cms.gov/measures/quality.

Centers for Medicare and Medicaid Services (CMS). 2017e. Medicare utilization for Part B. https://www.cms.gov/Research-Statistics-Data-and-Systems/Statistics-Trends-and-Reports/MedicareFeeforSvcPartsAB/MedicareUtilizationforPartB.html.

Centers for Medicare and Medicaid Services (CMS). 2016a. Hospital Outpatient Prospective Payment System: Payment system series. https://www.cms.gov/Outreach-and-Education/Medicare-Learning-Network-MLN/MLNProducts/downloads/HospitalOutpaysysfctsht.pdf.

Centers for Medicare and Medicaid Services (CMS). 2016b. March 2016 risk adjustment methodology white paper. https://www.cms.gov/CCIIO/Resources/.../RA-March-31-White-Paper-032416.pdf.

Experian. 2016. Stop claims denials now! Scrubbed claims = paid claims. http://www.experian.com/healthcare/claims-scrubber.html http://www.experian.com/healthcare/claims-scrubber.html.

National Uniform Billing Committee (NUBC). 2017. UB-04 data files. http://www.nubc.org/inc-NUBC/PDFs/Summary%20of%20UB-04%20Code%20Categories.pdf.

Noridian Healthcare Solutions. 2017. Revenue codes. https://med.noridianmedicare.com/web/jea/topics/claim-submission/revenue-codes.

Research Data Assistance Center (ResDAC). 2016a. Revenue center code. https://www.resdac.org/cms-data/variables/revenue-center-code.

Research Data Assistance Center (ResDAC). 2016b. Outpatient RIF. https://www.resdac.org/cms-data/files/op-rif.

Research Data Assistance Center (ResDAC). 2016c. Difference between RIF, LDS, and PUF data files. https://www.resdac.org/resconnect/articles/148.

Assessing Outpatient CDI Program Technology Options

Learning Objectives

- Explain the functionality of outpatient clinical documentation improvement software available in the healthcare marketplace.
- Describe the types of electronic health record software found in the outpatient setting and professional practice setting.
- Identify the clinical documentation features that support in-line clinical documentation.
- Discuss the features and benefits of natural language processing, computer-assisted coding, and personal mobile device query communication.
- Explain how to analyze clinical data using software that performs diagnosis suspecting.
- Identify the issues related to automatic evaluation and management code assignment.

Key Terms

Alerts
Big data
Claim adjustment reason code (CA or CARC)
Computer-assisted coding (CAC)
HCC suspecting
Overdocumentation
Prompts
Semantic reasoning
Tasks

The clinical documentation technology landscape is rapidly changing as many new software products are being developed to support specificity and accuracy in clinical documentation. Much of the technology available now appeals to physician users, who can use it to create accurate, concise, and specific clinical documentation for patient care and to collaborate with other providers. In addition, software tools increase the efficiency of the clinical documentation specialists (CDSs), allowing them additional time for provider education, data analysis, and thinking critically about how to improve the outpatient clinical documentation improvement (CDI) program.

The outpatient clinical documentation landscape includes a large variety of disparate electronic health records (EHRs), most of which lack interoperability. Therefore, CDSs should assess the functionality of each EHR used by providers involved in the outpatient CDI program. The CDS should also determine how each EHR is actually used for clinical documentation by shadowing the providers and other ancillary personnel documenting in the application. Once the CDS has a good understanding of how each system is used, he or she can collaborate with the stakeholders at each practice or clinic to make and evaluate workflow improvements.

A clear understanding of how various software systems function in the outpatient setting and how they are used by providers and other staff helps the CDS determine the root causes of system-related documentation gaps. The outpatient CDS should also be aware of other software tools in the marketplace so that he or she can recommend new technology if it is needed to resolve documentation gaps. Tools such as clinical editors and denials management systems can be used to identify the top areas of focus where CDI can improve the quality of patient care and the accuracy of reimbursement.

This chapter offers an overview of the technology in the healthcare marketplace as well as insight into how to effectively use the technology and bring the outpatient CDI program to the next level.

The Outpatient Clinical Documentation Technology Landscape

The technology used in the outpatient setting is expansive but often lacks interoperability. A health system or hospital may use one EHR for the inpatient and outpatient ambulatory setting as well as a variety of disparate EHRs in the various provider practices. To improve outpatient clinical documentation, the outpatient CDS must learn about each system from the clinical documentation and functionality perspective so that physician collaboration and education can be provided at the required level throughout the ambulatory and professional practice settings. The CDS may require training from the information technology (IT) department and may benefit from shadowing outpatient and professional practice coders. Analysis of patient accounts before the visit (pre-encounter review) and after the visit (postencounter review) can provide insight into the clinical documentation process (refer to chapter 6). Also, if possible, the outpatient CDS should observe the workflow of the physicians, nurses, and assistants as they document in the clinical record during the encounter.

Software functionality related to clinical documentation can be categorized into the following fundamental areas: EHR clinical record, natural language processing (NLP) enhancements, computer-assisted coding (CAC), Hierarchical Condition Category (HCC) suspecting, data analytics, claims processing, and query communication features, including features on personal mobile devices. Many users are unaware of the full range of features within each tool that might be used to significantly improve clinical documentation, reimbursement, and the quality of patient care. Because each function is important in its own right, the CDS should have a detailed understanding of all of them. Taking time to thoroughly learn these systems will provide a significant return on investment (ROI) to the outpatient CDI program.

EHR Functionality

EHR solutions in the physician practice setting typically have similar functionality to the EHRs used in the facility ambulatory setting, including patient look-up capability, problem lists, progress notes, provider report documentation, physician orders, nurses' notes, and medication records. The EHR has the ability to capture clinical documentation as well as the *International Classification of Diseases, Tenth Revision, Clinical Modification* (ICD-10-CM), Current Procedural Terminology (CPT), and Healthcare Common Procedure Coding System (HCPCS) code sets needed for claims submission.

Uses of EHRs for Clinical Documentation Improvement

If designed and used correctly, many EHR tools can expedite record keeping in the EHR, saving time, improving clinical documentation, and increasing the accuracy of code assignment. Provider education on the use of the EHR can help maximize its benefits and limit the risks of its misuse. First and foremost, the provider must understand how to use the EHR to ensure that the documentation in the clinical record reflects his or her clinical judgment. Only the provider can diagnose a problem and determine whether the condition is being monitored, evaluated, assessed, or treated during the visit. The following features can be of great assistance to the provider during the documentation process.

Templates and Drop-Down Menus

Templates can help providers in specialty clinics and practices to capture specific clinical information for commonly treated illnesses. For example, the following congestive heart failure (CHF) documentation suggestions could be built into an EHR template (AHIMA 2017a):

- Describe clinical signs and symptoms (exertional dyspnea, orthopnea, peripheral edema, pulmonary rales or crackles, jugular vein distention, etc.).
- Document workup (chest x-ray, EKG [electrocardiogram], Swan-Ganz [a catheterization procedure], echocardiogram, etc.).
- Document treatment (diuretics, ACE [angiotensin-converting-enzyme] inhibitors, digitalis, beta-blockers, O_2 [oxygen], morphine sulfate, monitoring input and output, daily weights, etc.).

- Etiology (valvular heart disease, renal failure with volume overload, congestive cardiomyopathy, myocardial ischemia, new-onset atrial fibrillation, etc.).
- Note LVEF [left ventricular ejection fraction], assessment for ACE inhibitor use, and contraindications for nonuse of ACE inhibitors.
- Note if CHF is valid by history. Chronic CHF may impact patient care, even in the absence of active treatment.

Drop-down menu options are intended to help providers add specificity to documentation. For example, when documenting a diagnosis of chronic obstructive pulmonary disease (COPD), the provider might select "acute exacerbation," "chronic," or "acute on chronic" COPD from a drop-down menu to add specificity to the record. This specificity, in turn, improves the coding of claims for reimbursement and other uses of clinical data.

Prompts and Alerts

Prompts automatically produce messages containing questions or additional information related to specific steps in the clinical documentation process; they are intended to help the provider ensure that all relevant information is recorded. For example, a prompt might remind the provider, "When smoking cessation counseling is conducted, document the details of the patient discussion." This feature may be especially helpful when providers continue to omit specific documentation even after group and one-on-one education have been conducted. The prompt can be set up to require a response from the provider.

Alerts are similar to prompts, but the alert appears when a specific patient's account is accessed. For example, if a patient has chronic conditions that require ongoing medication managed by the provider, an alert might be programmed to list the chronic conditions and corresponding medications with a statement such as, "The patient is being treated for these chronic illnesses and corresponding medications: (1) type 1 diabetes, U-500 insulin subcutaneously 2 to 3 times a day, approximately 30 minutes prior to start of a meal; (2) COPD, on home O_2 at 2 liters per minute. Please document any chronic conditions that are being monitored, evaluated, assessed, or treated during your visit with the patient."

In-line Documentation Functionality

Some EHR systems embed prompts into the EHR template to request specific documentation for HCCs or quality measures, or to capture other clinical data. Michael Marron-Stearns, a physician informaticist, health information technology (HIT) and healthcare compliance consulting professional, and chief executive officer and founder of Apollo HIT, LLC, shared the following observations about in-line documentation with the author (e-mail communication, 2017):

> In many, but not all, EHR applications, clinicians are required to record certain quality measures through processes that are not intrinsic to their normal workflow. For example, a provider may be seeing a patient with type 2 diabetes mellitus who has had a recent dilated retinal examination. To meet the requirements of this

diabetic quality measure, the provider is required to document the date and result of the recent eye examination. This [documentation] also needs to be stored as data that can be used for quality performance reporting. A common practice in most EHR applications involves having the provider open a separate reporting tool, such as a spreadsheet, to record information related to the measure. This often requires the clinician to deviate from their normal workflow solely for the purpose of data capture.

Providers also need to be reminded to address the measure, but they often ignore electronic alerts designed to perform this function. The combination of clinicians not remembering to document measure data, record it in a separate software module, and the additional time needed to complete this task can have an adverse impact on the practice's quality performance.

In-line documentation refers to the process of allowing the provider to document measure-related information within the body of a progress note template. The quality measure codes and supporting documentation are [substantiated] within the template. For example, if the provider chooses a diabetes template, the template requires that they address a quality measure from within the body of the progress note. Once they address the measure, the data are automatically stored in the EHR database and can be used for reporting.

This process accomplishes several goals, including reminding the provider to address the measure, documenting information related to the measure, and improving the efficiency of documentation by avoiding deviations from standard workflows.

In the diabetic eye examination example, the provider would be prompted to document information about the patient's most recent diabetic eye examination. They would be given a series of menu choices that will be mapped to the requirements for this measure. The provider may also be prompted to generate an ophthalmology referral or to document that the patient has declined the dilated eye examination, that the most recent examination took place within the specified time frame and was normal, or other findings that meet the measure requirement, including exclusions.

In-line documentation can lead to improvements in clinical care and efficiency while meeting reporting requirements for quality measures. It requires three elements: an EHR that supports measure-related data capture from templates, an individual proficient with making template modifications, and a thorough understanding of the requirements for each quality measure that the practice or organization has elected to report.

Clinical Documentation Risks Potentially Associated with EHRs

Although EHRs can be used to advance CDI, the poor design or misuse of EHR tools and programming errors can lead to serious problems, such as poor data quality, claims denials, decreased reimbursement, fraud, or patient harm. Specific risks associated with EHR functionality include the following:

Incorrect assignment of ICD-10-CM codes in older EHRs: Since October 1, 2015, US healthcare entities and providers have been required by the federal government to stop using the *International Classification of Diseases, Ninth Revision, Clinical Modification (ICD-9-CM)* code set and use ICD-10-CM instead. However, physician practice EHR software programmed before the conversion from ICD-9-CM to ICD-10-CM may still have embedded ICD-9-CM codes. For example, conversion tables (crosswalks) were sometimes used to transition from ICD-9-CM to ICD-10-CM codes. Errors in the crosswalk programming may generate incorrect

ICD-10-CM codes and be a root cause of medical necessity denials (Stearns 2014). If such a problem is suspected, an outpatient CDS with expertise in ICD-10-CM and billing should investigate. If the CDS identifies ICD-10-CM codes in the EHR that do not accurately correspond to the clinical documentation, the issues can be brought to the attention of the software vendor for correction.

Inappropriate automatic assignment of evaluation and management (E/M) codes: Most current EHR solutions include software to automatically suggest E/M codes that may be appropriate to assign to encounters (see chapter 3 for further discussion of E/M codes). This E/M coding functionality is a type of **computer-assisted coding (CAC)** software. CAC is the process of extracting and translating dictated and subsequently transcribed free-text data (or dictated and then computer-generated discrete data) into diagnostic and procedural codes from various classifications for billing and coding purposes. If EHRs are not programmed correctly (which may require customization for the facility or clinic), they may assign the wrong level of E/M code (for example, the EHR could assign a high-level E/M code that is unsupported by the clinical documentation of the patient encounter). To address this risk, the outpatient CDS should select a sample of cases and assign E/M codes to them based on the clinical documentation. The CDS should then compare those clinical documentation–based E/M level codes to the computer-generated E/M level codes for the same cases. If discrepancies are identified in the EHR's automated E/M coding, the system functionality should be evaluated. If the outpatient CDS cannot identify how E/M codes are assigned within the software, he or she should contact the vendor and discuss the system specifications for E/M assignment (Stearns 2013).

Insufficient documentation: Tools intended to aid in quick selections, such as problem lists and checkboxes, may contribute to insufficient documentation. For example, the Merit-Based Incentive Payment System (MIPS) offers reimbursement incentives related to smoking cessation, and the EHR may include a checkbox for smoking cessation counseling to help capture data for the MIPS measure. However, simply checking a box does not generate adequate documentation of the counseling process. The provider must also document in the clinical record what information was covered during the discussion between the provider and the patient. (As noted earlier, a prompt might help resolve this problem.)

Incorrect documentation: Tools intended to aid in quick selections may contribute to incorrect documentation and coding. For example, an EHR that offers a list of checkboxes to represent diagnostic options may not clearly or accurately label the options to reflect the complexity of the diagnostic criteria. In this situation, the provider might misunderstand the options and check a box for a diagnosis unsupported by the clinical documentation. Similarly, if the EHR generates E/M codes based on how a provider fills out a template and the template is poorly designed or not understood by providers because of a lack of training, the providers may enter the wrong data, and that will lead to the incorrect E/M code assignment.

Overdocumentation: Tools such as the copy/paste function, which is used to copy data from one source into another record or data field, and templates that autopopulate fields in the documentation may encourage **overdocumentation**, "the practice of inserting false or irrelevant documentation to create the appearance of support for billing higher level services" (OIG 2014). Overdocumentation can be a type of fraud that may be criminally prosecuted. It can also be the source of errors that cause patient harm.

Communication Tools in the EHR

The outpatient CDS can use tasks and notes to query providers or notify them of chronic illnesses or other potential clinical documentation gaps. **Tasks** are messages to remind the provider about a required action. For example, a task might state, "Ms. Jones is being followed for a series of chronic conditions, including CHF treated with furosemide 60 mg every 8 hours; acute on chronic COPD on home O_2 at 2 liters per minute. Please document any chronic conditions that are being monitored, evaluated, assessed/addressed, or treated during your visit with the patient." The provider must click the Task button to access tasks. Therefore, the use of tasks may not be the best option for those providers who tend to ignore system prompts.

The CDS may be able to use the Notes feature in the EHR instead of an e-mailed query to communicate with the provider or assistant. When the provider opens the patient account at the time of the visit, he or she sees the communication from the outpatient CDS. The Notes section can also be used to maintain a list of the patient's ongoing chronic illnesses or HCCs relevant to that patient's care that the provider should consider at the time of the visit. If notes are used in that way, the CDS is responsible for updating the note as new HCCs are identified or when chronic illnesses are resolved and should no longer be added to the documentation for the current episode of care.

Natural Language Processing

Natural language is a fifth-generation computer programming language that uses human language to give people a more natural connection with computers. Natural language processing (NLP) is a technology that converts human language (structured or unstructured) into data that can be translated and then manipulated by computer systems; it is a branch of artificial intelligence used to analyze the vast volumes of unstructured data in documentation so that the data can be used for coding, quality measurement, and big data purposes. Unstructured data are nonbinary, human-readable data (for example, a transcript of a discussion). On the other hand, structured data use a controlled vocabulary rather than narrative text. Structured data may also be referred to as *discrete data*. Discrete data represent separate and distinct values or observations; these data contain only finite numbers and have only specified values.

Between 2016 and 2021, the worldwide NLP market size is likely to expand dramatically, from $7.63 billion to $16.07 (Markets and Markets 2016). In healthcare, the demand for NLP is based on explosive growth in unstructured data from EHRs. The volume of data collected at each healthcare facility is so expansive that an efficient and effective review of all data requires the use of NLP. Without the support of NLP technology, the staff allocated to perform CDI and coding functions would simply not have enough time to identify problematic trends or query providers whenever more specific clinical information is needed.

> In the healthcare marketplace, NLP applications are processing "enormous amounts of data by utilizing high-end NLP technologies for information extraction, automatic speech recognition, machine translation, and dialogue systems" (Monegain 2015).

Big data refers to the concept of large volumes of complex and diverse data and is also a term for data sets that are so large or complex that traditional data processing applications are inadequate to process or analyze them. The challenge of big data analytics is further exacerbated by the increase of unstructured clinical data. Whereas databases can efficiently use discrete (structured) data to run reports and analyze trends, unstructured data cannot be used as efficiently. However, NLP software can review clinical records, such as discharge summaries and operative records, for key phrases and clinical indicators. For example, NLP software can scan unstructured data for evidence of acute respiratory failure. Within the data, NLP software may find multiple word combinations related to acute on chronic respiratory failure, such as the following:

- Evidence of acute on chronic respiratory failure
- Acute on chronic respiratory cannot be excluded
- Rule-out acute on chronic respiratory
- Acute on chronic respiratory failure in 2016

The term *semantics* refers to the meaning of a text (Tucker 2002), and the adjective *semantic* is used in a phrase to refer to the meaning of a word. For example, **semantic reasoning** refers to the use of software to make assertions or inferences based on a selected data within a data set such as an EHR (Maarala et al. 2016). During the process of semantic reasoning, the NLP software uses a database of similar terms to identify other texts related to the phrase. For example, the phrase *chronic kidney failure* might be described in the clinical record as *kidney failure, renal failure, chronic renal failure, chronic kidney failure, chronic kidney disease (CKD), renal insufficiency,* or *GFR (glomerular filtration rate) less than 15*, which is a clinical indicator for kidney failure (NKF 2015). Semantic reasoning in the NLP software evaluates all instances of the term in question (chronic kidney failure) by checking the associated database of key words and phrases, compares the phrases and words to data in the clinical record, and then displays the phrases and words for the user to see. This semantic reasoning process is valuable to the CDS because it provides a list of the phrases in a pop-up on the screen that is linked to the clinical documentation in the EHR, and the CDS can use this list rather than reading the entire record for key phrases, words, and clinical data. Thus, semantic reasoning software saves much time during the case review process.

An example use of semantic reasoning is the NLP assessing relationships among EHR key words and phrases to determine the true incidence of acute on chronic respiratory failure in a patient's clinical record. The system could compare the patient's laboratory values against a set of clinical indicators for respiratory failure, such as "$pCO_2 > 50$ mmHg with pH < 7.35, increase in baseline pCO_2 by 10 mmHg or $pO_2 < 60$ mmHg or $SpO_2 < 91\%$ on home oxygen flow" (Pinson and Tang 2017). The system would then display all identified key words and phrases that match the clinical indicator database for respiratory failure. By using the NLP engine, the CDS can access the autoreviewed records and identify cases that need further evaluation by a CDS. Rule-based NLP technology engines using semantic reasoning will help the CDS to perform functions related to CDI and CAC more effectively and efficiently.

NLP Applications for CDI

As noted, NLP applications can help with CDI. These applications are designed to perform clinical documentation–related tasks such as the following:

- *Speech recognition with in-line documentation prompts for specificity:* For example, when the provider documents CHF in the EHR, the software prompts the provider to include the appropriate level of specificity regarding the CHF diagnosis, such as systolic or diastolic, acute exacerbation, or chronic. The prompt can be either shown on the screen or a verbal prompt.
- *Data mining for key words and phrases:* This feature may be used for real-time CDI case review. For example, the NLP application scans the EHR for key phrases, such as "ejection fraction (EF) < 40%," which is suggestive of systolic heart failure, or "elevated EF > 70%," which is suggestive of diastolic heart failure. When these key words or phrases are found in the clinical documentation, the corresponding diagnostic options are displayed as a pop-up in the EHR for the user.

The CDI workflow with NLP is like that of the workflow in systems that do not use NLP. The daily CDI workflow tasks include the following (Hess 2015):

- Review the complete clinical record concurrently as provider entries are made.
- Identify signs, symptoms, and diagnostic test results that need further clarification for a more specific diagnosis.
- Identify missing diagnostic or procedural details that affect patient care, quality indicators, justification of medical necessity, and final coding of the record.
- Document case detail for use during the next concurrent review and for retrospective coding and final billing.
- Query the provider about documentation that is inadequate.
- Monitor the query submission and ensure that the provider responds.
- Track query activity and response times for use in program analytics and to support program success.

Although the steps in the CDI program are basically the same regardless of the use of NLP applications, such applications can improve efficiency and effectiveness of CDI. For example, NLP applications allow for rapid identification of key words and phrases corresponding to clinical indicators for specific diseases, and NLP applications can help the CDS identify specific diagnostic test results or other signs and symptoms that require a provider query to further clarify a specific diagnosis.

CAC Applications

CAC applications use NLP to identify possible diagnosis and procedure codes. The codes identified by the software are not final and should be reviewed by the coding department or CDS for adequate supporting documentation and to determine the need for provider queries. CAC is known in the healthcare industry as either "the savior of coding-based bottom lines" or the "automated destroyer of human coding jobs" (Crawford 2013). The major advantage of CAC is its efficiency; compared with a system that relies completely on humans to review and code documentation, CAC reduces the time required to review a clinical record and thus lowers costs. This advantage has become more significant since the implementation of ICD-10-CM, which requires greater specificity in clinical documentation for accurate code submission.

CAC can be built into encoder software, such as the 3M encoder. The CAC application uses a database of key terms, phrases, and clinical diagnostic criteria to search a patient's EHR for information that suggests a possible diagnosis or treatment. Then the CAC program associates the data it finds in the documentation with proposed ICD-10-CM, *International Classification of Diseases, Tenth Revision, Procedure Coding System* (ICD-10-PCS), or CPT codes and displays the results as a list for the coder or CDS to review. The clinical documentation in the EHR can be viewed within the CAC application, thus saving time through the use of one system for coding. Looking at the CAC results and the EHR documentation, the coder decides whether the documentation can be validated as having adequate specificity for final coding or requires further clarification from the provider. Because the coder is responsible for reviewing the proposed codes and deciding about their accuracy, use of CAC applications elevates the position of health information management coding professional to include an auditing function.

When paired with CDI technology, CAC can make code identification more accurate, which helps the CDS establish documentation requirements and collaborate with providers on concurrent CDI to support medical necessity and ensure HCC capture and accurate code assignment. The CAC-supported encoder can also be used when training new CDSs to identify specific key words and phrases needed for a complete clinical record.

HCC Suspecting

Under HCC guidelines, an HCC-related diagnosis can be credited and paid only once during a calendar year, but it can be reported on multiple claims during the year (CMS 2017a, CMS 2017b). **HCC suspecting** is the process of using an NLP engine to scan clinical documentation for potential chronic illnesses that are categorized as HCCs. Multiple vendors offer this solution. The process can include scanning historical data on patients within the current-year window so that HCCs that should be captured this year are identified and submitted on claims. For example, if the HCC suspecting report indicates that a patient was prescribed a diabetes medication during the current year but a corresponding ICD-10-CM code for diabetes has not yet been reported for the year, the physician practice can document the diabetes diagnosis in the clinical record and submit the code for the next patient encounter, so long as the monitor, evaluate, assess/address, or treat (MEAT) documentation is included in the provider note. This ICD-10-CM diagnosis supports the HCC capture for the year. Refer to chapter 3 of this textbook for more information on HCC documentation and coding.

HCC suspecting can also be performed for previous calendar years. For example, a report run for calendar years 2017 and 2018 can help identify patients with histories of chronic illnesses that may also qualify for HCCs in 2019. After reviewing the HCC suspecting information, the CDS can notify the provider of patients with records of chronic conditions. The provider may include the condition in the patient's current documentation if the condition meets the MEAT documentation requirements.

Many Medicare Advantage providers have applications to run HCC suspecting reports based on the ICD-10-CM codes, but the programs may not have NLP functionality. These reports are nevertheless valuable when used to identify past chronic conditions that may still exist in the current year. Examples of HCC reports generated by MedeAnalytics are highlighted in the following sections for illustrative purposes. MedeAnalytics is a company that licenses data analytics software in the healthcare industry. MedeAnalytics Revenue Integrity (RI) product is presented in this chapter as an example of software that can be used as part of an outpatient CDI program. The software offers HCC suspecting reports as well as other CDI-related data analytics reports referred to in this chapter.

To produce the reports mentioned in this chapter, the RI software receives an upload of the data after claims submission. Typically, the facility submits 837 healthcare claims files to MedeAnalytics for upload into the software. (Refer to chapters 3 and 10 for more information on 837 files.) The data are then used for data analytics and reporting purposes. The RI software is presented here for illustration purposes; the discussion of this software is not an endorsement.

Patient HCC Capture Report

The outpatient CDS can use the MedeAnalytics Patient HCC Capture report to evaluate HCCs and Medicare risk adjustment factor (RAF) scores for patients from the current year and the previous two years (MedeAnalytics 2017). A variance between the two previous years raises the possibility that a chronic condition with a corresponding HCC was not captured during year 2. The year-to-date (YTD) variance alerts the outpatient CDS to possible chronic conditions associated with HCCs that have not yet been documented in the current year. The report also provides the specific HCCs that have been captured over the three-year period. Users of the MedeAnalytics reports can select the desired report from a MedeAnalytics software menu and run them with various filters and options to further focus the report based on the user specifications.

Figure 7.1 shows an example of a report that provides a detailed list of patients with corresponding claims containing HCC codes. The data in the report are fictional and used for illustrative purposes only. The report provides individual patient HCC volumes in the second, third, and fourth columns for the inpatient (IP), outpatient (OP), and professional practice (pro-fee) settings, respectively. The report also provides the RAF score for 2015, 2016, and 2017 (YTD). This report helps the outpatient CDS identify opportunities for HCC capture by displaying when a patient's RAF score for the current year is lower than the scores for the previous two years. By clicking a patient's medical record (MR) number, the user can see the graphical depiction (right side of the report) for the HCC capture for that patient over the three years.

Figure 7.1. Patient HCC Capture (MedeAnalytics 2017)

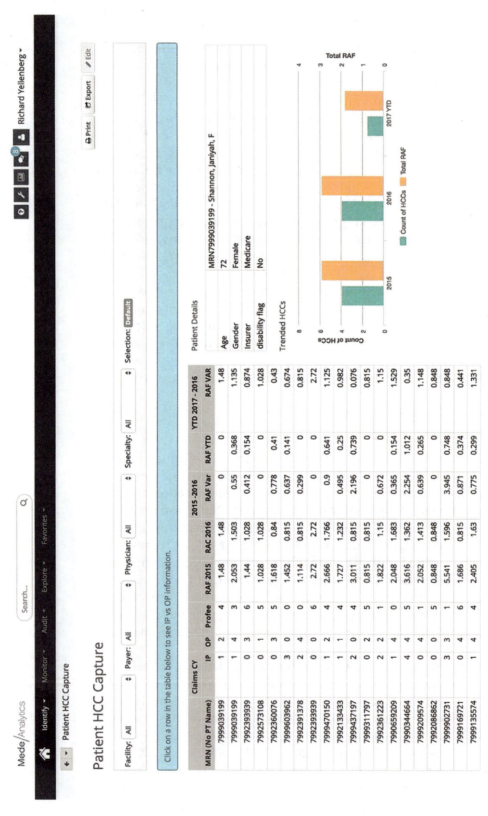

Source: MedeAnalytics 2017. Reprinted with permission. The example screenshots and dashboards for Revenue Integrity were provided by MedeAnalytics, Inc. MedeAnalytics offers a cloud-based analytics platform that aggregates and normalizes data across multiple sources, delivering it in an intuitive format that inspires clear and actionable insights into healthcare organizations' revenue, cost, quality, and risk. MedeAnalytics and Revenue Integrity are registered trademarks of MedeAnalytics, Inc. All rights reserved.

Patient HCC Profile Report

The Patient HCC Profile report provides information on a specific patient and lists all HCCs, with descriptions for those captured during a three-year period that includes the current year (MedeAnalytics 2017). The RAF scores are listed for each year along with the variance. In figure 7.2, the report shows that HCC 111 (COPD) was reported in 2015, 2016, and 2017 with the same RAF score for each year. However, for HCC 17 (diabetes mellitus [DM] with acute complications), the HCC was captured in 2016 but not in 2017. This report therefore points out an opportunity for the outpatient CDS to query the provider regarding the diabetes complication that was present in 2016 and whether it should be captured in documentation for the current year (2017).

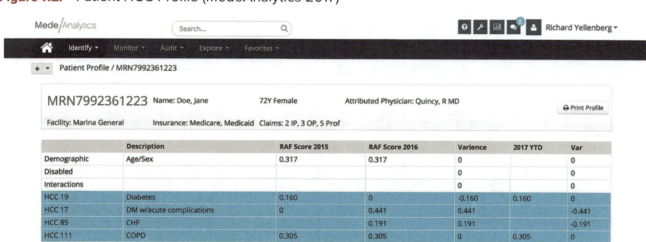

Figure 7.2. Patient HCC Profile (MedeAnalytics 2017)

Source: MedeAnalytics 2017. Reprinted with permission. The example screenshots and dashboards for Revenue Integrity were provided by MedeAnalytics, Inc. MedeAnalytics offers a cloud-based analytics platform that aggregates and normalizes data across multiple sources, delivering it in an intuitive format that inspires clear and actionable insights into healthcare organizations' revenue, cost, quality, and risk. MedeAnalytics and Revenue Integrity are registered trademarks of MedeAnalytics, Inc. All rights reserved.

Physician HCC Capture Report

The Physician HCC Capture report (figure 7.3) provides a snapshot of the physician names, total claims, and RAF scores for each of the most recent two years, including the current year (MedeAnalytics 2017). The report presents the number of HCCs captured by the provider practice over the two-year period in graphical format. The high-volume HCCs captured by the provider practice are listed for the two-year period. The report also includes a graphical depiction of the E/M code distribution compared with the HCC capture by a physician. There is a direct correlation between these two metrics, as higher E/M levels are typically associated with higher HCC capture. The outpatient CDS can use this comparative analysis to identify physicians who have high E/M-level scores but low HCC capture. When that occurs, the CDS should educate physicians related to HCC code documentation. The CDS may also improve the clinical documentation workflow by recommending technology solutions such as drop-down lists and NLP applications.

Figure 7.3. Physician HCC Capture (MedeAnalytics 2017)

Physician HCC Capture

Facility: All   Payer: All   Physician: All   Specialty: All   Selection: Default

Click on a row in the table below to see IP vs OP information.

Attributed Physician	Claims CY	RAF 2015	RAC 2016	RAF Var	RAF YTD	RAF VAR
		2015-2016			**YTD 2017 - 2016**	
Love, Sheryl, O	120	0.803	2.173	-1.37	0.967	1.206
Roberts, Ryan, O	57	0.118	1.472	-1.354	1.472	0
Tuttle, Norman, U	103	0.298	0.289	0.009	0.434	-0.145
Frazier, Eddie, R	82	0.3	0.446	-0.146	0.727	-0.281
Mangum, Max, A	68	0.341	0.455	-0.114	0.322	0.133
Sullivan, Nancy, U	101	0.337	0.501	-0.164	0.534	-0.033
Davidson, Jan, A	201	0.352	0.384	-0.032	0.484	-0.1
Bland, Michelle, L	147	0.317	0.344	-0.027	0.481	-0.137
Wise, Matthew, I	74	0.192	0.192	0	0.812	-0.62
Patel, Geoffrey, A	93	0.479	0.638	-0.159	0.441	0.197
Houston, Martin, O	35	0.286	0.405	-0.119	0.182	0.223
Wrenn, Gordon, R	10	0.462	0.493	-0.031	0.452	0.041
Cross, Norma, R	85	0.283	0.386	-0.103	0.469	-0.083
Conner, Regina, O	160	0.315	0.511	-0.196	0.338	0.173
Rich, Marian, I	43	0.315	0.448	-0.133	0.523	-0.075
Bryant, Priscilla, R	57	0.355	0.517	-0.162	0.471	0.046
Nixon, Melvin, I	153	0.098	0.283	-0.185	0.92	-0.637
Nelson, Mike	82	0.177	0.227	-0.05	0.283	-0.056
Callahan, Nathan, A	52	0.864	1.01	-0.146	0.425	0.585
Sawyer, Gloria, A	168	0.787	0.854	-0.067	0.214	0.64

Top Reported HCCs

	2015	2016	2017
1st HCC	42	35	16
2nd HCC	15	111	58
3rd HCC	111	17	111
4th HCC	85	18	17
5th HCC	12	40	96
6th HCC	18	96	18
7th HCC	96	85	85
8th HCC	58	12	12
9th HCC	58	58	40
10th HCC			

Source: MedeAnalytics 2017. Reprinted with permission. The example screenshots and dashboards for Revenue Integrity were provided by MedeAnalytics, Inc. MedeAnalytics offers a cloud-based analytics platform that aggregates and normalizes data across multiple sources, delivering it in an intuitive format that inspires clear and actionable insights into healthcare organizations' revenue, cost, quality, and risk. MedeAnalytics and Revenue Integrity are registered trademarks of MedeAnalytics, Inc. All rights reserved.

Personal Mobile Device Query Options

Numerous applications for personal mobile devices are used in communication among providers. For example, physicians often use e-mail and text messaging to communicate via mobile devices; however, these modes of communication do not allow for a streamlined query response and clinical record addenda. Other software tools are available to facilitate direct communication with the provider related to queries and in-application addenda to the EHR clinical documentation.

DocEdge Communicator is a first-of-its-kind software tool developed by Provident (Provident 2017). The tool has been selected for discussion in this chapter based on its functionality and application to the outpatient clinical documentation workflow; this discussion is not a product endorsement.

The DocEdge Communicator is designed to interface with the facility EHR. The tool has interface capabilities with multiple EHR platforms and can receive 837-file feeds on an ongoing basis to provide concurrent query communication between the CDS and the provider. Using templates, provider communication is enhanced not only for CDI queries and clinical documentation addenda but also for care management and utilization review to improve patient authorization, ambulatory care management, transition of care, readmission management, and bundled payment processes.

Templates within the DocEdge tool guide coders and CDSs as they create concise and accurate queries that the provider can easily view on a mobile device. The provider can respond with a few clicks, and the response is then added to the clinical record in the EHR via HL7 interfaces that are compliant with the security requirements of the Health Insurance Portability and Accountability Act. (Refer to chapter 2 for additional information on HL7.) The following is an outline of the process:

- The CDS reviews the clinical documentation for a specific patient concurrently with the patient encounter.
- Where a query is needed, the CDS enters the clinical scenario and the compliant query options into the software.
- The CDS sends the query through software to the provider's personal mobile device.
- The provider receives the query via the personal mobile device and reads the case scenario and query options.
- The provider answers the query by selecting one of the options or by typing specific wording to update the clinical record. Most queries are answered by selecting from a list of standard queries based on the facility's diagnosis-specific query formats. These formats are preloaded into the software and are available as query options.
- When the provider sends the query response, the clinical information from the query is documented in the EHR at a designated location determined by the facility during the software implementation process. For example, if the facility has decided to include the query as a provider progress note, the information in the query response is documented in the EHR as a progress note with the current date.

The software saves time and eliminates the need for the provider to open the EHR and add the clinical documentation. Figure 7.4 provides an example of the personal mobile device screen layout for a query communicated via the DocEdge tool.

Figure 7.4. Personal mobile device screen layout for a DocEdge Communicator query

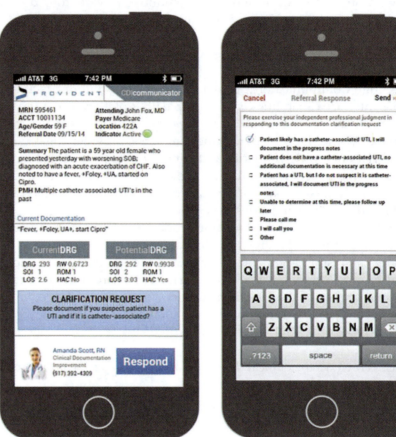

Source: Provident 2017

The clarification (query) request in template format is easy to read, and the provider response is automatically transferred to the clinical record in the EHR. This process eliminates the need for the provider to go back into the EHR to create an addendum to the clinical record. In the example in figure 7.5, the provider adds the specificity of "acute on chronic systolic heart failure" by checking one button and the response is then added to a progress note in the EHR.

Preformatted query templates may be loaded into the DocEdge tool to ensure compliance with American Health Information Management Association (AHIMA) query guidelines. These guidelines are found in the AHIMA Query Toolkit (AHIMA 2017b). Also, refer to chapter 15 of this text for more information on the compliant query process. The HCC query screen in figure 7.6 shows how the outpatient CDS can use the DocEdge tool to submit queries the physician. The figure shows an oncology example and is specific to a patient with a history of malignancy. The screen displays the patient demographics and a summary of the case. The clarification request is a standard statement: "Based on the clinical indicators and your professional judgment, please complete by selecting one of the options below." The screen then outlines the response options, which include a request for further explanation, an option for inability to determine, and acknowledgment that no further clarification is needed. The provider may use the "Messaging" or "Please Call" options to further communicate with the CDS regarding the case.

Figure 7.5. Example of a clinical record addendum created via the DocEdge Communicator tool

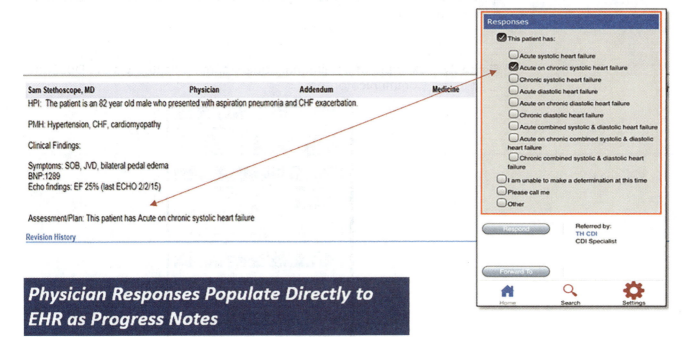

Source: Provident 2017

Figure 7.6. Example of an oncology query: history of malignancy communicated via the DocEdge Communicator tool

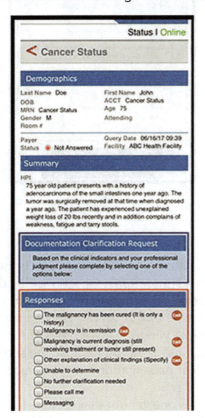

Source: Provident Edge 2017

Figure 7.7 shows a pulmonary medicine query specific to pneumonia. The query has the same layout as the oncology query example, but the response options have changed.

Figure 7.7. Example of a pulmonary query communicated via the DocEdge Communicator tool

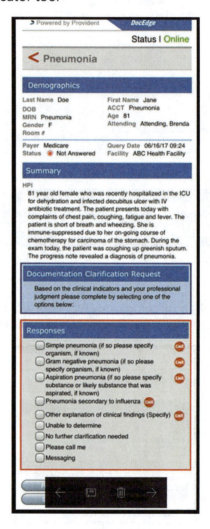

Source: Provident 2017

Denials Tracking

One of the most useful databases for outpatient CDI is the denials database. This database may be kept as a simple spreadsheet tracking denials by payer, denial type, provider, coder, service, diagnosis, and treatment or procedure. However, the use of a denials software tool is a more efficient method for tracking denials. Available from multiple vendors, these types of tools are recommended for effective denials tracking and trending because the software can produce line-item reports and graphical presentations about denials trends such as denials by type, service, or provider.

The Wellington Group is one vendor that licenses healthcare claims software. Its offerings include a denials management (DenialsNavigator) module for use by facilities and provider practices. The software is described here for illustration purposes only, to show how denials management software may be used by CDI teams to improve clinical documentation; this discussion does not constitute a product endorsement.

Figure 7.8 provides a report created with Wellington Group software to summarize denials by **claim adjustment reason code (CA or CARC)**. CA/CARC codes are standardized within the insurance industry, and a complete list may be found on the X12 website (X12 2017). By analyzing this report, the outpatient CDS can determine the most frequent types of denials and those with a high financial impact. For example, the report indicates an adjustment of $97,190 as a result of CA code B12. These services were not reimbursed because they were not documented in the patient's clinical record. With further analysis of a sample of these claims, the CDS can determine the type of service being denied and whether the denial is based on a lack of specificity in the procedure note. Perhaps the provider of the service was unaware of the specificity required to describe the procedure in question. After the root-cause analysis is done, the CDS can offer CDI suggestions and provide education about the clinical documentation issue to the relevant parties.

Figure 7.8. Claim adjustment reason code summary

Top Ten Claim Denial CAS Reason Codes						Top Ten Zero Paid CAS Reason Codes					
CAS Reason Code	Total Claims	Total Remits	Reason Count	Denied Amount	Percent of Total	CAS Reason Code	Total Claims	Total Remits	Reason Count	Denied Amount	Percent of Total
23 - The impact of prior payer(s) adjudication including payments and/or adjustments.	17	17	17	$647,087	21.62%	16 - Claim/service lacks information or has submission/billing error(s) which is needed for adjudication.	59	64	1,006	$2,023,941	37.81%
22 - This care may be covered by another payer per coordination of benefits.	9	9	56	$583,224	19.48%	45 - Charge exceeds fee schedule/maximum allowable or contracted/legislated fee arrangement.	58	58	59	$772,965	14.44%
18 - Exact duplicate claim/service.	12	12	69	$397,056	13.26%	139 - Contracted funding agreement - Subscriber is employed by the provider of services.	32	32	32	$651,857	12.18%
16 - Claim/service lacks information or has submission/billing error(s) which is needed for adjudication.	4	4	42	$243,939	8.15%	197 - Precertification/authorization/notification absent.	47	48	429	$407,112	7.61%
252 - An attachment/other documentation is required to adjudicate this claim/service.	8	8	29	$212,925	7.11%	A1 - Claim/Service denied.	13	15	255	$354,027	6.61%
31 - Patient cannot be identified as our insured.	7	7	7	$130,772	4.37%	96 - Non-covered charge(s).	11	11	194	$309,785	5.79%
A1 - Claim/Service denied.	6	6	84	$116,601	3.90%	B13 - Previously paid. Payment for this claim/service may have been provided in a previous payment.	29	29	30	$199,821	3.73%
B12 - Services not documented in patients' medical records.	4	4	4	$97,190	3.25%	18 - Exact duplicate claim/service.	15	15	165	$134,668	2.52%
197 - Precertification/authorization/notification absent.	7	7	7	$93,398	3.12%	39 - Services denied at the time authorization/pre-certification was requested.	5	5	53	$105,960	1.98%
27 - Expenses incurred after coverage terminated.	5	5	5	$84,518	2.82%	252 - An attachment/other documentation is required to adjudicate this claim/service.	7	7	72	$104,566	1.95%
Total	105	106	516	$2,993,335		Total	237	255	2,695	$5,352,647	

Source: Wellington Group, LLC

Figure 7.9 presents a report generated with Wellington Group software that provides information on the total claims and denials revenue by payer type over a three-month period. This type of trend report can be used to track increasing and decreasing numbers of denials and total charges over a period. Figure 7.9 shows a decreasing number of total denied claims and a decline in the total denied charges during the three-month period, which might reflect improvements made through denials management by the outpatient CDS and other stakeholders working on specific root causes for denials. The outpatient CDS can also drill down into a section of the report, such as indemnity insurance for the month of January, and review the claims denials for the 51 cases included in January for that category.

Figure 7.9. Report on denied claims by payer category

Payer Category	Trend Period (Monthly)	Total Claims	Total Charges	Total Denied Claims	Total Denied Charges	Percent Claims Denied	Percent Denied Charges
Indemnity Insurance	2016 March	8	$7,029.97	1	$1,377.00	12.50%	19.59%
	2016 February	38	$61,294.42	17	$27,085.17	44.74%	44.19%
	2016 January	51	$223,934.27	15	$104,633.74	29.41%	46.73%
	Total	97	$292,258.66	33	$133,095.91	34.02%	45.54%
Medicare Part A	2016 March	3,736	$11,464,704.17	51	$346,376.84	1.37%	3.02%
	2016 February	5,126	$20,101,385.10	92	$521,316.55	1.79%	2.59%
	2016 January	4,865	$23,874,164.16	98	$1,006,230.11	2.01%	4.21%
	Total	13,727	$55,440,253.43	241	$1,873,923.50	1.76%	3.38%
Total		13,824	$55,732,512.09	274	$2,007,019.40	1.98%	3.60%

Denied Claims by Payer Category - Trending
Wellington General
Claims From 1/1/2016 - 4/13/2016

Source: Wellington Group, LLC

The report in figure 7.10 provides the total number of denials, related revenue, and CA reason code by CPT code. This information can be used by the CDS to determine areas of focus for an outpatient CPT-related root-cause analysis. For example, if the outpatient CDS has been working on denials improvement in revenue code category 302, this report for the first quarter (1/1/16–4/11/16) could be compared to a report for the second quarter to see whether the number of denials and corresponding revenue loss increases, decreases, or stays the same. In the first quarter, there were five accounts for CPT code 86703 with corresponding revenue loss per instance of $265. If the outpatient CDS is able to reduce the number of denials for code 86703 for the second quarter, the success can be celebrated by all stakeholders who participated in the redesign project.

Figure 7.10. Line denials by revenue, CPT/HCPCS, and claim adjustment reason code

Line Denials by - Revenue, CPT/HCPCS, CAS Codes
Wellington General
Claims From 1/1/2016 - 4/11/2016

Revenue Code	CPT/HCPCS	CAS Code	Number Claims	Occurrences	Line Denied Amount	Line Paid	Average Denied Amount
301	Total		465	620	$79,393.00	$0.00	$128.05
302	86301	50	1	1	$82.00	$0.00	$82.00
		Total	1	1	$82.00	$0.00	$82.00
	86304	50	4	4	$328.00	$0.00	$82.00
		Total	4	4	$328.00	$0.00	$82.00
	86592	50	6	6	$216.00	$0.00	$36.00
		Total	6	6	$216.00	$0.00	$36.00
	86703	50	5	5	$265.00	$0.00	$53.00
		Total	5	5	$265.00	$0.00	$53.00
	Total		17	22	$2,270.00	$0.00	$103.18
323	Total		1	2	$7,690.00	$0.00	$3,845.00
352	Total		3	3	$10,103.00	$0.00	$3,367.67
410	Total		2	2	$255.00	$0.00	$127.50
Total			483	649	$99,711.00	$0.00	$153.64

Source: Wellington Group, LLC

Clinical Editors

Clinical editors may be included as part of the health information system's claims scrubber or encoder, or they may be stand-alone tools such as the ones discussed in this section. A clinical editor tool is valuable for determining reasons for denials, claims delays, or improper payments. A clinical editor uses rules that analyze clinical data to determine potential errors in claims submission. These errors are referred to as *edits*. For example, the clinical editor could compare the number of units for a drug entered into a patient's record against the standard drug dosage for a patient of that age; if the number of units in the patient record did not match the standard dosage, the editor would flag the possible inconsistency in clinical data (the edit), which might lead to a claim being denied. Cases that are flagged with potential errors must be reviewed by an auditor or CDS to validate that the edit is truly an error. The outpatient CDS should become familiar with the reports that these systems generate so that audits, root-cause analysis, workflow redesign, and provider and coder education can be conducted. Refer to chapter 6 of this text for additional information on claims edits.

Multiple clinical editors, including the Wellington Group's Ambulatory Revenue Manager, are available in the marketplace. Their features vary; the Wellington Group's clinical editor tool identifies the potential lack of payment for missing blood administration components, component injection and infusion codes, and missing payable medications. Discussion of this tool does not imply a product endorsement.

Figure 7.11 shows a screen from the Ambulatory Revenue Manager claims editor (Wellington 2017). It points to a possible missing charge based on an

Figure 7.11. Claims editor showing drug dosage units below expected volume edit

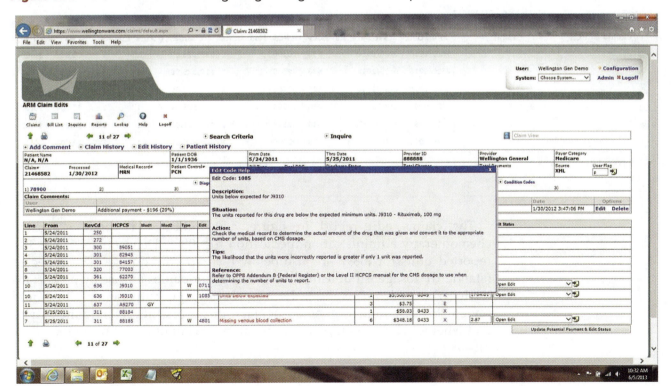

Source: Wellington Group, LLC

edit for "units below expected" for HCPCS code J9310, Rituximab, 100 mg. This edit means that for a specific patient, the drug rituximab was provided at a dosage below what is standard. If this edit seems to be part of a trend, the outpatient CDS should audit a sample of relevant claims to determine whether there is an actual claims error and, if so, determine its root cause. A trend is identified when a pattern is noted over time; for example, a series of "units below expected" edits for rituximab over several months for a specific provider or service line would constitute a trend. When such a trend occurs, further investigation is needed to determine the root cause of the issue identified by the edit.

The report in figure 7.12 provides insight into clinical edits related to HCPCS code J2505, Injection, pegfilgrastim, 6 mg. Pegfilgrastim is a long-acting medication that stimulates the flow of neutrophils to help fight infection and reduces fever in patients undergoing chemotherapy. The report shows several claims where the charge amount of $10,875 for one unit of J2505 was not paid. Further investigation of the patient's clinical record may reveal that the claims for pegfilgrastim were denied because they lacked the diagnosis specificity required by Local Coverage Determination (LCD) or National Coverage Determination (NCD) guidelines. Refer to chapter 2 for more information on LCDs and NCDs.

Figure 7.12. Claims edit summary by claims edit codes

Claim#	PCN	Patient	From Date	Svc Date	Rev Code	HCPCS	Mod	Units	Charges	Occurs	Claims	Est Pay	Ave Pay
			7/20/2016	7/20/2016	636	J2505		1	$10,875.00	1	1	$0.00	$0.00
			6/29/2016	6/29/2016	636	J2505		1	$10,875.00	1	1	$0.00	$0.00
			6/22/2016	6/22/2016	636	J2780		2	$50.00	1	1	$0.00	$0.00
			6/8/2016	6/8/2016	636	J2505		1	$10,875.00	1	1	$0.00	$0.00
			6/2/2016	6/2/2016	636	J2505		1	$10,875.00	1	1	$0.00	$0.00
			5/26/2016	5/26/2016	636	J2505		1	$10,875.00	1	1	$0.00	$0.00

Report Range: 12/23/2016 - 2/12/2017
Edit Code: 0718

Source: Wellington Group, LLC

The claims edit report in figure 7.13 indicates a possible missing chemotherapy administration medication for J0897, Denosumab, 1 mg. The reported units for J0897 are also below the expected dosage. The expected (standard) dosage is published by the drug companies for use by physicians during the patient-specific ordering process. The outpatient CDS should review this case to determine the actual number of units given to the patient and whether chemotherapy administration was omitted from the record by mistake.

Figure 7.13. Ambulatory Revenue Manager claims edit report

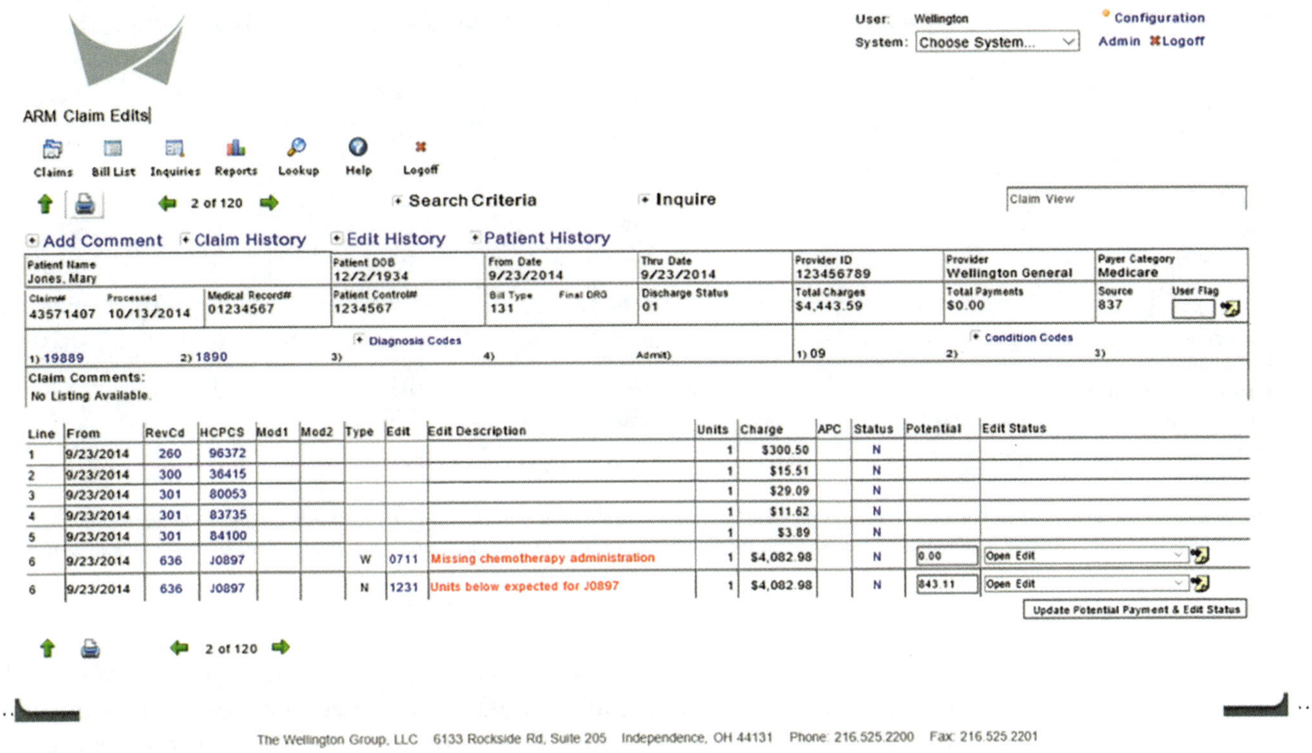

Source: Wellington Group, LLC

Figure 7.14 shows a top revenue risk report generated by MedeAnalytics software and filtered to include outpatient facility claims. It reveals a number of missed charge opportunities that the outpatient CDS could investigate further. The following are examples of charge capture gaps that might warrant further investigation:

- Missing radiology payment in fracture care
- Missing blood or administration charge
- Missing hemophilia clotting factors
- Observation services billed for 7 hours
- Missing organ transplant
- Missing ultrasounds with multi-gestation diagnosis
- Missing implantable
- Missing mesh implantation when mesh supply is present
- Missing trauma activation charges
- Missing ablation in conjunction with cardiac electrophysiology studies

182 Chapter 7 Assessing Outpatient CDI Program Technology Options

Figure 7.14. Revenue risk/top revenue risks (missing charges)

Risk Category	Volume	% of Total	Average Charges	Avg Commercial/Other Pmts	Avg Medicaid Pmts	Avg Medicare Pmts
Missing Charges						
Review for Missing Radiology Payment in Fracture Care (224)	4,863	44.00%	$2,385	$724	$0	$54
Review for missing blood or admin charge (185)	2,520	22.80%	$11,156	$3,714	$0	$326
Review for Missing Hemophilia Clotting Factors (206)	2,493	22.55%	$115,792	$34,373	$0	$6,201
Review for Observation Services billed for 7 hours (225)	814	7.36%	$7,021	$1,804	$0	$130
Review for Missing Organ Transplant (205)	111	1.00%	$8,270	$3,125	$0	$0
Review for Missing ultrasounds with multi-gestation diagnosis (201)	57	0.52%	$1,747	$457	$0	$0
Review for missing implantable (189)	42	0.38%	$21,716	$11,963	$0	$1,090
Review for Missing Mesh implantation when mesh supply present - Pelvic Floor Defect (198)	36	0.33%	$35,907	$12,738	$0	$757
Review for Missing trauma activation charges (196)	31	0.28%	$17,487	$3,851	$0	$27
Review for Missing ablation in conjunction with cardiac electrophysiology studies (199)	24	0.22%	$35,695	$14,021	$0	$490

Source: MedeAnalytics 2017. Reprinted with permission. The example screenshots and dashboards for Revenue Integrity were provided by MedeAnalytics, Inc. MedeAnalytics offers a cloud-based analytics platform that aggregates and normalizes data across multiple sources, delivering it in an intuitive format that inspires clear and actionable insights into healthcare organizations' revenue, cost, quality, and risk. MedeAnalytics and Revenue Integrity are registered trademarks of MedeAnalytics, Inc. All rights reserved.

Reports on top revenue risks can also be used to review procedure-related issues, bundled payments, unit counts, noncovered services, and diagnosis-related issues. For example, figure 7.15 highlights a common error: Review coding for add-on codes without primary code. This error occurs when claim for a procedure omits a required procedure code. The error code highlighted in this example shows 278 claims where a secondary procedure code was submitted but the primary code was omitted from the claim.

Figure 7.15. Top revenue risks (procedure related)

Risk Category	Volume	% of Total	Average Charges	Avg Commercial/Other Pmts	Avg Medicaid Pmts	Avg Medicare Pmts	Average Pmts
Proc Related							
Review for Billing with Incorrect Drug Revenue Code (215)	5,083	41.65%	$4,586	$1,451	$0	$85	$1,536
Review for Mutually Exclusive Edits (192)	4,646	38.07%	$13,802	$1,954	$0	$1,125	$3,079
Review Age of patient is inconsistent with CPT code description (167)	741	6.07%	$8,832	$3,096	$0	$0	$3,096
Review Principal Procedure for Medical Necessity Modified Barium Swallow (168)	374	3.06%	$1,561	$278	$0	$79	$357
Review Procedure code on Medicare IP-only list conducted as OP (188)	298	2.44%	$27,942	$3,690	$0	$245	$3,935
Review coding for Add On codes used without Primary code (260)	278	2.28%	$12,607	$2,109	$0	$741	$2,850
Review for Billing with unacceptable principal diagnosis code (216)	214	1.75%	$44,690	$9,633	$0	$4,185	$13,818
Review Procedure Code for New vs. Established Patients (193)	171	1.40%	$1,073	$422	$0	$75	$497
Review Inpatient Percutaneous vertebral augmentation (Kyphoplasty) (103)	170	1.39%	$58,978	$9,044	$0	$6,514	$15,558
Review for Medical Necessity Complex Cataract Removal (270)	67	0.55%	$10,406	$1,031	$0	$871	$1,902
Review for Medical Necessity Sacral Neurostimulation (273)	65	0.53%	$22,817	$4,205	$0	$6,127	$10,332
Review for Medical Necessity Blepharoplasty (268)	50	0.41%	$9,254	$1,765	$0	$1,095	$2,861

Source: MedeAnalytics 2017. Reprinted with permission. The example screenshots and dashboards for Revenue Integrity were provided by MedeAnalytics, Inc. MedeAnalytics offers a cloud-based analytics platform that aggregates and normalizes data across multiple sources, delivering it in an intuitive format that inspires clear and actionable insights into healthcare organizations' revenue, cost, quality, and risk. MedeAnalytics and Revenue Integrity are registered trademarks of MedeAnalytics, Inc. All rights reserved.

Similar reports can be run using MedeAnalytics or comparable software for professional practice claims and may include the following categories: CPT guidelines, global package, modifier usage, noncovered services, procedure-related, and service count. In most claims editors, the outpatient CDS should review a sample of claims in the high-volume, high-risk categories to evaluate the charge gap and determine its root cause. The report in figure 7.16 provides a snapshot of categories that should be reviewed based on the total amount at risk (noted in the fourth column from the left). The following categories should be considered:

- CPT guidelines, which include charge capture issues as well as possible coding compliance issues:
  - Age of patient is inconsistent with code description
  - Coding for add-on codes used without primary code
  - Coding for new versus established patients
- Global package, a category that points to possible compliance risks:
  - Potential duplicate billing during a global period (a specified period pre- or postoperatively where only one procedure code may be submitted for payment)
  - Potential duplicate billing for ultrasound or diagnostic procedures that should not be billed separately from antepartum care because they are part of a packaged service for maternity patients

Figure 7.16. Top Professional Practice Revenue Risks report

Risk Category	Line Items	% of Total	Total Amt at Risk	Total Pmts	Avg Pmts	Medicare Pmts	Avg Medicare Pmts	Medicaid Pmts	Avg Medicaid Pmts
CPT Guideline									
Review Age of patient is inconsistent with code description (16)	30,322	82.59%	6,054,865	758,347	25	58	0	99,932	3
Review coding for Add On codes used without Primary code (23)	859	2.34%	308,102	59,047	69	18,535	22	3,183	4
Review coding for New vs. Established Patients (18)	5,456	14.86%	1,653,883	202,965	37	48,316	9	17,298	3
Review Service Counts exceeded Initial Infusion Chemotherapy or IV Hydration per day (15)	79	0.22%	152,801	2,991	38	0	0	0	0
Total : CPT Guideline	**36,716**	**26.95%**	**8,160,464**	**1,023,350**	**28**	**66,910**	**2**	**120,414**	**3**
Global Package									
Global vs TC/PC (17)	111	0.21%	35,369	4,905	44	23	0	292	3
Review for potential duplicate billing for Global Days Post Op (21)	49,344	93.32%	40,057,003	7,778,895	158	2,056,311	42	88,465	2
Review for potential duplicate billing for Global Days Pre Op (22)	3,293	6.23%	5,996,123	188,135	57	44,486	14	9,514	3
Review for potential duplicate billing Ultrasound or diagnostic procedures should not be billed separately from antepartum care (35)	128	0.24%	71,341	23,569	184	0	0	5,311	41
Total : Global Package	**52,876**	**38.81%**	**44,259,127**	**7,995,503**	**151**	**2,100,820**	**40**	**103,582**	**2**
Modifier Usage	16,684	12.25%	27,366,911	5,674,082	340	993,089	60	46,484	3
Non Covered Service	16,896	12.40%	3,586,900	1,500,233	89	611,577	36	71,347	4
Proc Related	737	0.54%	163,644	21,410	29	6,189	8	140	0
Service Count	12,329	9.05%	4,956,847	379,238	31	12,176	1	612	0
Total : Selected Filter(s)	**136,238**	**100.00%**	**88,493,893**	**16,593,816**	**122**	**3,790,761**	**28**	**342,578**	**3**

Source: MedeAnalytics, 2017. Reprinted with permission. The example screenshots and dashboards for Revenue Integrity were provided by MedeAnalytics, Inc. MedeAnalytics offers a cloud-based analytics platform that aggregates and normalizes data across multiple sources, delivering it in an intuitive format that inspires clear and actionable insights into healthcare organizations' revenue, cost, quality, and risk. MedeAnalytics and Revenue Integrity are registered trademarks of MedeAnalytics, Inc. All rights reserved.

Risk target dashboards, such as the one shown in figure 7.17, can be used in discussions during CDI steering committee or taskforce meetings to point out program successes and areas for improvement. The dashboards can be filtered to include some or all facilities (for multifacility health systems or specific payers).

184   Chapter 7   **Assessing Outpatient CDI Program Technology Options**

Figure 7.17.   Risk target dashboard

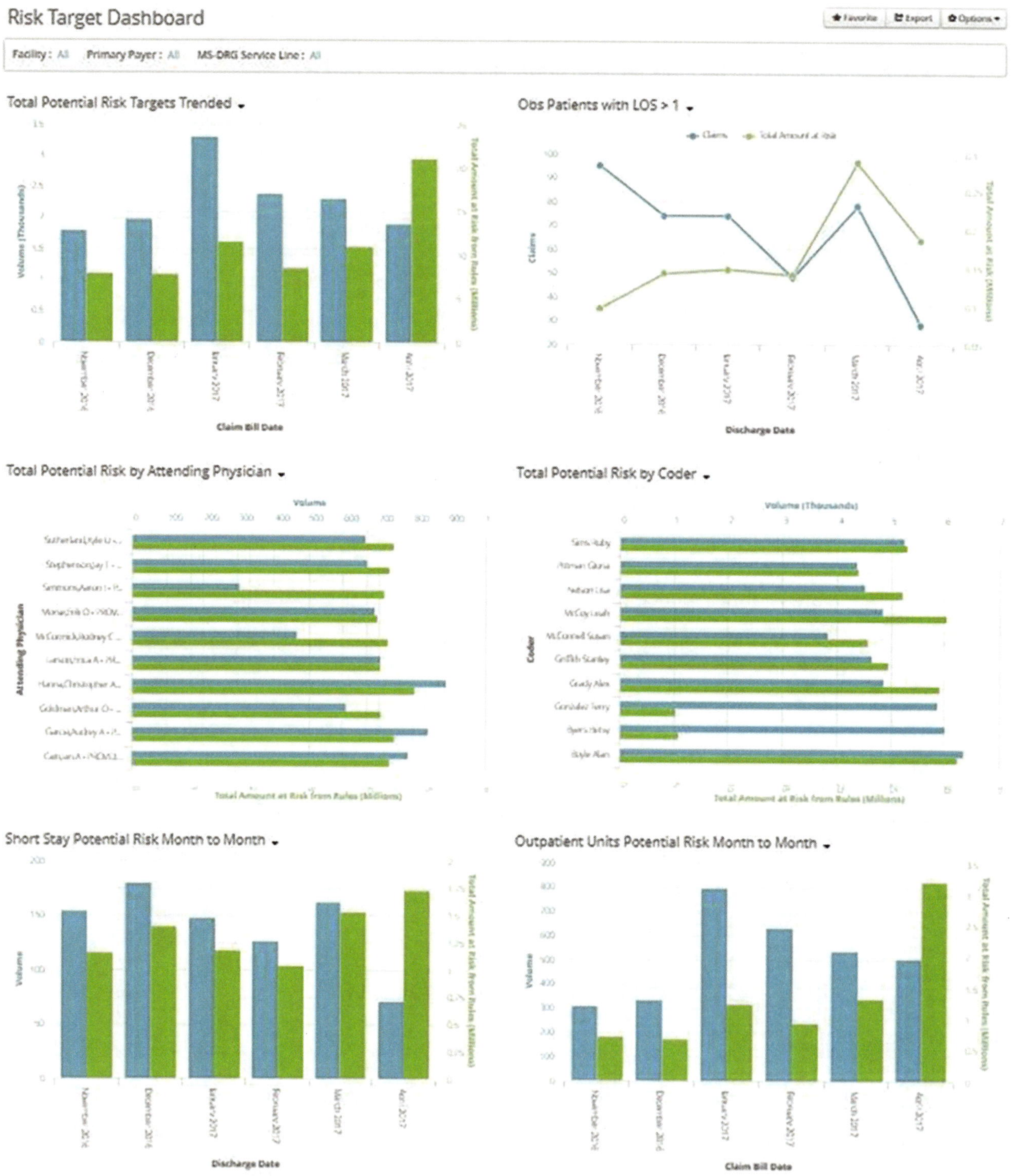

Source: MedeAnalytics, 2017. Reprinted with permission. The example screenshots and dashboards for Revenue Integrity were provided by MedeAnalytics, Inc. MedeAnalytics offers a cloud-based analytics platform that aggregates and normalizes data across multiple sources, delivering it in an intuitive format that inspires clear and actionable insights into healthcare organizations' revenue, cost, quality, and risk. MedeAnalytics and Revenue Integrity are registered trademarks of MedeAnalytics, Inc. All rights reserved.

The reports in this chapter are offered as illustrations so that the CDS can conceptualize the report presentation and use of the report in CDS practice. In each instance, more than one company offers the type of product discussed. The reports highlighted are example reports and corresponding data items and edits that can be used to select areas of focus for outpatient clinical documentation improvement activities.

Chapter 7 Review Exercises

1. Tools such as clinical editors and _____ systems can be used to identify the top areas of focus where CDI can improve quality patient care and assist in accurate reimbursement.
   a. Pharmacy formulary
   b. Denials management
   c. Computer assisted coding
   d. Revenue cycle management

2. EHRs offer tools such as the copy/paste function, templates, and auto-populating fields that can help with clinical documentation. However, the misuse of these tools could lead to false or irrelevant documentation that seems to support billing higher-level services or services that were not provided. This potential risk is known as _____.
   a. Overdocumentation
   b. Insufficient documentation
   c. Incorrect assignment of ICD-10-CM codes
   d. Inappropriate automatic assignment of E/M codes

3. The Patient HCC Capture report can be used by the outpatient CDS to determine the _____ for the previous two years.
   a. RAF score
   b. RVU average weight
   c. Calculated outpatient average charge rate
   d. Percentage of HCC capture errors in previous years

4. Clinical editors may be stand-alone tools or included as part of the health information system's claims scrubber or _____.
   a. Encoder
   b. Operating room database
   c. Denials management system
   d. Evidence-based medicine database

5. Most denials management tools can produce reports or graphical depictions of denials trends by denial type, service, and _____.
   a. Provider
   b. HCC code
   c. RVU weight
   d. Unstructured data element

6. The prevalence of NLP software usage in the healthcare industry is expected to increase dramatically in the coming years. Which of the following *best* explains the rise in NLP usage?
   a. The workforce who would manually process data continues to shrink.
   b. The growing use of EHRs has created an abundance of unstructured data.
   c. Data is processed more economically with NLP software than by a salaried staff.
   d. Healthcare facilities are increasingly interested in avoiding human error when processing data.

7. HCC suspecting is the process of using _____ to scan clinical documentation for potential chronic illnesses that are categorized as HCCs.
   a. A claims editor
   b. An NLP engine
   c. EHR scanning software
   d. A disease classification system

8. During the process of semantic reasoning, an NLP engine uses a database of _____ to identify other text related to a specific phrase.
   a. Similar terms
   b. Disparate adjectives
   c. Cross-functional data
   d. Correlated clinical elements

9. Misuse of EHR tools and programming errors can lead to serious problems. Specific risks are associated with EHR functionality. One risk includes incorrect ICD-10-CM assignment because of _____ errors from embedded ICD-9-CM codes.
   a. Crosswalk
   b. Copy/paste
   c. Template design
   d. Translation and transcription

10. Upon accessing a patient's EHR, the provider receives an automatically generated message giving information about the patient's chronic illnesses and corresponding medications. The notification the provider has received would *best* be described as a(n):
    a. Note
    b. Task
    c. Alert
    d. Prompt

References

American Health Information Management Association (AHIMA). 2017a. Congestive heart failure (CHF) [documentation suggestions]. http://library.ahima.org/doc?oid=60161#.WQpLiIWcE2w.

American Health Information Management Association (AHIMA). 2017b. Query toolkit. http://bok.ahima.org/PdfView?oid=302140.

Centers for Medicare and Medicaid Services (CMS). 2017a. Risk adjustment. https://www.cms.gov/Medicare/Health-Plans/MedicareAdvtgSpecRateStats/Risk-Adjustors.html.

Centers for Medicare and Medicaid Services (CMS). 2017b. Medicare Managed Care Manual. Chapter 7: Risk adjustment. https://www.cms.gov/Regulations-and-Guidance/Guidance/Manuals/Internet-Only-Manuals-IOMs-Items/CMS019326.html.

Crawford, M. 2013. Truth about computer-assisted coding: a consultant, HIM professional, and vendor weigh in on the real CAC impact. *Journal of AHIMA* 84(7):24–27. http://bok.ahima.org/doc?oid=106663#.Wd_1U2hSw2w.

Hess, P. 2015. *Clinical Documentation Improvement: Principles and Practice*. Chicago: AHIMA.

Maarala, A., X. Su, and J. Riekki. 2016. Semantic reasoning for context-aware internet of things applications. *Internet of Things Journal*. https://arxiv.org/ftp/arxiv/papers/1604/1604.08340.pdf.

Markets and Markets. 2016. Natural language processing market by type. http://www.marketsandmarkets.com/Market-Reports/natural-language-processing-nlp-825.html.

MedeAnalytics. 2017. http://medeanalytics.com.

Monegain, B. 2015 (August 14). Natural language processing in high demand. Healthcare IT News. http://www.healthcareitnews.com/news/natural-language-processing-demand.

National Kidney Foundation (NKF). 2015. A to Z health guide: Glomerular filtration rate (GFR). https://www.kidney.org/atoz/content/gfr.

Office of Inspector General (OIG). 2014. US Department of Health and Human Services. CMs and its contractors have adopted few program integrity practices to address vulnerabilities in EHRs. https://oig.hhs.gov/oei/reports/oei-01-11-00571.pdf.

Pinson, R. and C. Tang. 2017. *2017 CDI Pocket Guide.* Brentwood, TN: HCPro.

Provident. 2017. http://www.providentedge.com.

Stearns, M. 2014 (June 9). EHRs and the ICD-10 transition: Planning for 2015. http://www.physicianspractice.com/icd-10/ehrs-and-icd-10-transition-planning-2015.

Stearns, M. 2013 (December). EHRs and E/M coding: Warnings, pitfalls, and best practices. *AAPC Cutting Edge*. http://www.michaelstearnsmd.com/wp-content/uploads/2013/12/Stearns-E-M-EHR-Article-Cutting-Edge-Dec-2013.pdf.

Tucker, A.B. 2002. Semantics—meaning representation in NLP. http://www.bowdoin.edu/~allen/nlp/nlp6.html.

The Wellington Group. 2017. https://www.wellingtonware.com.

X12. 2017. Claim adjustment reason codes. X12 External Code Source 139. http://www.x12.org/codes/claim-adjustment-reason-codes.

PART II
Implementing an Outpatient Clinical Documentation Improvement Program

Moving Forward with a CDI Program

8

Learning Objectives

- Describe the importance of buy-in from key executive decision makers when developing a new clinical documentation improvement (CDI) program.
- Differentiate the responsibilities of the CDI steering committee and CDI taskforce during development of an outpatient CDI program.
- Learn how to create the CDI program vision, mission, goals, and objectives.
- Identify the best practices for CDI program organizational communication.

Key Terms

CDI steering committee
CDI taskforce
Goals
Governance structure
Mission statement

Objectives
Specific, measurable, attainable, relevant, time-bound (SMART)
Vision statement

Moving forward with an outpatient clinical documentation improvement (CDI) program is no small task, but it is achievable. The concept for a CDI program could originate as part of any number of scenarios. For example, someone at the executive level, such as the chief executive officer (CEO) or chief financial officer (CFO) may approach the health information management (HIM) director or coding team to determine whether outpatient CDI can benefit the health system and whether the program potentially could have a positive return on investment (ROI); then, the CFO requests that the team move forward with preliminary exploration. Alternatively, the HIM director or coding team may propose the program to the executive officers, and the executives give the team the green light to start putting together a project plan, interviewing stakeholders, and convening the committees that will govern and manage the project.

The decision to move forward should be carefully thought out and discussed among key stakeholders (CFO and CDI program leader); this decision must align with the organization's overall vision, goals, and objectives. If the key stakeholders agree that a program could be worthwhile, the next step is to create the governance structure, goals, and objectives for the program. An initial assessment of the likely ROI is important to ensure that executives and other key decision makers have an idea about the funding and resources needed to support the program on an ongoing basis. In this initial assessment, the potential financial benefit of CDI is compared to the estimated cost of the program staff and contractor support. If the ROI seems promising, further, more detailed analysis can be done to create a budget and refine financial projections. The staffing and contract costs can be included in the overall program budget that is monitored by the governance committee. The budget will include not only the cost of monthly resources but also the financial benefits realized from the program during and after implementation.

This chapter provides insight into the initial phase of organizing and communicating the program. First, the key health-system decision makers—for example, the CFO—must select a CDI leader. The key decision makers will next create a governance committee that will develop the program vision, mission, goals, and objectives. This committee, which may be called the CDI steering committee, will determine the best way to communicate the new program to the medical staff and other leaders within the health system and select the implementation model that will be the best fit for the health system. There are several options, including new program implementation, program redesign, and outsourced CDI. The governance committee will also discuss the options for recruiting qualified staff to manage and operate the program. See chapter 11 for additional discussion on CDI program staffing, including recruitment and outsourcing.

Key Decision Makers

The first step in the creation of a new outpatient CDI program is the development of a vision and mission statement, goals, and objectives. This step requires the participation of the executive leadership that will sponsor the CDI program within the organization. The executive leadership must be actively engaged in discussion and decisions as well as periodic review and updates of proposals.

Each institution will have its own distinctive organizational structure and political environment; however, in general, participants in this phase will include chief executives as well as the leaders that manage the day-to-day operations in the clinical areas, revenue cycle, finance, quality, HIM and coding, care management, and compliance.

An outpatient CDI program director should be selected by the executive leaders. In some organizations, the program may be incorporated into the inpatient CDI program. However, in larger institutions where there are multiple large ambulatory clinics with separate ambulatory services leadership, the outpatient CDI program may best be organized under the executive leaders in the ambulatory setting because the extensive tasks required in the outpatient CDI program may be too time-consuming for the existing inpatient CDI program to take on. The HIM director or other CDI program oversight executive should carefully consider who will fill this position. The selection of the program director will be based on skill sets and knowledge requirements related to ambulatory reimbursement, coding, and clinical documentation, as well as multisystem electronic health record (EHR) functionality and clinical documentation requirements. The outpatient CDI program director may be selected from existing facility staff, hired through a recruiting process, or a consultant contracted on an interim basis.

Once the outpatient CDI program director is selected, he or she should contact key decision makers within the health system to discuss the importance of the program and why each member is a vital part of the program's success. A meeting of the key stakeholders will be held to discuss the program vision, mission, goals, and objectives. The list of relevant leaders may vary depending on the organization, but the following are typical:

- Chief operating officer (ambulatory clinic)
- Chief medical officer (CMO)
- CFO
- Chief information officer (CIO) (or appropriate representative from information technology [IT])
- Chief compliance officer
- Chief nursing officer (ambulatory clinic)
- Physician specialty clinic and physician practice leaders
- Clinic administrators
- Director of HIM
- Director of quality
- Director of admitting or central scheduling
- Director of care management
- Emergency department (ED) director

Governance Structure

After the CFO or CEO has selected an outpatient CDI program director, a governance structure should be established to oversee the program. A **governance structure** provides a framework for the leadership and oversight of the new outpatient CDI program. The two primary parts of the governance structure are the CDI steering committee and the CDI taskforce. The **CDI steering committee** is the higher-level oversight committee and is made up of the facility or health system executive-level leaders and selected department directors (that is, the key stakeholders identified in the previous section of this chapter). The purpose of the steering committee is to provide visibility for the program and resources needed to implement and maintain the program functions. The steering committee chair can be appointed by the senior executive (CEO or CFO) providing oversight for the program or can be elected by the steering committee membership.

The **CDI taskforce** is the day-to-day working committee of those members actively involved in the clinical documentation process. It oversees and creates workplan tasks for the CDI program, and its members are those responsible for the day-to-day management of the clinic and professional practice operations and corresponding support departments. Recommended outpatient CDI taskforce members are as follows:

- HIM director
- Outpatient CDI program director
- Clinic administrator
- Clinic manager
- Medical staff specialty leader
- Clinic or practice nursing representative
- Representative for the clinic or practice clinical documentation specialists (CDSs)
- Admitting or central scheduling director
- Care management director

In large clinics and practices, more than one CDI taskforce may be needed to ensure that the various departments are represented but the taskforce does not become too large. The ideal number of members on the taskforce is between 5 and 10. When the taskforce is larger than that, meetings may become more of a presentation by the chair than a discussion among the group.

Responsibilities of the Steering Committee

The steering committee is responsible for creating the program vision, mission, goals, and objectives, as well as monitoring the progress of the program implementation and removing operational roadblocks that may occur if the clinic or medical staff leaders do not adopt the CDI program.

The committee has the following five primary responsibilities (Hess 2015):

- *Obtain and maintain medical staff support*. The steering committee should encourage support of the outpatient CDI program by both formal and informal medical staff leaders in the outpatient setting.
- *Create a chain of command to manage uncooperative physicians*. If physicians do not adapt to CDI initiatives, the CDI taskforce may request that steering committee leadership have one-on-one meetings with these physicians to answer questions, provide information on goals and objectives, and encourage adoption of the program.

- *Support the program financially.* The steering committee ensures that adequate resources such as office space, computer equipment, program managers, and CDS staff are available to implement the program throughout the ambulatory clinic and professional practice settings.
- *Determine key metrics to be reviewed at the strategic level.* To assess the ROI and sustainability of the CDI program, the committee will want to monitor ambulatory CDI targets such as Hierarchical Condition Category (HCC) capture rates, lower denial rates, and decreased charge capture issues as related to the quality of clinical documentation.
- *Provide feedback to the CDI taskforce.* The steering committee can provide strategic insights into issues such as CDI program communication efforts, medical staff adoption progress, and resource allocation.

Table 8.1 presents a detailed task list for the steering committee discussions; it uses a phased approach and identifies the frequency of committee meetings during each phase. By dividing the tasks into phases, the committee members can recognize accomplishments at the end of each phase and encourage participants in the CDI program to move on to the next phase. After the full implementation of the CDI program in all clinics and practices, the steering committee should continue to meet on a quarterly basis to monitor program metrics, review new focused CDI targets, discuss roadblocks, and develop high-level recommendations for program expansion and solutions.

Table 8.1. Phases in outpatient CDI steering committee task discussions

Phase	Tasks	Frequency of Meetings
Establish governance and oversight committee	Invite stakeholders to steering committee meetings	Monthly
	Introduce committee members	
	Discuss a group vision	
	Create a mission statement	
	Set measurable goals	
	Identify objectives	
Develop workplan	Agree on necessary steps	Monthly
	Craft a detailed workplan	
	Assign workplan responsibilities	
	Identify additional resource requirements	
Implement CDI in pilot site	Implement CDI program at pilot site	Monthly
	Discuss achievements and challenges	
	Revise goals and objectives as needed	
Implement CDI in additional clinic and physician practices	Implement programs in remaining clinics and professional practices	Bimonthly
	Monitor progress (metrics)	
	Implement redesign as required	
Monitor the ongoing outpatient CDI program	Continual oversight of the outpatient CDI program	Quarterly

Responsibilities of the Outpatient CDI Taskforce

The seven major responsibilities of the outpatient CDI taskforce are as follows (Hess 2015):

- *Hire and train the outpatient CDS manager and staff.* This responsibility includes making decisions about the skill sets and credentials necessary for the outpatient CDS job description (see chapter 12 for sample job description).

- *Oversee the training of physicians and other clinicians in the clinic as well as the physician practice.* To ensure physician adoption of the program, the taskforce engages physicians through initial one-on-one discussions and observes the clinic or practice clinical documentation process and charge capture workflow.

- *Implement and oversee activities to obtain high-quality clinical documentation.* Members of the taskforce participate in activities such as physician shadowing; previsit, concurrent, and postvisit case review; and metrics data collection and reporting. Refer to chapter 12 for more information on the CDS case review process.

- *Evaluate the program against its metrics and establish new areas of CDI focus.* Committee members review program data analyses to assess whether outcomes achieve program goals, and they discuss concurrent and future areas of CDI focus as certain issues are resolved and a new set of focused targets in the outpatient CDI workflow are selected.

- *Supervise the design of functions to audit and improve clinical documentation.* The taskforce oversees the establishment of an internal monitoring and external audit program to ensure the accuracy of code assignments, charge capture, and high-quality clinical documentation.

- *Supervise the design of follow-up training for physicians.* The methodology used for physician education is critical for program success. Considerations include who will be the educator (physician colleague, CDS, or both); whether education will be done one-on-one or in a specialty group setting; and the approval process for program content (prior approval by a specialty-specific physician leader is recommended).

- *Report on key metrics to the governance committee.* This should include preparing a slide presentation with an executive overview and pertinent detail with supporting metrics and graphics in a dashboard format.

The phases outlined previously for the steering committee also apply to the CDI taskforce. However, the level of detail in the CDI taskforce's task list is greater, and its work steps more extensive. These work steps are discussed in detail in chapter 9.

The frequency of CDI taskforce meetings will vary depending on the phase of implementation (see table 8.2). The meeting frequency may be revised to accommodate the tasks and challenges incurred during the implementation process.

Table 8.2. Taskforce meeting frequency

Meeting Frequency	Implementation Phase
Weekly	I: Establishment of taskforce
Weekly	II: Workplan development
Weekly	III: Pilot site implementation
Weekly	IV: Full clinic and physician practice rollout
Monthly	V: Ongoing monitoring of outpatient CDI program

CDI Program Vision, Mission, Goals, and Objectives

Each new program to be rolled out at a hospital or health system should have a corresponding vision, mission, goals, and objectives. Even if the outpatient CDI program is being added to an existing inpatient CDI program, an outpatient CDI vision statement is needed because outpatient CDI differs from inpatient CDI in terms of organizational reach, stakeholders, workplan tasks, and program areas of focus.

One of the most substantial challenges when creating the vision, mission, goals, and objectives of the outpatient CDI program is bringing together a group of leaders to discuss the process. Once the leaders are gathered in one room, it is incumbent on the CDI steering committee chair to ensure that the meeting is organized, interesting, and fruitful—which is not always an easy task. The chair's role is not to tell the group exactly what the vision, mission, goals, and objectives will be, but to facilitate a discussion that leads to a shared philosophy and methodology for moving forward. The University of Maine Cooperative Extension (2004) has published a methodology for this process to make the group productive and not only create a vision, mission, goals, and objectives but also develop a practical plan of action. At the start of the meeting, all participants should introduce themselves. These introductions help the steering committee see how its various members can effect change within the organization.

Vision Statement

After introductions, a good way to begin the meeting is to discuss the purpose of the meeting and how the steering committee will achieve the goal of a new outpatient CDI program. This discussion can be orchestrated by encouraging the steering committee members to address the following questions (University of Maine Cooperative Extension 2004):

- Where have we been?
- Where are we now?
- Where do we want to be?
- How do we want to get there?
- How will we know when we have arrived at our destination?

Although these questions are fairly simplistic, they are thought-provoking and will allow each committee member to share his or her insights into the current state of clinical documentation and ideas about how the CDI program can move forward. As the discussion progresses, participants should begin to see themselves as a group and realize that this group has the power to realize their ideas and aspirations together.

The first task that the steering committee will tackle is the development of a vision statement: "The vision embodies people's highest values and aspirations. It inspires people to reach for what could be and to rise above their fears and preoccupations with current reality" (University of Maine Cooperative Extension 2004). The **vision statement** clearly and concisely describes the purpose of the group and why that purpose is important, is directional and future-focused, reflects the values of each stakeholder, and includes images that "bring the vision to life" (University of Maine Cooperative Extension 2004). The vision statement may be short or long, depending on the desires of the committee. An example of a vision statement for the outpatient CDI program could be as follows:

> Clinical documentation is at the core of every patient encounter. To be meaningful, the documentation must be accurate and timely and reflect the scope of services provided. Successful clinical documentation improvement (CDI) programs facilitate the accurate representation of a patient's clinical status that translates into coded data. Coded data are then translated into quality reporting, physician report cards, reimbursement, public health data, and disease tracking and trending. The convergence of clinical, documentation, and coding processes is vital to a healthy revenue cycle and, more importantly, to a healthy ambulatory services patient. To that end, outpatient CDI has a direct impact on patient care in the ambulatory setting by providing clinical information to all members of the care team, as well as those downstream who may be treating the patient at a later date (AHIMA 2017a).

The chair of the CDI steering committee is responsible for facilitating the development of the vision statement. At the stakeholder meeting, the attendees can break into smaller groups to discuss and document their ideas about how to word the vision statement. After they put their ideas down on paper, each group then presents them for discussion by everyone at the meeting. The vision statement could also include a visual depiction of the program vision. An example of this type of graphic is shown in figure 8.1. The figure displays the CDI program surrounded by the various tenets of outpatient CDI, such as a clinical record that is legible, reliable, precise, complete, consistent, clear, timely, and patient-centered (see chapter 1). The final selection of the vision statement should be made via committee vote, with final approval by the executive decision maker (CEO or CFO).

Mission Statement

A **mission statement** is "a written statement that sets forth the core purpose and philosophies of an organization or group; [it] defines the organization or group's general purpose for existing" (AHIMA 2017b). Like a vision statement, a mission statement looks at the big picture, but a mission statement expresses the vision in more concrete, outcome-oriented terms that are intended to inspire people to action (Center for Community Health and Development 2017). In other words, it explains, in general terms, how the group or organization will

Figure 8.1. CDI across the continuum of care

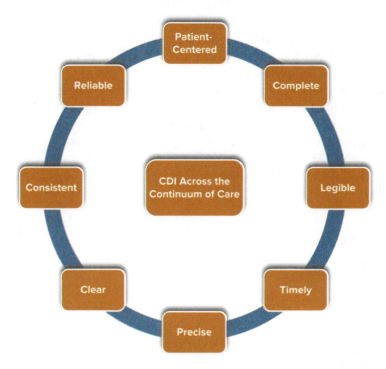

achieve a shared vision with regard to the following three objectives (University of Maine Cooperative Extension 2004):

- What will be done
- For whom will it be done
- How will it be done

Thus, the mission statement sets the direction for the CDI program and reflects the values and beliefs of its leadership. The statement should be clear, concise, realistic, inspirational, and action-oriented. For example, a mission statement for the outpatient CDI program might be, "The mission of the Memorial Hospital CDI program is to improve the quality of clinical documentation in the ambulatory setting so as to facilitate provider collaboration and ensure that the clinical information needed to achieve high-quality care and accurate reimbursement is shared throughout the EHR network." The wording of the mission statement should be chosen via a committee vote, with final approval by the executive decision maker (CEO or CFO).

Goals and Objectives

Goals are statements that explain what the program will accomplish. A goal is a destination rather than a measurement of the program's achievements. Goals present the results of program activities but do not provide extensive details. Goals provide a direction for the program and can be considered a foundation for the objectives development process (MNDOH 2017).

The outpatient CDI steering committee should create goals that are broad enough to include the overall mission ahead but also concise and inclusive of the short-, intermediate-, and long-range goals for the program. These goals should be "believable, attainable, and based on identified needs" (University of Maine Cooperative Extension 2004). For example, a broad goal for the outpatient CDI program could be to communicate the importance of high-quality clinical documentation for the purposes of improving quality of patient care and provider collaboration, reflecting accurate patient severity, and ensuring accurate billing and reimbursement.

Objectives are specific, measurable, achievable steps to meet the goal within a given time frame (MNDOH 2017). Objectives focus on changing behavior, circumstances, and establishment of a process to meet specific goals (University of Maine Cooperative Extension 2004).

A helpful mnemonic used for making objectives more powerful and measurable is called **SMART** (Tulane University School of Public Health and Tropical Medicine n.d.):

- Specific
- Measurable
- Attainable
- Relevant
- Time-bound

Case Example

After establishing the vision and mission for the CDI program, the steering committee meets in January to discuss the program goals and objectives. The executive leadership expects the program to have a tight time frame, so the committee chair encourages the members to set all goals and objectives in this meeting, if possible. After discussion, committee members agree that the primary goal will be to develop and implement a program to improve clinical documentation in the ambulatory setting by December of the current year.

Next, the committee turns to the task of defining objectives for this goal. Committee members use the SMART mnemonic and the following questions to discuss each objective thoroughly.

- What will be done?
- To what extent?
- By whom? (Who is involved in meeting the objective?)
- By when?

Each of these questions offers direction for the group discussion and encourages a thorough consideration of the objective and how to achieve it. Through this exercise, the group can identify specific, measurable, and obtainable objectives. After the discussion, the committee arrives at the following objectives to meet the goal they have set.

- Create a taskforce to oversee the outpatient CDI program by May.
- Develop a vision and mission statements and corresponding goals and objectives by June.
- Create an action plan for outpatient CDI program implementation that aligns with the vision and mission statements provided by the steering committee by July.

- Identify three pilot clinics or physician practices and begin the CDI program implementation in August.
- Clarify the implementation tasks and complete implementation of the new outpatient CDI program in the three pilot clinics or practices by October.
- Develop the rollout plan for CDI in the remaining clinics and practices by November.
- Begin implementation of CDI program in the remaining clinics by December.

Each program will customize its goals and objectives to fit the organization, practice patterns, clinic operational workflow, and political environment. Setting target completion dates helps to achieve goals and objectives because key stakeholders can track them on their calendars.

As the previous case example shows, goals can involve short-, intermediate-, and long-term objectives. These categories should be considered during the planning stage of the program. The participants in the goal-setting process should understand that intermediate- and long-term objectives will be planned from the outset; however, based on resources and factors that may be outside the control of the participants, these longer-term objectives may need revision.

Case Example

The CDI steering committee sets a goal is to develop an effective outpatient CDI process in all facility-owned provider practices within a one-year period. Then, in the sixth month of the program, a major payer changes the reimbursement methodology to a risk-based plan, and revenue at the health system drops unexpectedly and significantly. To address this financial shortfall, the CFO freezes hiring for outpatient CDI staff positions. Because of these unforeseen events, the CDI program goals and objectives must change.

Organizational Communication

As discussed in other chapters, buy-in by leaders in the clinic, professional practice, and supporting departments is essential to successfully improve the clinical documentation workflow and establish effective communication to clinic staff and providers about CDI. Therefore, one of the primary responsibilities of the outpatient CDI steering committee is effective, strategic communication about CDI to those people within the facility, health system, and network of clinics and professional practices who will be affected by the program.

The most considerable challenge in a CDI program is effective communication to the medical staff. Without medical staff adoption, the program will not be effective. For this reason, careful consideration should be given to how the communication will occur. The organization should consider the following three key concepts in communication (Hess 2015):

- *Who communicates?* Typically, the communication announcing the new outpatient CDI program will come from the CEO of the organization to the department directors and medical staff leaders. In addition, the CMO may also communicate details and support of the program to the medical staff. As the program proceeds, periodic communications from executive leaders about CDI will demonstrate their commitment to high-quality clinical documentation and sustain a high level of visibility for the program. For example, progress reports from the executive leaders communicated during existing department and medical staff meetings, as well as in newsletters and on the intranet, can continue the momentum started at the beginning of the program.

- *How will information be communicated?* The program may be communicated in a variety of ways and through various media, such as a formal letter to the medical staff, announcements in the facility newsletter or on the intranet, and discussions at key department and medical staff meetings.
- *What is communicated?* To encourage adoption of the CDI program, the specific information that is communicated should address why the program is being established; the vision, mission, goals, and objectives of the program; who will be affected by the program; high-level steps; and the time frame for program rollout. Publication of program metrics by specialty or clinic can encourage healthy competition among departments and providers. Above all, communications to promote adoption of the CDI program should stress the benefits of CDI and address specialty-specific concerns. Narratives such as the ones in figure 8.2 can be used in newsletters, flyers, meeting agendas, and the intranet to encourage provider buy-in of the new process.

Figure 8.2. Benefits of outpatient CDI

Benefits of Outpatient CDI

Improved quality of clinical documentation for patient care using rapid feedback loop: The Outpatient CDI program workflow allows for rapid communication with the provider to improve the quality of the clinical record by adding diagnostic and treatment specificity. The use of customized provider communication via e-mail, personal mobile device, EHR menus, prompts, alerts, tasks, and notes presents the query at the time of the outpatient encounter.

Improved charge capture, accurate claims submission and reimbursement. The Outpatient CDI process identifies root cause for missing charges due to lack of clinical record specificity, coding, or charge capture issues and develops a streamlined provider-friendly solution. Accurate billing and reimbursement benefit both patients and providers.

Improved care coordination. Quality clinical documentation improves the patient experience throughout the continuum of care from the inpatient, outpatient, physician practice, and other healthcare settings. Inconsistencies in diagnostic and treatment information are corrected, resulting in an accurate complete clinical record.

In addition to identifying the benefits of CDI, communications to encourage medical staff adoption should address the staff's apprehensions about the potential downsides of CDI. Providers may believe that insufficient resources, time, and staff make CDI impractical or impossible. Communications about the CDI program should reassure them that every possible effort will be made to streamline the case review and query process according to the provider specifications and without major disruptions in the provider and staff workflow.

Along with messages from organization executives, communication among colleagues can foster the success of the CDI program. Physician advisors to the CDI program, as well as informal medical staff leaders, should be invited to provider discussion groups so that they can share their experiences and encourage other physicians to embrace the benefits of CDI. Many providers would welcome an improved workflow but may not be aware of the various options available to help them with clinical documentation.

Outpatient CDI Program Implementation Strategies

As the CDI program's steering committee and taskforce begin the process of setting goals and objectives for the outpatient CDI program, their strategies will be shaped by whether the program is completely new, a customization of an inpatient program or an ongoing outpatient program, or the expansion of an existing outpatient program to include additional clinics or practices.

Where outpatient CDI has not been previously implemented at a facility, a complete CDI program implementation is required. Refer to chapter 10 for more information about this process.

Customization of an Existing CDI Program

Healthcare entities that have an existing inpatient CDI program have several options for customizing the program to include the outpatient setting. To select the best option, the following issues about the type of CDI program needed going forward, as well as the organizational and governance structure that will best support the program, must be evaluated:

- Will the outpatient CDI program be incorporated into the existing inpatient CDI program?
- Who will lead the outpatient CDI program?
- If the outpatient CDI program is separate from the inpatient program, will it include both outpatient facility clinics and outpatient professional practices, or will the program be further subdivided?
- Will the program expand into other outpatient facility departments such as the ED or observation services?

The answers to these questions will be based largely on the size of the organization and the complexity of the clinics and practices within it. If an outpatient clinic is part of a large health system and is run as a separate operation, it may be more feasible to separate the inpatient and outpatient CDI programs. If a large outpatient clinic operates under a separate faculty practice plan or other physician network, it may be more effective to separate the outpatient clinic and professional fee CDI programs. However, because the billing and clinical documentation processes in different settings often overlap, consideration should be given to combining programs where day-to-day workflows and documentation processes are integrated.

As discussed in chapter 6, a CDI program often begins in a few pilot clinics or professional practices before being rolled out to all clinics and practices. After the CDI program is successfully implemented in all outpatient clinics and professional practices in a health system, a logical next step may be to expand CDI to the ED and observation services department. High-quality documentation in these settings not only improves outpatient clinical documentation but also improves inpatient clinical documentation when patients are admitted through the ED or observation department. Refer to chapter 16 of this text for more information on CDI in the ED and observation department.

Decisions about customizing the implementation and ongoing management of the outpatient CDI program should be based on an assessment of the available resources and the maturity of the program itself. The CDI taskforce can determine the appropriate model based on the answers to the following questions:

- Is this a new or existing outpatient CDI program?
- What are the existing and proposed components of the program? (For example, outpatient clinic, facility-owned physician practice, private practice, ED)
- How long has each component program been in existence?
- Is the component program effective?
- If it is ineffective, what are the primary challenges?
- What are the primary payers and types of contracts? (For example, risk-based HCC, physician fee schedule, or bundled services)
- What is the annual outpatient volume for each clinic, provider, and practice by payer?
- What are the provider types by specialty and clinic location?
- Are adequate outpatient CDS staff available to cover all clinics and practices?
- What are the skill sets of existing CDS staff and which clinics or practices do they cover?
- What is the process and timing of CDS case review?
- What is the process for CDS staff physician queries?
- Who tracks the query responses to ensure timely billing?

After these questions are answered and discussed, a decision can be made by the CDI steering committee and executive decision makers (CEO or CFO) regarding the outpatient CDI program support required.

Implementation of a Redesigned Outpatient CDI Program

Where an existing outpatient CDI program is in place, a program redesign may be required to expand the program to additional clinics and physician practices. In this scenario, the governance structure of the program should already be in place, and the basic CDI processes for education, data collection, and analytics tracking may also be in place. However, the volume and type of services, as well as the payer mix, in the additional clinics and practices must be evaluated to determine the type of case review required as well as the number of CDS staff and types of skill sets needed. In addition, development of specialty-specific educational materials and clinic- or practice-specific case review and query processes may be required.

Whether the program is new, ongoing, or redesigned, the implementation strategies should always reflect the vision and mission established by program leadership. Figure 8.3 depicts the path to CDI program success, beginning with the creation of a shared vision. The chapters that follow elaborate on other steps along this path.

Figure 8.3. Path to CDI program success

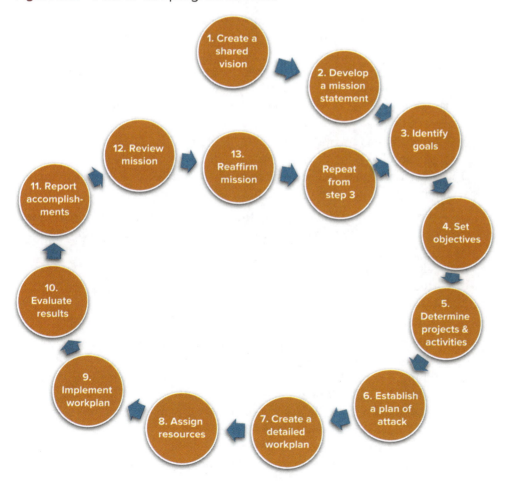

Chapter 8 Review Exercises

1. The CDI steering committee, also called the *governance committee*, is responsible for determining the CDI program implementation model that best suits the organization or health system. Which of the following does *not* represent an implementation model from which the CDI steering committee may choose?
   a. Hybrid model
   b. Program redesign
   c. Outsourced model
   d. New program implementation

2. A meeting of the key stakeholders should be held to discuss the program vision, mission, goals, and objectives. The list of participating leaders may vary depending on the organization but may include the CFO and the _____.
   a. CMO
   b. Chief marketing officer
   c. Director, strategy and budget
   d. Vice president, network development

3. The members of a healthcare facility's CDI taskforce have been meeting regularly for several months. The taskforce has recently agreed to significantly reduce the frequency of these meetings. What is the *most* likely explanation for this change?
   a. Several unexpected challenges related to program implementation have recently arisen.
   b. The taskforce has deemed frequent meetings to be an ineffective component of the CDI program.
   c. The facility has encountered a financial shortfall and CDI program implementation has been deprioritized.
   d. The CDI program has been successfully rolled out and the less demanding program-monitoring phase has commenced.

4. Once the stakeholder leaders are gathered in one room, it is incumbent on the steering committee chair to make the meeting organized, interesting, and _____.
   a. Brief
   b. Virtual
   c. Fruitful
   d. Normative

5. The difference in the implementation phases for the two primary parts of the governance structure is _____.
   a. Nothing. There are no differences in the phases for the steering committee and the CDI taskforce.
   b. The CDI taskforce will have a more detailed task list, and the work steps of the CDI taskforce will be more extensive.
   c. The steering committee will have a more detailed task list, and the work steps of the steering committee will be more extensive.
   d. The steering committee will cease meeting once the program is fully implemented, whereas the CDI taskforce will continue to meet quarterly.

6. Which of the following is likely to present the *most* substantial challenge to creating vision, mission, goals, and objectives of the outpatient CDI program?
    a. Writing SMART objectives
    b. Establishing a methodology for creation
    c. Bringing together a group of leaders to discuss the process
    d. Asking thought-provoking questions to encourage insights into the current state

7. One possible strategy for implementing outpatient CDI is to customize an inpatient CDI program or ongoing outpatient program, and certain questions can help guide the decision-making process about the customization options. Answers to these questions will be based primarily on _____.
    a. The governance structure to be decided
    b. Expansion to the ED and observation services department
    c. The maturity of the inpatient program or already established outpatient program
    d. The size of the organization and the complexity of the clinics and practices involved

8. The mission statement offers a solution to how a group or organization will achieve its shared vision. The statement is a tool that will achieve three objectives: what will be done, for whom will it be done, and _____.
    a. How will it be done
    b. Why it will be done
    c. When it will be done
    d. By whom it will be done

9. Even if there is an existing inpatient CDI program and the outpatient component is being added, there remains a need for an outpatient CDI _____ statement, as the components and stakeholders in outpatient CDI are very different in terms of organizational reach, workplan tasks, and program areas of focus.
    a. Vision
    b. Values
    c. Cost-benefit
    d. Strategic planning

10. After goals have been established and objectives have been set, the next step in a CDI program that is on the path to success is to _____.
    a. Assign resources
    b. Create a detailed workplan
    c. Review its mission statement
    d. Determine projects and activities

References

American Health Information Management Association (AHIMA). 2017a. Clinical documentation improvement: Overview. http://www.ahima.org/topics/cdi.

American Health Information Management Association (AHIMA). 2017b. *Pocket Glossary of Health Information Management and Technology.* 5th ed. Chicago: AHIMA.

Center for Community Health and Development, University of Kansas. 2017. Chapter 8, Section 2: Proclaiming your dream: Developing vision and mission statements. In: *The Community Tool Box.* http://ctb.ku.edu/en/table-of-contents/structure/strategic-planning/vision-mission-statements/main.

Hess, P. 2015. *Clinical Documentation Improvement: Principles and Practice.* Chicago: AHIMA.

Minnesota Department of Health (MNDoH). 2017. SMART objectives. http://www.health.state.mn.us/divs/opi/qi/toolbox/objectives.html.

Tulane University School of Public Health and Tropical Medicine. Tulane Center of Excellence in Maternal and Child Health. n.d. Tips for writing goals and objectives. https://www2.tulane.edu/publichealth/mchltp/upload/Tips-for-writing-goals-and-objectives.pdf.

University of Maine Cooperative Extension. 2004. Vision, mission, goals & objectives...Oh My! Group Works: Getting Things Done in Groups bulletin 6107. https://extension.umaine.edu/publications/wp-content/uploads/sites/82/2015/04/6107.pdf.

Creating Interdisciplinary CDI Leadership Teams in the Outpatient Healthcare Setting

Learning Objectives

- Describe why an interdisciplinary team approach is required for outpatient clinical documentation improvement (CDI).
- Reinforce the roles of the key stakeholders in the CDI program.
- Discuss how to create a collaborative CDI team.
- Identify the primary functions of the interdisciplinary CDI team.

Key Terms

Chief financial officer (CFO)
Chief information officer (CIO)
Chief medical officer (CMO)
Executive sponsor
Interdisciplinary team
Practice plan administrator

The success of the outpatient clinical documentation improvement (CDI) program requires an **interdisciplinary team** of subject matter experts and leaders that represent the many specialties, locations, and types of healthcare delivery settings involved in clinical documentation. "Interdisciplinary teamwork is increasingly prevalent, supported by policies and practices that bring care closer to the patient and challenge traditional professional boundaries" (Nancarrow et al. 2013). Chapter 8 introduced the governance structure of the CDI program, including the responsibilities of the CDI steering committee and taskforce. This chapter looks more closely at how these interdisciplinary teams are built. This endeavor involves the sharing of information, collaboration among team members, and effective communication with providers, clinicians, managers, and ancillary staff involved in the day-to-day clinical documentation, coding, and charge capture activities.

Making the Case for an Interdisciplinary Team

> Interdisciplinary team work is a complex process in which different types of staff work together to share expertise, knowledge, and skills to impact on patient care (Nancarrow et al. 2013).

Because the ultimate goal of high-quality clinical documentation is improved patient care, it stands to reason that the interdisciplinary team is essential to an effective outpatient CDI program. When building the specific type of interdisciplinary team for the program, many factors should be considered including the "skill mix, setting of care, service organization, individual relationships, and management structures" (Nancarrow et al. 2013).

The following definition of the interdisciplinary healthcare team helps shed light on its value for CDI programs (Xyrichis and Ream 2008):

> A dynamic process involving two or more health professionals with complementary backgrounds and skills, sharing common health goals and exercising concerted physical and mental effort in assessing, planning, or evaluating patient care. This is accomplished through interdependent collaboration, open communication and shared decision-making. This in turn generates value-added patient, organizational and staff outcomes.

The need for an interdisciplinary CDI team is further reinforced by the following points (Nancarrow et al. 2013):

- CDI programs must recognize that job functions in the healthcare setting tend to be highly specialized, and each job requires a complex combination of skills and knowledge. Historically, healthcare generalists covered many specialties. In contrast, few healthcare workers today perform broad job functions, and knowledge is fragmented among specialists. Therefore, an interdisciplinary team works best to capture all relevant perspectives. For example, a nurse manager who has worked primarily in cardiology may not have the knowledge base to advise the CDI taskforce on workflow and physician practice patterns in the oncology clinic. Also, a CDI program in a neurology clinic will benefit from including an outpatient clinical documentation specialist (CDS) who has worked in the clinic and has a strong neurology coding background.
- CDI that supports the continuity of care from the inpatient to ambulatory settings requires team members capable of making continuous

improvements in both clinical documentation quality and operational efficiency. For example, because healthcare systems and providers focus on the continuum of patient care from the hospital admission through the patient's transition to the rehabilitation facility and periodic visits back to the outpatient clinic, complete and specific clinical records championed by the outpatient CDS benefit the quality of care in all settings and improve efficiency.

- CDI teams need experts who can review the array of technology options that offer new forms of service delivery and resolve interoperability challenges. For example, the outpatient CDS can contribute to CDI by identifying interoperability problems and working with the stakeholders in information technology (IT), informatics, and clinical sites to improve workflow and develop streamlined solutions.
- Interdisciplinary CDI teams can help overcome changes in organizational values and generational gaps among healthcare professionals and providers that pose challenges to provider practice workflows and the allocation of resources for CDI. For example, as budget-conscious and resource-strapped health systems require that providers see a higher volume of patients than in the past, CDI can demonstrate a return on investment (ROI) by ensuring that providers can work faster, be more efficient, and use fewer resources without compromising the quality of care.

Identifying CDI Team Leaders in the Outpatient Healthcare Organization

The U.S. Bureau of Labor Statistics (BLS) reports that healthcare management is a rapidly growing field. "Employment of medical and health services managers is projected to grow 17 percent from 2014 to 2024, much faster than the average for all occupations," and the fastest growth is to be expected in the outpatient clinic and physician practice settings (BLS 2015). Given the pace of change, the outpatient CDI program must be aligned with other strategic planning and development activities within the hospital or health system so that the program is prepared to provide CDI services as needed for the future. Healthcare organizations today must plan for tasks that are much larger in scope and more complex than any individual can manage. CDI is most effective when it involves an interdisciplinary team of subject matter experts, including those who are familiar with operations and strategy in their areas; those who are experts in their fields of study; and those who can advise about regulatory guidelines, CDI tools, and available IT solutions. During any health system implementation of CDI, those who manage the project should focus on the external and internal domains that will affect the decisions and tasks at hand (Buchbinder and Shanks 2012). Examples of external domains applicable to the outpatient CDI program are regulations for Medicare and Medicaid programs and the rules set by managed care organizations and insurers to govern the claims submission process and reimbursement for services rendered. Examples of internal domains pertinent to new program development are staffing, budget, quality control, physician relationships, financial performance, and technology within the hospital or health system (Buchbinder and Shanks 2012). Notably, individuals with the required expertise in these domains may be found in management positions below the executive or director level. Therefore, when developing the interdisciplinary CDI team, it is important to understand the functional responsibilities that the key leaders will need to represent so that everyone needed on the team can be invited to join.

The organization size and type affect the strategy for the outpatient CDI program. It is incumbent upon the CDI program leadership to understand each organizational level, its roles, and how each part of the organization must work together to ensure organization-wide performance and CDI program organizational viability (Buchbinder and Shanks 2012). Leadership structures at healthcare entities can vary widely based on their patient volumes; specialty case mixes; number and types of facilities, clinics, and practices; and their missions, goals, and objectives. Compared with smaller organizations, larger organizations tend to have more leadership staff and more complex reporting relationships. For example, an academic medical center's leadership organization chart is typically much more complex than that of a community medical center or small hospital. In the academic medical center, the CDI department may be managed by a CDI director who reports to a senior director of health information management (HIM), who reports to a revenue cycle vice president, who reports to the **chief financial officer (CFO)**. The CFO is the executive financial officer for the health system or facility and may also be referred to as the senior vice president (SVP) of finance. In the community medical center, the CDI department may be managed by a supervisor or manager who reports to the HIM director, who reports to the CFO.

Figure 9.1 presents a very high-level organization chart for a moderately complex healthcare entity. The organizational structure is fairly straightforward, with a chief executive officer (CEO) leading a group of SVPs, who lead the major functional groups: internal audit, finance, marketing and sales, operations, human resources, and legal affairs. In this example, the outpatient CDI program could become a part of the revenue integrity department, which reports directly to the CFO, or it could be part of the outpatient clinic organization under the **chief medical officer (CMO)**. The CMO is the chief executive of the medical staff. It is also common to see the outpatient clinics and owned physician practices under an SVP of ambulatory services. In academic hospital settings, physician practices are also often organized under the faculty practice plan leadership. An owned physician practice is one that is owned by the health system or facility rather than by the physicians. Under the organization structure outlined in figure 9.1, the CDI steering committee could include the CEO, SVP of finance, SVP of administrative operations, SVP of hospital operations, CMO, and leaders from revenue integrity, IT, HIM, clinic operations, and quality standards and medical audit (reporting to the SVP of hospital operations). The CDI taskforce could include leaders in HIM, managers of clinic operations, physician practice managers, and physician specialty leaders (see chapter 8 for an overview of the distinctions between the CDI steering committee and CDI taskforce).

Figure 9.2 is another organizational chart that shows the specific departments under each executive leader. In this example, the HIM department reports to the

Figure 9.1. High-level organizational chart for a moderately complex healthcare entity

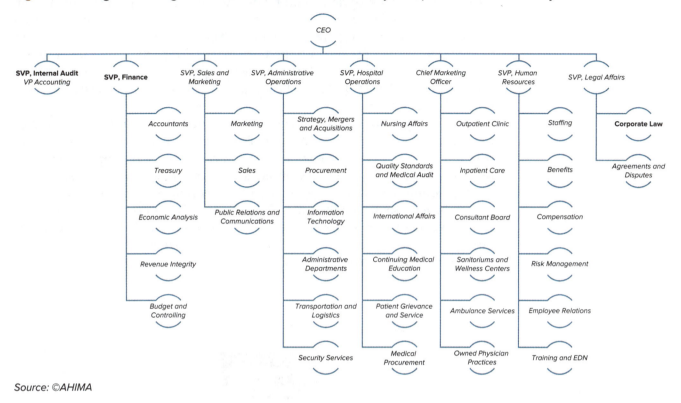

Source: ©AHIMA

Figure 9.2. Healthcare entity organizational chart with dotted-line reporting relationship for the CDI program

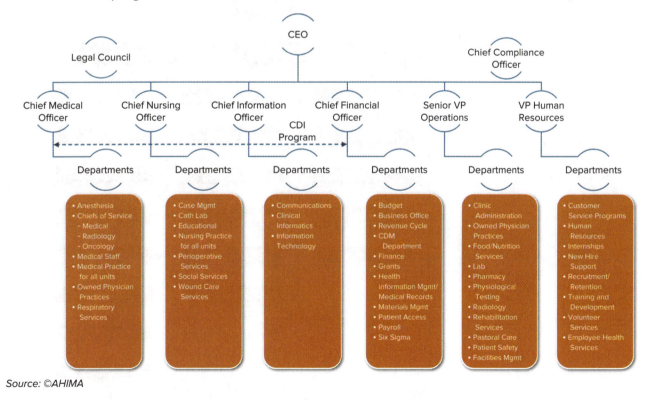

Source: ©AHIMA

SVP of finance, and the clinics report to a different leader, the CMO. Therefore, the outpatient CDI program could report through either organizational leader. If the inpatient and outpatient CDI programs are going to be integrated, the CDI program may be best organized under the CFO, with a dotted-line relationship to the CMO. When there is a dotted-line relationship, the subordinate (HIM director) would report, for administrative purposes, to one of the two senior leaders. But for day-to-day operations, the subordinate would closely collaborate with both leaders.

Figure 9.3 provides an organizational overview of a multihospital, multipractice network that includes rehabilitation centers, skilled and long-term care (LTC) facilities, a dialysis center, and a surgical center. Building an interdisciplinary team that can effectively implement an outpatient CDI program in this setting requires careful consideration of the key roles and responsibilities that need to be represented on the team. The most effective governance model might be to have an overarching steering committee at the health system operations group level and create separate CDI taskforces and subgroups at each hospital and corresponding physician network.

Figure 9.3. Example of an organizational chart for an integrated health system

```
                        Integrated Health System
                                 |
                      Health Systems Operations Group
                                 |
        ┌────────────────────────┼────────────────────────┐
   Hospital Group           LTC Facility Group        Clinic Office Group
        |                        |                        |
    Hospital A               Rehab Center A              Clinic 1
    Hospital B               Rehab Center B              Clinic 2
    Hospital C               Skilled Nursing X           MD Office A
    Trauma Center X          Skilled Nursing Y           MD Office B
    Pediatric Center Y       LTC Facility D              MD Office C
                             LTC Facility E              MD Office D
                                                         Dialysis Ctr A
                                                         Surgical Ctr A
```

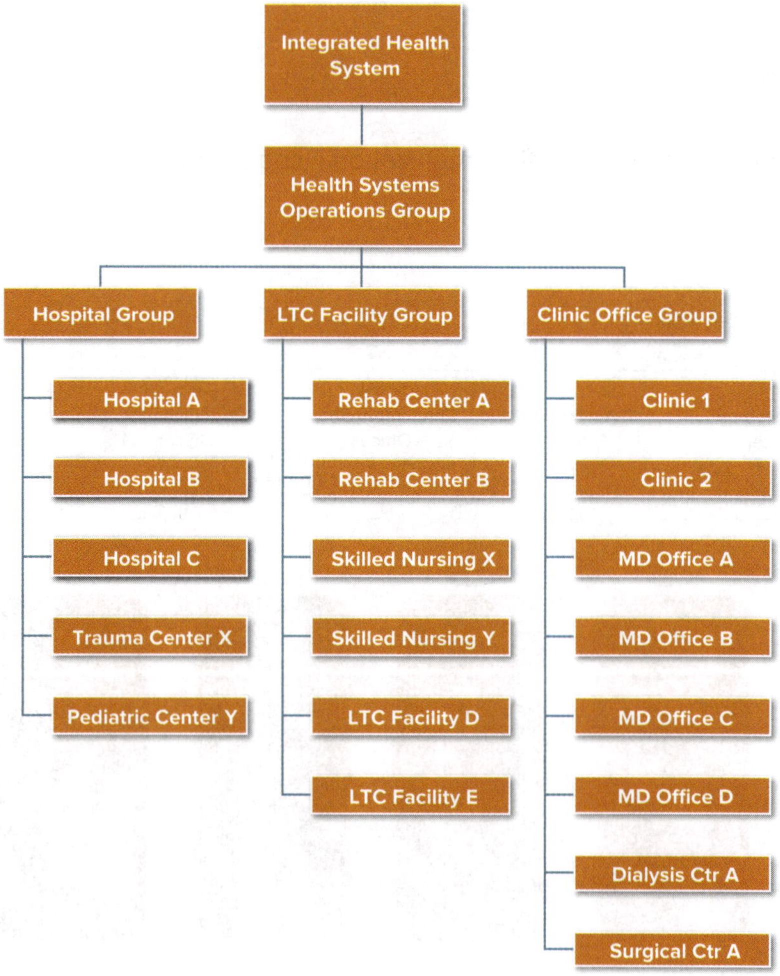

Source: ©AHIMA

Team Member Selection and Roles

Recruitment of the required talent is the first step in the development of the interdisciplinary CDI team, and the availability of each candidate is a formidable consideration when selecting team members. If a key stakeholder is spread too thin and cannot actively contribute to the team's efforts to achieve goals and objectives set forth by the CDI governance structure, that person may not be a suitable team member. Another committed and energetic leader in a similar but lower-level role may be a better choice. For example, the outpatient coding manager may be a good fit if the outpatient HIM director is not available.

Succession planning is also a consideration in team building. The outpatient CDI leader should have a backup committee chair who can lead the team in case the chair is unavailable or needs assistance for specific tasks during the implementation.

Selecting Steering Committee Members

As discussed in chapter 8, the CDI steering committee is an oversight group responsible for ensuring that outpatient CDI program goals and objectives are met and that required resources are available for program success. This committee is also responsible for monitoring the program at a high level and will review executive-level metrics and dashboards to assess the program's success and sustainability. The steering committee members may be asked to intervene on a one-on-one basis when the program encounters roadblocks from the medical staff. The following list describes the steering committee members and their roles on the committee:

- Executive sponsor: The **executive sponsor** can be any one of the organization's top leaders, such as the CEO, chief operations officer (COO), CFO, or HIM director. The executive sponsor provides high-level visibility and endorsement for the program and keeps everyone on track through periodic progress reports. The executive sponsor may also chair the CDI steering committee.
- *Outpatient CDI leader and CDI taskforce chair:* The outpatient CDI leader may also be the leader of the inpatient CDI program when both programs are integrated. If the program is being implemented by a large health system, the systemwide HIM director or vice president is the recommended leader. The HIM director is also recommended as the oversight leader for CDI in a medium to small facility because the director will be the person most likely to have the required expertise in the functionality and integration of multiple electronic health record (EHR) systems, coding, clinical documentation requirements and practice, medical staff collaboration, and other operational issues related to program implementation.
- *CMO:* The participation of the top medical executive in the steering committee serves to foster collaboration with the medical staff. The CMO represents the medical staff's perspectives to the committee, shows the staff why they should support the CDI program, and can intervene and resolve challenges involving changes to provider practice

workflow. The CMO can offer valuable insight into the best way to approach the medical staff about the new program and anticipate challenges so that solutions may be developed before, not during, the implementation.

- **Chief information officer (CIO)** *or IT director*: The CIO is the leader of IT services within the health system or facility. The outpatient CDI steering committee should provide oversight and monitor the progress of IT enhancements, and the IT director or CIO's role on the steering committee is to understand the technological systems related to CDI and how they interface with each other. He or she can assess the functionality of the EHR as well as possible system enhancements, such as templates, alerts, tasks, and notes, that can be used to guide the entry of clinical documentation by physicians and otherwise improve clinical documentation. If outpatient CDI involves multiple EHR systems within the clinic and physician practices, the IT director or CIO can outline any interoperability challenges and explain how the IT department's development team may be able to improve functionality.
- *Ambulatory clinic administrator:* The primary executive leader of clinical operations is essential to the CDI program's success. The clinic administrator can introduce the concept to the clinic managers and encourage cooperation, provide additional resources as needed, and make suggestions about how best to communicate with the medical staff.
- *Provider* **practice plan administrator**: Where there is a separate medical staff practice plan or network, the leader of this organization is critical to the new outpatient CDI program. This executive is a subject matter expert in the operations of the owned medical practice, works collaboratively with the physician specialty leaders, and has a working relationship with most of the physicians in the network. These relationships are valuable during meetings where the outpatient CDI program is being discussed and during one-on-one physician and provider conversations regarding program challenges.
- *HIM director:* As noted above, the HIM director is often the outpatient CDI program leader. Even if that is not the case, the participation of the HIM director on the steering committee is essential because he or she has expertise in coding workflows and guidelines. The HIM director can also help establish the best communication and educational processes between the outpatient CDI program and the coding staff.
- *Quality and compliance director:* This person can offer subject matter expertise on regulatory guidelines for clinical documentation and coding practices as well as recommendations on the program auditing and reporting process.

Selecting CDI Taskforce Members

As discussed in chapter 8, the CDI taskforce is responsible for oversight of the outpatient CDI workplan during implementation, using metrics and reports from individual clinics and practices to monitor program progress on a detailed level, and removing organizational and operational roadblocks that could impede successful implementation. The taskforce should include 5 to 10 members. A group that is too large may make interaction and discussion among the members unwieldy. A group that is too small may not include the subject matter expertise needed for a substantive discussion. In complex healthcare organizations with multiple, large specialty clinics and practices, multiple taskforces may be formed.

The following list describes the CDI taskforce members and their roles on the committee:

- *Outpatient CDI program leader and CDI taskforce chair:* A member of the steering committee, such as the HIM director, should lead the operations of the taskforce. The person in this role is responsible for keeping abreast of all program activities and challenges on a day-to-day basis, scheduling taskforce meetings, developing presentation materials, reporting on the progress of the program at taskforce and steering committee meetings, and recommending solutions for issues facing the program.
- *Clinic administrative manager:* The clinic administrative manager plays a prominent role in the success of the outpatient CDI program and will be a liaison between the taskforce and the medical, nursing, and CDS staff at the clinics. The CDI leader should meet with the clinic administrative manager one-on-one before the taskforce meeting to explain goals and objectives and discuss concerns and potential challenges to operationalizing the program.
- *Clinic nurse manager:* The clinic nurse manager may also be the clinic administrative manager. Where these functions are separate, the clinic nurse manager will communicate with the nurses in the outpatient clinic and provide support to the CDI program as it relates to nursing care. Nurses play a significant role in clinical documentation as they assist with the query process and communication between the physicians and CDSs. In the CDI program, nurses may help identify the patients to include in the case review process. Refer to chapter 6 of this text for more information on the case review process. For example, if smoking cessation is being captured as a Merit-Based Incentive Payment System (MIPS) measure, the nurse can identify patients who smoke, remind the provider to document details of discussions with the patient about tobacco use, and notify the outpatient CDS to perform a postvisit case review. Refer to chapter 4 for more information about the MIPS program.
- *Provider practice manager:* Where the provider practice manager and clinic administrative manager are separate roles, the provider practice manager will lead the efforts to implement the outpatient CDI program in the practice. The CDI leader should meet with the provider practice manager one-on-one to present the program concepts and discuss streamlined operationalization of the program in the practice. The buy-in of the provider practice manager is essential to success because the practice workflow may be redesigned to accommodate the CDI program, and the practice manager can help ensure that these changes are accepted by the providers and practice staff.

- *HIM director:* As noted earlier, even if the HIM director is not the outpatient CDI leader/taskforce chair, he or she should be a member of both the taskforce and the steering committee. In large facilities, the director may delegate representation of the HIM department at taskforce meetings to the coding manager.

- *Coding manager:* The coding manager is, of course, a key stakeholder in the outpatient CDI program because the focus of the program is to improve clinical documentation, charge capture, and the accuracy of claims submission. The coding manager will spearhead efforts to improve specificity in clinical documentation, manage system edits, reduce claims denials, and educate coding staff. He or she will also provide feedback from the coding staff about root causes of documentation problems.

- *Representatives of the outpatient CDS staff:* If multiple CDSs work in a clinic or practice, at least one representative from the group should attend the taskforce meetings to provide insight into the day-to-day operations, effectiveness, and efficiency of the CDI program. To ensure a full range of perspectives, CDSs representing specific areas and specialties can participate in meetings on a rotating basis. The outpatient CDS may provide education to coders and physicians and should be part of the planning for group educational sessions.

Fostering Collaborative Team Dynamics

Collaboration among team members is the most important component of the team process (Nancarrow et al. 2013), but it may be particularly challenging on an interdisciplinary team that represents many points of view and has potentially divergent priorities. To build a collaborative team, the outpatient CDI leadership should model and encourage in team members the attitudes and behaviors that are most likely to help the team establish a positive group identity and culture. Some attributes for leaders to foster in team members are competency, confidence, commitment to the project's mission and the team, respect for other people and their points of view, trust, patience, relationship building, shared decision-making skills, and a willingness to share leadership responsibilities (Nancarrow et al. 2013). If team members have worked together closely in the past, they may already respect and trust each other and recognize one another's competencies. However, even if that is the case, it will take time and work to build positive relationships among all team members and create a collaborative and supportive group dynamic.

Ten characteristics of a good outpatient CDI team are shown in figure 9.4. The outpatient CDI leadership can use these characteristics as a guide to team development and education as the group works together over time. As with any group, the CDI team will inevitably engage in "give and take" during the decision-making process. The outpatient CDI leadership must be able to facilitate difficult conversations when committee members do not agree or where objectives are at cross-purposes. Having a collaborative group will promote a good outcome when these challenges arise.

Figure 9.4. Ten characteristics of a good CDI team

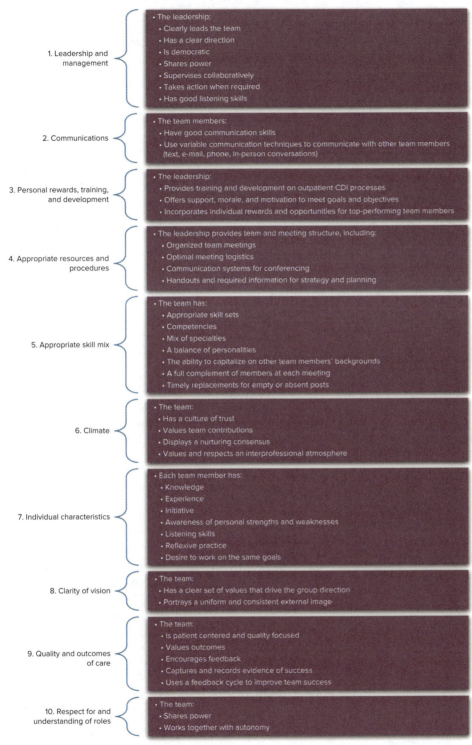

1. Leadership and management
   - The leadership:
     - Clearly leads the team
     - Has a clear direction
     - Is democratic
     - Shares power
     - Supervises collaboratively
     - Takes action when required
     - Has good listening skills

2. Communications
   - The team members:
     - Have good communication skills
     - Use variable communication techniques to communicate with other team members (text, e-mail, phone, in-person conversations)

3. Personal rewards, training, and development
   - The leadership:
     - Provides training and development on outpatient CDI processes
     - Offers support, morale, and motivation to meet goals and objectives
     - Incorporates individual rewards and opportunities for top-performing team members

4. Appropriate resources and procedures
   - The leadership provides team and meeting structure, including:
     - Organized team meetings
     - Optimal meeting logistics
     - Communication systems for conferencing
     - Handouts and required information for strategy and planning

5. Appropriate skill mix
   - The team has:
     - Appropriate skill sets
     - Competencies
     - Mix of specialties
     - A balance of personalities
     - The ability to capitalize on other team members' backgrounds
     - A full complement of members at each meeting
     - Timely replacements for empty or absent posts

6. Climate
   - The team:
     - Has a culture of trust
     - Values team contributions
     - Displays a nurturing consensus
     - Values and respects an interprofessional atmosphere

7. Individual characteristics
   - Each team member has:
     - Knowledge
     - Experience
     - Initiative
     - Awareness of personal strengths and weaknesses
     - Listening skills
     - Reflexive practice
     - Desire to work on the same goals

8. Clarity of vision
   - The team:
     - Has a clear set of values that drive the group direction
     - Portrays a uniform and consistent external image

9. Quality and outcomes of care
   - The team:
     - Is patient centered and quality focused
     - Values outcomes
     - Encourages feedback
     - Captures and records evidence of success
     - Uses a feedback cycle to improve team success

10. Respect for and understanding of roles
    - The team:
      - Shares power
      - Works together with autonomy

Source: Adapted from Nancarrow et al. 2013.

Chapter 9 Review Exercises

1. Healthcare management is a rapidly growing field and is projected to grow much faster than the average for all occupations. In which of the following settings is the fastest growth expected?
    a. Urgent care
    b. Inpatient care
    c. Walk-in clinic
    d. Outpatient clinic

2. The executive sponsor of the steering committee can be any one of the organization's top leaders, such as the CEO or COO. Which of the following individuals would be *best* suited for the executive sponsor role on the steering committee?
    a. Chief medical officer
    b. Chief financial officer
    c. Chief marketing officer
    d. Chief medical informatics officer

3. Which of the following individuals provides high-level visibility and endorsement for the outpatient CDI program and keeps everyone on track through periodic progress reports?
    a. HIM director
    b. Executive sponsor
    c. Outpatient CDI leader
    d. Provider practice plan administrator

4. Who among the following would be included on the steering committee for his or her subject matter expertise on the regulatory guidelines related to clinical documentation and coding practices?
    a. IT director
    b. HIM director
    c. Coding manager
    d. Quality and compliance director

5. In a collaborative team, certain attitudes and behaviors help the team to establish a positive group identification and culture. Which of the following characteristics is demonstrated by a team that shares power and works together while maintaining autonomy?
    a. Climate
    b. Clarity of vision
    c. Leadership and management
    d. Respect for and understanding of roles

6. Where there is a separate medical staff practice plan or network, the provider practice plan administrator should be part of the outpatient CDI program's _____.
    a. Taskforce
    b. Steering committee
    c. Both the taskforce and steering committee
    d. Neither the taskforce nor the steering committee

7. How a CDI team communicates is one of the characteristics that determine the team's quality. A good CDI team includes members who _____.
   a. Communicate primarily via e-mail
   b. Use variable communication techniques
   c. Limit communication about low-importance topics
   d. Hold postgraduate degrees in communications or a related field

8. Positive quality and outcomes of care are among the characteristics that define a good CDI team. A team that exemplifies this characteristic will be patient centered and quality focused, value outcomes, encourage feedback, capture and record evidence of success, and _____.
   a. Share power
   b. Have experience
   c. Provide training and development
   d. Use a feedback cycle to improve team success

9. The CDI taskforce should include _____ members. A larger group may result in lack of true interaction and discussion among the members.
   a. 2–3
   b. 3–5
   c. 5–10
   d. 12–15

10. Due to factors such as increasingly complex organizational operations, evolving technology, and specialization of job functions, an effective outpatient CDI program should emphasize _____ teamwork among its staff.
    a. Interactive
    b. Interpersonal
    c. Interdisciplinary
    d. Interdepartmental

References

Buchbinder, S. and N. Shanks. 2012. *Introduction to Health Care Management*. Burlington, MA: Jones & Bartlett Learning.

Nancarrow, S.A., A. Booth, S. Ariss, T. Smith, P. Enderby, and A. Roots. 2013. Ten principles of good interdisciplinary team work. *Human Resources for Health* 11:19. doi: 10.1186/1478-4491-11-19.

U.S. Bureau of Labor Statistics (BLS). 2015. Quick facts: medical and health services managers. Occupational Outlook Handbook. https://www.bls.gov/ooh/management/medical-and-health-services-managers.htm.

Xyrichis A. and E. Ream. 2008. Teamwork: a concept analysis. *Journal of Advanced Nursing* 61(2):232–241. doi: 10.1111/j.1365-2648.2007.04496.x.

Project Management Using a CDI Workplan

10

Learning Objectives

- Illustrate how to communicate and update the clinical documentation improvement (CDI) workplan.
- Explain the value of a workplan for effective project management.
- Describe the tasks required for a robust outpatient CDI program.
- Identify stakeholder responsibilities and the value of deadlines.
- Discuss how the workplan keeps the project on track.

Key Terms

Case review
High-level technology assessment
Ongoing program monitoring
Physician collaboration
Project kickoff meeting

Project management
Project manager (PM)
Project workplan (workplan)
Rapid redesign

Project management is the process of defining project tasks, goals, and objectives; developing and tracking the project timeline; managing project resources; and planning and conducting activities that result in a successful project. It is a familiar process in the healthcare industry today.

Most large projects establish a project management office and appoint a **project manager (PM)** to lead the project activities and keep the project on time and delivered as established in the project workplan. The PM is tasked with identifying and garnering agreement among the stakeholders on the specific tasks and goals that govern the project. He or she must estimate time frames, delegate responsibilities among stakeholders, document completion dates, and provide alternatives to planned tasks as needed to keep the project on track. Chapter 5 reviews the process and components of the outpatient clinical documentation improvement (CDI) assessment. Whereas that chapter provides an overview of the assessment process so that the reader can understand the assessment as a separate component of the CDI program, this chapter focuses on the responsibilities of the PM, including the development of a detailed workplan for the CDI program. The workplan is created at the start of a facility-specific CDI program and is used to keep the project on track. As the project moves forward and evolves, the PM adds additional tasks to the workplan. The CDI team and CDI committees can refer to the workplan when discussing these additional tasks and assessing the progress of the program.

Project Management for the Outpatient CDI Program

In response to increasing operational complexities, many of which are created through rapidly evolving technology solutions, healthcare organizations use project management methodologies as a standard tool for day-to-day operations as well as new program development. Selecting the right PM improves the organization and efficiency with which the program is implemented. The outpatient CDI program PM, who may be an existing employee of the health system or facility or may be a consultant hired to fill this role, may be chosen before the program begins and before the steering committee and taskforce are created, or he or she may be selected after these committees are already functioning.

The PM should have experience in project management and in CDI as a manager or clinical documentation specialist (CDS). He or she always serves as a member of the CDI steering committee and CDI taskforce and may be the leader of either or both committees.

Having a PM helps a project run smoothly from an organization and scheduling perspective. However, not all programs have a PM. In those cases, the CDI program leader (director or manager) will take on the responsibility of project management. The PM or other person charged with project management may have other day-to-day responsibilities, but he or she must have adequate time to focus on the project tasks at hand and be available for the ongoing implementation of the CDI program.

The PM should follow the following steps to ensure that the project runs smoothly, meets goals and objectives, and finishes on time:

- Establish an initial workplan with achievable objectives. (These objectives will be approved by the governance team.)
- Communicate the workplan to all stakeholders.
- Maintain project scope and schedule as much as possible to stay on budget.
- Include key stakeholder executives, medical staff, directors, and managers.
- Provide ongoing communication on project status and achievements with steering committee, taskforce, and key stakeholders.
- Conduct steering committee and taskforce meetings only as necessary (see chapter 8 for information on the frequency of meetings).
- Use metrics to measure project success, and share this information with key stakeholders.
- Maintain and update the project workplan to document task completion and compliance with due dates.

The Project Workplan

The essential tool that holds the project together is the **project workplan**, which is used to list tasks, assign responsibility, and monitor task deadlines. It helps the outpatient CDI manager and PM to control and manage the project. The plan, which should be formally reviewed and accepted by the stakeholders on the CDI steering committee and CDI taskforce, provides a basis for all the tasks associated with the project and documents changes in tasks as they occur during the life of the project.

The workplan tasks and commentary should be clear, concise, and accurate. The workplan is updated as new tasks are added and original tasks are closed. Thus, the plan provides a complete history of the project: what, who, when, and how. The plan can be created using spreadsheet software, such as Microsoft Excel, or project management software, such as Microsoft Project. The plan assists the PM in holding stakeholders responsible for activities and helps ensure that project deadlines are met. The project workplan can be set up in any number of formats, depending on the facility and how much detail the PM and stakeholders would like to record about the project progress.

Figure 10.1 is an excerpt of a sample project workplan created in Excel that can be used as a starting point for planning a new outpatient CDI program. The complete sample workplan is available as appendix 10A. The columns listed in the plan include the following:

- *Task #:* Each major milestone is assigned a task number. Subtasks are assigned a subnumber. For example, the first subtask in the Task # column is 1.a.
- *Task:* The name of the top-level task is entered in the topic column.
- *Subtasks:* This column lists all subtasks. Subtasks may be added as needed.

Figure 10.1. Excerpt from a project workplan

Medical Center CDI Workplan

Task #	Task	Subtasks	Status Notes	Priority / Disposition	Consultant Responsible Party	Facility Responsible Party	Start Date	Due Date	Project Timeline (Dec Jan Feb Mar Apr May)
PHASE I: CDI PROGRAM ASSESSMENT									
1	**Data Analytics**								
1.a.		Submit data requests for 835/837 files, CDM, fee schedules.		Complete	Project Mgr		Dec 1	Dec 5	

Source: ©AHIMA

- *Status Notes:* This column includes an update of any delays or barriers, issues, or information needed to understand the progress related to a subtask.
- *Disposition:* The disposition column notes the status of each subtask as priority, pending, or complete. The filter function can be used to view only pending or priority subtasks.
- *Consultant Responsible Party:* This column is used when an outside consulting firm is managing the project. This column is not required when the project is managed internally.
- *Client Responsible Party:* This column is used to document the internal stakeholder(s) responsible for ensuring completion of each subtask.
- *Start Date:* This is the date that work on the subtask begins.
- *Due Date:* This is the date that the subtask should be complete.
- *Project Timeline:* The project timeline section displays the months during which each subtask is being completed. This timeline may change over time as deadlines are revised. To further clarify the timeline, a completion date may be added to the workplan in addition to using arrows to mark the start-and-stop time frame.

The example in figure 10.1 shows the first topic, Data Analytics, with subtask Submit Data Requests for 835/837 files, CDM [charge description master], fee schedules. The subtask has been completed by the PM. The start and due dates are December 1 and December 5, respectively. The projected time frame was December 1 to January 1.

Example of an Outpatient CDI Program Workplan

The following example of a workplan documents the basic tasks required for completing an outpatient CDI implementation project. Each major task is listed along with example subtasks.

Phase I, Task 1: Data Analytics

This task focuses on the initial collection and analysis of data that will help identify potential focus areas for the CDI program (refer to the section titled "Step 2: Gather Data and Identify Areas of Focus" in chapter 5). Subtasks are managed by the PM and CDI program manager and include the following:

- Submit data requests to the information technology (IT) department and other departments that capture relevant data, such as 835/837 claims files, the CDM, professional practice fee (pro-fee) schedules, denials reports, claims scrubber reports, coding audit reports, and the payer-mix matrix (a list of payers and corresponding patient volumes). The electronic remittance advice, or 835, is "the electronic transaction which provides claim payment information in the HIPAA [Health Information Portability and Accountability Act] mandated ACSX12 005010X221A1 format. These files are used by practices, facilities, and billing companies to autopost claim payments into their systems" (United Healthcare 2017). The EDI 837 healthcare claim is "the transaction set that is formatted and established to meet HIPAA requirements for the electronic submission of healthcare claim information" (1EDIsource n.d.). Chapter 3 also discusses 837. Note that this subtask assumes that the CDI program will use software licensed from a vendor to perform the data analysis. If data analytic tools, such as claims scrubbers, are built into the facility electronic health record (EHR) or health information system, the data for those tools will already be resident in the EHR/health information system software modules and will not need to be requested. (See chapter 7 for more information on CDI-related technology.)

- If denials management or outpatient claims editor tools from a vendor are used, submit the 835/837 files to the vendor for analysis. These tools provide insight into denials by categorizing the data on reports by claims adjustment reasons (CAs) code and clinical claims edit (refer to chapter 7). In some facilities, the files will be submitted to the vendor by the IT department instead of by the PM or CDI program manager.
- Gather all requested information to be used to assess focus areas for the CDI program.

Figure 10.2 is a spreadsheet that includes the workplan contents for task 1. It can be used as a model to create and customize a facility outpatient CDI workplan. Although these tasks can be performed by a PM who is employed by the facility, figure 10.2 assumes that the PM is an outside consultant and, therefore, the term "work client" is used to refer to stakeholders in the facility.

Phase I, Task 2: On-Site Kickoff Meeting and Interviews

After the data identified in task 1 have been requested, received, and analyzed, the **project kickoff meeting** and stakeholder interviews are conducted. The kickoff meeting is a presentation by the project leaders and a discussion by the key stakeholders of the outpatient CDI program. The participants in the kickoff meeting are the executive leaders, medical staff leaders, health information management (HIM) director, CDI PM, and CDI program manager. The meeting is hosted by the executive leaders to provide visibility for the outpatient CDI program within the facility. A formal presentation is given by the PM or CDI program manager during the kickoff meeting. The presentation in Microsoft PowerPoint format is available as appendix 5A of this text. The kickoff meeting presentation should include the findings from the initial data analytics review along with recommendations for areas of focus for the ongoing outpatient CDS case review and query process. A **case review** is the process of reviewing the clinical record and assessing the completeness and specificity of the clinical documentation. The project vision, mission, goals and objectives, project workplan, and timeline, as well as the stakeholder interview process, are presented during the kickoff meeting. Stakeholder interviews discuss the interviewee's challenges to complete specific clinical documentation and their perceptions of an improved process and workflow.

The subtasks included in task 2 are as follows:

- Schedule on-site week with client (applicable when an external consultant is managing the project for the client hospital or health system).
- Prepare kickoff meeting presentation to include initial findings from data analytics.
- Prepare list of stakeholders to interview.
- Conduct on-site project kickoff meeting and stakeholder interviews.

Figure 10.3 shows a spreadsheet that includes the workplan contents for task 2.

Figure 10.2. Task 1 workplan

Medical Center CDI Workplan

Task #	Task	Subtasks	Status Notes	Disposition	Priority: Pending / Complete	Consultant Responsible Party	Facility Responsible Party	Start Date	Due Date	Project Timeline: Dec	Jan	Feb	Mar	Apr	May
PHASE I: CDI PROGRAM ASSESSMENT															
1	**Data Analytics**														
1.a.		Submit data requests for 835/837 files, CDM, fee schedules.		Complete		Project Mgr		Dec 1	Dec 5	↑					
1.b.		Upon receipt of 835/837 files, submit to IT for the denials and ambulatory claims manager tool update.	835/837 files received. Analytics review is under way.	Complete		Project Mgr		Dec 1	Dec 5	↑					
1.c.		Gather additional information as needed from client for project assessment.	Files gathered during on-site review: Chargemaster, fee schedules, and payor contract matrix.	Complete		Project Mgr		Dec 1	Dec 15	↑					
1.d.		Analyze data and identify trends for focused outpatient audits and physician, CDI, and coder education. These findings and recommendations will be included in assessment report.	Focused targets complete.	Complete		Project Mgr		Dec 1	Dec 15		↑				

Source: ©AHIMA

Figure 10.3. Task 2 workplan

Medical Center CDI Workplan

Task #	Subtasks	Status Notes	Priority: Pending / Complete	Disposition	Consultant Responsible Party	Facility Responsible Party	Start Date	Due Date	Project Timeline: Dec Jan Feb Mar Apr May
PHASE I: CDI PROGRAM ASSESSMENT									
2	**On-site Kickoff Meeting and Interviews**								
2.a.	Schedule on-site week with client.			Complete	Project Mgr		Dec 5	Dec 15	↑
2.b.	Prepare kickoff meeting presentation to include initial findings from data analytics.	Kickoff meeting presentation held.		Complete	Project Mgr		Dec 5	Dec 15	↑
2.c.	Prepare stakeholder interview client list and deliver to client.			Complete	Project Mgr		Dec 5	Dec 15	↑
2.d.	Conduct on-site project kickoff meeting and stakeholder interviews.	Interviews held with all stakeholders.		Complete	Project Mgr	HIM Dir	Dec 15	Jan 15	— ↑

Source: ©AHIMA

Phase I, Task 3: CDI Program Governance and Oversight

Task 3 includes the development of the executive oversight steering committee and CDI taskforce. There may be more than one taskforce, depending on the size and complexity of the facility or health system. The steps in task 3 are as follows:

- Validate the CDI project leader after the project scope and time frame are discussed by executive leaders of the facility or health system.
- Establish a CDI steering committee.
- Establish a CDI taskforce.
- Validate the vision, mission, goals, and objectives of the program.

Figure 10.4 shows a spreadsheet that includes the workplan contents for task 3.

Phase I, Task 4: Outpatient and Professional Practice Case Review

Task 4 includes the professional practice and outpatient facility case review for clinical documentation and coding issues. The review will include the following (refer to chapter 6 for additional information on the case review process):

- Assessment of the clinical record to determine gaps in high-quality clinical documentation
- Review of coding accuracy, including *International Classification of Diseases, Tenth Revision, Clinical Modification* (ICD-10-CM), Current Procedural Terminology (CPT), and Healthcare Common Procedure Coding System (HCPCS)
- Review of Hierarchical Condition Category (HCC) assignment and related clinical documentation gaps for all sites of services (inpatient, outpatient, and pro-fee)

Once the review is completed by the CDS, the PM should review the results and discuss with the program's executive sponsor—in this case, the HIM director (see chapter 9 for further discussion of the role of the executive sponsor). The findings are next presented to the outpatient CDI taskforce. After the taskforce has discussed the information, a formal presentation to the CDI steering committee will be given by the project manager or HIM leader.

The subtasks included in task 4 are as follows:

- Obtain system access for outpatient or pro-fee CDS case reviewers.
- Review focused cases in all settings for missing documentation that affects payment but is inconsistent across the continuum of care. An example would be diagnoses that are listed in the acute care inpatient record but not in the primary care physician's office records.
- Prepare detailed and summary audit reports.
- Discuss detailed and summary audit report with the executive sponsor and obtain approval for presentation to the taskforce.
- Prepare a formal presentation to the outpatient CDI steering committee and CDI taskforce. The presentation should be limited to 15 minutes or less and include a summary of the cases review findings and issues, clinical examples, and recommendations.

Figure 10.5 is a spreadsheet that includes the workplan contents for task 4.

Figure 10.4. Task 3 workplan

Medical Center CDI Workplan

Task #	Task	Subtasks	Status Notes	Priority: Pending / Complete	Disposition	Consultant Responsible Party	Facility Responsible Party	Start Date	Due Date	Project Timeline: Dec	Jan	Feb	Mar	Apr	May
PHASE I: CDI PROGRAM ASSESSMENT															
3	**CDI Program Governance and Oversight**														
3.a.		Validate CDI project leader.			Complete	Project Mgr	HIM Dir	Dec 23	Dec 23	↑					
3.b.		Establish outpatient CDI steering committee.			Complete	Project Mgr		Jan 2	Jan 15		↑				
3.c.		Establish outpatient CDI taskforce.			Complete	Project Mgr		Feb 1	Feb 15			↑			
3.d.		Discuss and validate the mission, vision, goals, and objectives for the program.			Complete	Project Mgr		Feb 1	Feb 15			↑			

Source: ©AHIMA

Figure 10.5. Task 4 workplan

Medical Center CDI Workplan

				Priority					Project Timeline					
				Pending										
				Complete										
Task #	Task	Subtasks	Status Notes	Disposition	Consultant Responsible Party	Facility Responsible Party	Start Date	Due Date	Dec	Jan	Feb	Mar	Apr	May
	4	**PHASE I: CDI PROGRAM ASSESSMENT**												
		Outpatient and Professional Practice Case Review and Report												
4.a.		Obtain system access for outpatient and pro-fee CDS case reviewers.		Complete	Project Mgr	HIM Dir	Feb 1	Feb 15			↑			
4.b.		Review focused cases in all settings for missing documentation that impacts payment but is not consistent across continuum of care.	We will review clinical documentation in all settings (inpatient, outpatient, and pro-fee) to include the professional practice EHR when we perform the pro-fee and outpatient case review. We will determine if there are missing diagnoses and MCC/CCs on the inpatient side using the pro-fee and outpatient record. This was completed during the HCC audit. These findings were reported on 3/30.	Complete	CDS Consultant		Jan 1	Mar 30		⌐		↑		
4.c.		Prepare detailed and summary audit report.		Complete	Project Mgr		Mar 15	Mar 15				↑		
4.d.		Discuss detailed and summary audit report with program sponsor and obtain approval for presentation to the taskforce.		Complete	Project Mgr	HIM Dir	Mar 15	Mar 15				↑		
4.e.		Prepare formal PowerPoint presentation to the CDI steering committee and outpatient CDI taskforce.		Complete	Project Mgr		Mar 15	Mar 30				↑		

Source: ©AHIMA

Phase I, Task 5: High-Level Technology Assessment

Task 5 requires a high-level assessment of technology to support the outpatient CDI program. The **high-level technology assessment** should be conducted by the PM in conjunction with the IT department and include a review of current software tools to support the denials management; software to perform HCC suspecting (HCC capture); and tools to support outpatient coding and coding compliance (an encoder). A review of EHR interoperability issues should also be performed. Chapter 7 further discusses technology to support the outpatient CDI program.

After the assessment is complete, the PMCU along with the IT director or chief information officer should provide recommendations to the CDI taskforce about technology improvements needed to enhance the access to analytics and clinical information needed to track compliance edits for the outpatient CDI program. The IT department is responsible for identifying specific products available in the marketplace, making recommendations about which to consider licensing, issuing requests for proposals (RFPs), and creating a budget for the software tools.

Figure 10.6 is a spreadsheet that includes the workplan contents for task 5.

Phase I, Task 6: Outpatient Clinical Documentation Assessment

Task 6 includes the completion of an outpatient assessment report by the project manager or CDI manager that makes recommendations for areas of focus during the new outpatient CDS case review process. The findings will address clinical documentation gaps, communication barriers, coding issues, charge capture issues, and technology requirements. The report will outline the proposed previsit, concurrent visit, and postvisit review process to be conducted by the outpatient CDSs. The report should be presented to the project's executive sponsor in draft form so that revisions can be made as needed. It is important for the project sponsor to agree with the content of the assessment report. A presentation on the report findings will be made to both the executive steering committee and the CDI taskforce. Figure 10.7 is a spreadsheet that includes the workplan contents for task 6. The steps outlined in the workplan are as follows:

- Develop draft outpatient assessment report to include results of the outpatient physician practice case review, high-level technology assessment, findings during stakeholder interviews, and recommendations for next steps to be presented to the CDI taskforce.
- Present and discuss draft assessment report with the CDI taskforce to approve for discussion.
- Present report to the executive steering committee.

Phase II, Task 7: Rapid Redesign of Clinical Documentation Workflow at Pilot Clinics

Task 7 is the first in Phase II, CDI program implementation. **Rapid redesign** refers to the process of evaluating and revising the workflow of the CDI program over a short period (usually during a one- to two-day discussion

Figure 10.6. Task 5 workplan

Medical Center CDI Workplan

Task #	Task	Subtasks	Status Notes	Disposition	Consultant Responsible Party	Facility Responsible Party	Start Date	Due Date	Project Timeline Dec Jan Feb Mar Apr May
PHASE I: CDI PROGRAM ASSESSMENT									
5	**High-Level Technology Assessment**								
5.a.		Conduct an assessment of the tools available to support denials management, EHR interoperability, HCC suspecting, and ambulatory coding compliance edits.		Complete	Project Mgr		Feb 15	Mar 15	
5.b.		Make recommendations to the CDI taskforce on any gaps identified.		Complete	Project Mgr		Feb 15	Mar 15	
5.c.		Defer the recommendations to the IT department, who will be responsible to search for specific products available in the marketplace, make recommendations about which to consider licensing, issue RFPs, and create a budget for the software tools.		Complete	Project Mgr		Feb 15	Mar 15	

Priority: Pending / Complete

Source: ©AHIMA

Chapter 10 Project Management Using a CDI Workplan

Figure 10.7. Task 6 workplan

Medical Center CDI Workplan

Task #	Task	Subtasks	Status Notes	Disposition	Priority (Pending / Complete)	Consultant Responsible Party	Facility Responsible Party	Start Date	Due Date	Project Timeline (Dec / Jan / Feb / Mar / Apr / May)
PHASE I: CDI PROGRAM ASSESSMENT										
6	**Outpatient Clinical Documentation Assessment Report**									
6.a.		Develop draft outpatient assessment report to include results of outpatient and pro-fee case review, high-level technology assessment, findings during stakeholder interviews, and recommendations for next steps if desired by client.		Complete		Project Mgr		Feb 1	Mar 30	
6.b.		Presentation and discussion of draft assessment report with client to approve for final presentation.		Pending		Project Mgr		Feb 1	Mar 30	
6.c.		Presentation of report to executive steering committee and taskforce (as recommended).		Pending		Project Mgr	HIM Dir	Mar 30	Mar 30	

Source: ©AHIMA

group). This task includes the steps to visit the pilot clinic(s) and evaluate the clinical documentation workflow. A pilot clinic is where the outpatient CDI program will first be implemented (see chapter 5). During this step, the new outpatient CDI program is explained by the CDI program manager or CDS staff to the clinic managers, nursing staff, and providers. The PM and outpatient CDI program manager will observe the providers as they document in the EHR. The options for an outpatient CDI query process will be discussed and agreed upon by the project team (CDI program manager and CDS staff), clinic manager, nurses, and providers. The project team will finalize the workflow process. An implementation start date and time will be set. The project team will implement the process by shadowing the providers on the agreed-upon start date. Figure 10.8 is a spreadsheet that includes the workplan contents for task 7.

The steps outlined in the workplan for task 7 are as follows:

- Schedule on-site week with pilot sites to observe the outpatient clinical documentation workflow.
- Consider outpatient and pro-fee audit findings from root cause analysis process when planning the rapid redesign of workflow and education of coders and physicians scheduled during Phase II Implementation.
- Evaluate clinical documentation, charge capture, and coding processes at pilot sites.
- Redesign workflow based on findings from professional practice and outpatient facility reviews performed during the assessment. The workflow redesign should include improved methods for communicating a query to the physicians, as well as templates, menus, or drop-down lists to assist the physician during the documentation process (refer to chapter 16 for more information on the physician query process).
- Set CDI implementation project start date.
- Begin new clinical documentation process with redesigned outpatient CDS query workflow.

Phase II, Task 8: Physician Collaboration and Education during Outpatient CDI Program Implementation

Task 8 is an essential part of the CDI program. **Physician collaboration** refers to the process used to communicate with the physicians. This process could be through e-mail, one-on-one meetings, group education, or delivery of educational materials such as newsletters and intranet blogs. Physician education related to clinical documentation in the outpatient and pro-fee setting will improve the CDI program outcomes by reducing the number of queries required to address documentation gaps. (Refer to chapter 13 for more information on physician education programs.) The programs should be short (no more than 30 minutes), and the content should be specific to the specialty area invited to the meeting. Colleague-to-colleague education is often more effective than other methods. If a physician advisor

Figure 10.8. Task 7 workplan

Medical Center CDI Workplan

Task #	Task	Subtasks	Status Notes	Disposition	Priority: Pending / Complete	Consultant Responsible Party	Facility Responsible Party	Start Date	Due Date	Project Timeline Dec	Jan	Feb	Mar	Apr	May
PHASE II: CDI PROGRAM IMPLEMENTATION															
7	**Rapid Redesign of Pilot Clinic Workflow**														
7.a.		Schedule on-site week with pilot sites for outpatient workflow.	Review workflow for four clinics complete.	Complete		Project Mgr	HIM Dir	Mar 1	Mar 5				↑		
7.b.		Include outpatient and pro-fee audit findings in root cause analysis process with rapid redesign of workflow and education of coders and physicians scheduled during Phase II implementation.	Determine specific root cause based on NCD, LCD medical necessity edits, coding errors, chargemaster issues, electronic record order documentation issues, and clinical documentation specificity.	Complete		Project Mgr		Mar 1	Apr 30					↑	
7.c.		Evaluate clinic clinical documentation, charge capture, and coding processes at pilot sites.		Complete		Project Mgr	Clinic Mgr	Mar 1	Apr 30					↑	
7.d.		Workflow redesign based on findings from professional practice and outpatient facility reviews performed during the assessment.	Redesign of workflow and shadowing completed for pilot sites.	Complete		Project Mgr	Clinic Mgr	Mar 1	Apr 30					↑	
7.e.		Set project start date.		Complete		Project Mgr	Clinic Mgr	Mar 1	Mar 21					↑	
7.f.		Begin new clinical documentation process with outpatient CDS query workflow.		Complete		Project Mgr	Opt CDS	May 1	May 30						↑

Source: ©AHIMA

or champion is available, he or she should be considered as presenter or co-presenter.

The following steps outlined in task 8 (figure 10.9) are completed by the CDI program manager:

- Meet with physician champions and clinic managers to develop a physician education program tailored by specialty that includes HCC, outpatient, and pro-fee case review findings and recommendations.
- Develop specialty-specific slide presentations with actual examples for physician education.
- Invite an outside or internal physician leader to participate during presentations (if appropriate and feasible).
- Provide physician education on pro-fee, HCC, and outpatient audit findings.

Phase II, Task 9: Rapid Redesign of Clinical Documentation Workflow in Remaining Clinics

Task 9 is a continuation of the CDI program rollout to the remaining clinics in the project. It requires essentially the same steps as the pilot program, except the timing will depend on the number of facilities, distance to remote clinics, and available staff resources (see chapter 5). While setting the timing and assignments, it is a good time to incorporate lessons learned from the pilot rollout that will make the rollout for the remaining clinics more efficient. Figure 10.10 is a spreadsheet that includes the workplan contents for task 9.

Phase III, Task 10: Ongoing Program Monitoring

Task 10 is the first step in Phase III. It includes steps to ensure the sustainability of the outpatient CDI program. Figure 10.11 is a spreadsheet that includes the workplan contents for task 10. **Ongoing program monitoring** refers to the process of analyzing program effectiveness through the use of metrics related to HCC capture, coding gaps, and denials management. It includes discussions with key stakeholders on the progress the teams have made and the areas of focus for future improvements.

The PM or program sponsor should conduct monthly calls with the taskforce and other stakeholders to ensure that the program is progressing as planned. These calls should discuss the improvements noted in the areas of focus and newly identified focus areas that are gathered from the denials reports, clinical editors, and coding and HCC audits.

Steps outlined in task 10 are as follows:

- Conduct monthly conference calls with the taskforce and other stakeholders to review program metrics, identify clinical documentation gaps, and discuss recommendations for improvement.
- Visit sites as needed to coordinate program activities.
- Develop a "going forward" plan, and secure client approval for ongoing sustainability.

Figure 10.9. Task 8 workplan

Medical Center CDI Workplan

Task #	Task	Subtasks	Status Notes	Disposition	Priority: Pending / Complete	Consultant Responsible Party	Facility Responsible Party	Start Date	Due Date	Project Timeline Dec	Jan	Feb	Mar	Apr	May
8	**Physician Collaboration and Education**														
		PHASE II: CDI PROGRAM IMPLEMENTATION													
8.a.		Meet with physician champions and clinic managers to develop a physician education program offering education by specialty and to include HCC, outpatient, and pro-fee case review findings and recommendations.	Discussion with taskforce included key physician specialty leaders.	Complete		Project Mgr	Physician Leaders, Clinic Mgr	Apr 1	Apr 1					↑	
8.b.		Develop specialty-specific PowerPoint presentations with actual examples for physician education.	Protected health information and physician names removed from presentations.	Complete		Project Mgr		Apr 1	Apr 15					↑	
8.c.		Invite outside or internal physician leader to participate during presentations.		Complete		Project Mgr		Apr 1	Apr 15					↑	
8.d.		Provide physician education on pro-fee, HCC, and outpatient audit findings.	Schedule specialty group or one-on-one meetings.	Pending		Physician Advisor		Apr 15	Apr 30						↑

Source: ©AHIMA

Figure 10.10. Task 9 workplan

Medical Center CDI Workplan

Task #	Task	Subtasks	Status Notes	Priority: Complete / Pending	Disposition	Consultant Responsible Party	Facility Responsible Party	Start Date	Due Date	Project Timeline — Dec	Jan	Feb	Mar	Apr	May
9					**PHASE II: CDI PROGRAM IMPLEMENTATION**										
	Rapid Redesign of Remaining Clinics Workflow														
9.a.		Schedule on-site time for remaining sites for outpatient workflow.	Review workflow for all clinics complete.		Complete	Project Mgr	HIM Dir	May 15	Ongoing						↑
9.b.		Include outpatient and pro-fee audit findings in root cause analysis process with rapid redesign of workflow and education of coders and physicians scheduled during Phase II implementation.	Determine specific root cause based on NCD, LCD medical necessity edits, coding errors, chargemaster issues, electronic record order documentation issues, and clinical documentation specificity.		Complete	Project Mgr		May 15	Ongoing						↑
9.c.		Evaluate clinical documentation, charge capture, and coding processes.			Complete	Project Mgr	Clinic Mgr	May 15	Ongoing						↑
9.d.		Workflow redesign based on findings from professional practice and outpatient facility reviews performed during the assessment.	Redesign of workflow and shadowing completed.		Complete	Project Mgr	Clinic Mgr	May 15	Ongoing						↑
9.e.		Set project start date.			Complete	Project Mgr	Clinic Mgr	May 15	Ongoing						↑
9.f.		Begin new clinical documentation process with outpatient CDS query workflow.			Complete	Project Mgr	Opt CDS	May 15	Ongoing						↑

Source: ©AHIMA

Figure 10.11. Task 10 workplan

Medical Center CDI Workplan

Task #	Task	Subtasks	Status Notes	Disposition	Consultant Responsible Party	Facility Responsible Party	Start Date	Due Date	Project Timeline Dec Jan Feb Mar Apr May
				Priority					
				Pending					
				Complete					
PHASE III: Ongoing Program Monitoring									
10	**Program Monitoring**								
10.a.		Conduct monthly conference calls with taskforce and stakeholders to review program metrics, identify gaps, and discuss recommendations for improvement.		Pending	Project Mgr	Stakeholders	Dec 1	Ongoing	
10.b.		On-site visits by project manager as needed to coordinate program activities.		Pending	Project Mgr		Dec 1	Ongoing	
10.c.		Develop go-forward plan and client approval for ongoing sustainability.		Priority	Project Mgr	Stakeholders	May 15	May 30	

Source: ©AHIMA

Chapter 10 Review Exercises

1. A high-level technology assessment should be conducted by the PM in conjunction with which of the following parties?
   a. IT department
   b. Executive sponsor
   c. Steering committee
   d. Physician champion or advisor

2. Completion of an outpatient assessment report should be included in a workplan to provide findings addressing clinical documentation gaps, charge capture and coding issues, as well as technology requirements. This report should be presented to whom among the following?
   a. PM
   b. CIO
   c. Executive sponsor
   d. CDI taskforce and steering committee

3. Which of the following outpatient CDI tasks includes meeting with physician champions and clinic managers to develop a physician education program?
   a. Program monitoring
   b. Physician collaboration
   c. High-level technology assessment
   d. Rapid redesign of clinic workflow

4. Preparing detailed and summary audit reports is a subtask involved in which of the following tasks?
   a. Ongoing program monitoring
   b. High-level technology assessment
   c. Outpatient and professional practice case review
   d. Rapid redesign of clinical documentation workflow at pilot clinics

5. Which of the following is the primary purpose of an outpatient CDI project workplan?
   a. Complete history of the project
   b. Financial overview of the project
   c. Review of software and tools to be used for the project
   d. Discussion of challenges associated with completing the project

6. Project stakeholders require access to the 835/837 claims files, CDM, professional practice fee schedules, denial reports, claims scrubber reports, and _____.
   a. Disease index
   b. Coding audit reports
   c. Operating room supply item list
   d. Emergency department encounter forms

7. The following facility software applications and technology tools should be included during the assessment process: denials management, EHR interoperability, HCC suspecting, and _____.
   a. Pharmacy system
   b. Clinical operating system
   c. Computer-assisted coding software
   d. Outpatient coding compliance edits

8. After executive and medical staff leaders meet with the HIM director and CDI PM to review findings from the initial data and learn of the project vision, mission, goals, and objectives, the very next step in the workplan should be _____.
   a. Conducting data analytics
   b. Initiating stakeholder interviews
   c. Developing an executive oversight steering committee
   d. Assessing the clinical record to identify gaps through case review

9. Validating the vision, mission, goals, and objectives for the program are crucial steps for _____.
   a. Data analytics
   b. Case review and report
   c. CDI program assessment
   d. CDI program governance and oversight

10. Physician education programs should include content specific to the specialty area invited to the meeting. What is another objective of the outpatient CDI education program?
    a. Limit meeting to no more than 30 minutes.
    b. Include physician names and credentials in the presentation materials.
    c. Evaluate clinical documentation, charge capture, and coding processes during the education program.
    d. Arrange for follow-up meetings with the physician champion and clinic managers after the program has been developed.

References

1EDISource, Inc. n.d. EDI 837 Healthcare Claim. https://www.1edisource.com/resources/edi-transactions-sets/edi-837.

United Healthcare. 2017. EDI 835: Electronic Remittance Advice (ERA). Electronic Remittance Advice 835. https://www.uhcprovider.com/en/resource-library/edi/edi-835.html.

Program Staffing Options

11

Learning Objectives

- Explain the sources of physician champion, project manager, and clinical documentation specialist (CDS) staffing.
- Describe the key decision points for outsourcing models.
- Identify the required skills for the outpatient CDS.
- Discuss the role of the physician advisor.
- Describe how to convert an outsourced project to an internal staffing model.

Key Terms

AHIMA Registered HIM Apprenticeship Program

Outsourcing

Preceptorship

When planning an effective and timely staffing model for a new outpatient clinical documentation improvement (CDI) program, the healthcare organization's structure, management style, political environment, and recruiting abilities should be considered. Consideration should also be given to the availability of the CDI program manager or director to jumpstart an organization-wide program with such a broad reach. It may be the case that the leader can manage the program after it is established and operating efficiently but does not have the available time to organize the program or assign personnel and allocate resources for its implementation. This chapter provides insight into these considerations and options for staffing a new CDI program.

Organizational Considerations

Before staff and resources are allocated to the CDI program, the executives in the healthcare entity must decide where in the organizational structure the program should report. Many facilities have a functional inpatient CDI program that reports through either the health information management (HIM) department under the revenue cycle vice president (VP) and chief financial officer (CFO) or the nursing, care management, or quality division. Any of these structures can successfully support CDI program efficiency, effectiveness, and sustainability in the inpatient setting. In some circumstances, it will make sense to incorporate an outpatient CDI program covering the outpatient clinic and physician practice organizations into the existing inpatient program; in other contexts, it might be best to manage outpatient CDI under a separate organizational structure. See chapter 9 for figures presenting overviews of various organizational structures.

The following questions can help guide stakeholder discussions about the reporting structure for the outpatient CDI program:

- What would be the advantages and disadvantages of expanding the inpatient CDI program to include outpatient CDI?
- What would be the advantages and disadvantages of placing the inpatient and ambulatory CDI programs under separate leadership?
- If the inpatient and outpatient CDI programs are under separate leadership and in different parts of the organization, how will the programs be managed so that all CDI activities are coordinated to encourage collaboration by key stakeholders who are part of the inpatient, outpatient, and physician practice CDI components?
- Which organizational leader (executive sponsor) has the required broad reach, can provide high-level program visibility, and can allocate resources needed for the outpatient CDI program?
- Which additional organization leaders should be included in the planning, oversight, and day-to-day operational support of the program?
- Which organizational leaders have the greatest insight into the appropriate clinical documentation, claims submission, regulatory guidelines, electronic health record (EHR) technology considerations, and operational workflows in the inpatient and outpatient settings? Consideration should also be given to where the clinical documentation specialists (CDSs) are placed within the organizational structure.

The organizational charts presented in the following sections provide options based on these considerations. Facilities and healthcare systems can adapt the proposed models to suit their existing organizational structures.

Example 1: Integrated Inpatient and Outpatient CDI Programs

In the example shown in figure 11.1, an integrated CDI program for the inpatient clinic, outpatient clinic, and physician practice settings reports through HIM to the revenue cycle VP and ultimately the CFO. The advantages of this organizational structure are that (1) the CDI program will be well integrated under one manager, and (2) the HIM director, revenue cycle VP, and CFO have high-level visibility in the organization and are authorized to allocate the required resources. The disadvantage is that the CDI program manager, who has been primarily working with executives and leaders in the inpatient facility areas, will now need to develop collaborative relationships with leaders in the outpatient setting, who report to the chief medical officer (CMO).

Figure 11.1. Organizational chart for an integrated CDI program for inpatient and outpatient settings

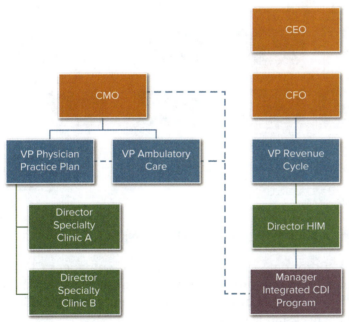

Source: ©AHIMA

Example 2: Separate Inpatient and Outpatient CDI Programs

In the organizational chart in figure 11.2, the inpatient and outpatient CDI programs are entirely separate. The inpatient program is under the director of care management, VP of compliance, and chief nursing officer (CNO), and the outpatient program is under the CMO and ambulatory HIM director. The ambulatory HIM director has a dotted-line reporting relationship to the VPs of the physician practice plan and ambulatory care. The managers of ambulatory and inpatient CDI work collaboratively to integrate the programs and ensure that data and metrics are shared with key stakeholders in both organizational structures. Many of the key stakeholders in both organizations will be included in the steering committees and CDI taskforces for both the inpatient and ambulatory CDI programs to ensure continuity of CDI throughout the continuum of care (see chapters 8 and 9 for additional information on steering committees and taskforces).

The advantage of this organizational structure is that the new outpatient CDI program leader is organizationally aligned with a smaller group of executives and leaders in the outpatient setting, making their collaboration less complex. The disadvantage of this structure is that the goals and objectives for inpatient and outpatient CDI may be more likely to diverge if they are not part of an integrated program, and the two programs may therefore be at cross-purposes when tasks are assigned or resources are allocated.

Figure 11.2. Organizational chart for separate outpatient and inpatient CDI programs

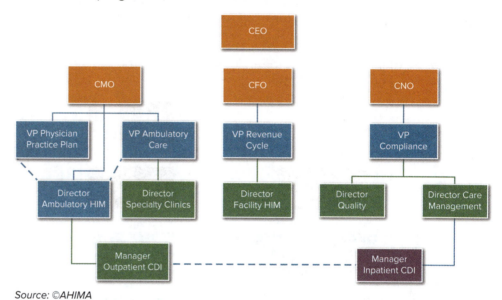

Source: ©AHIMA

Selecting a Program Staffing Model

To select an appropriate staffing model for the outpatient CDI program, the steering committee and program manager must assess multiple variables, including the availability of qualified staff or outsourcing options, cash flow issues, and medical staff leadership.

Availability of Qualified Program Staff

Outpatient CDI requires skills that are not easily found in the marketplace; therefore, it is not always possible to hire and train in-house CDS staff for the CDI program. The outpatient CDS should have an in-depth understanding of *International Classification of Diseases, Tenth Revision, Clinical Modification* (ICD-10-CM) and Current Procedural Terminology/Healthcare Common Procedure Coding System (CPT/HCPCS) coding; Outpatient Prospective Payment System (OPPS) guidelines; project management; workflow redesign; physician practice, emergency department, and ambulatory clinic clinical documentation requirements and processes; risk-based payer methodologies (for example, Hierarchical Condition Categories [HCCs]); and value-based purchasing models. If time permits, existing employees with all or most of the required skills can be trained by the CDI manager to work on the outpatient program.

When choosing a staffing model, consideration should be given to how the department will cover paid time off and holidays. Backup contractor CDSs may be a good option for coverage during these times to ensure that the momentum of the program is not lost.

At the beginning of a new program or when staff turnover occurs in a well-established program, CDI leaders may also choose to contract with outpatient CDSs who can fill in for or train new staff members. The use of contractors is discussed in further detail later in this chapter.

Staff recruitment may be especially difficult for facilities located in rural areas, facilities in states with limited options in HIM education, and facilities located in areas with a high cost of living. For example, if a state does not have a bachelor-degree-level HIM program to prepare students to sit for the registered health information administrator (RHIA) examination, a facility in that state will have to rely on recruiting HIM professionals from programs in other states. Two-year associate-degree HIM programs prepare students for registered health information technician (RHIT) certification, but these programs are challenged to meet the needs of CDI programs, which need staff with at least bachelor degrees and skills in hospital administration, health system technology strategic planning, data analytics, privacy and security, clinical informatics, and other hospital administrative functions. States with a high cost of living may also experience a shortage of HIM and CDI practitioners because the salary scales for those positions may not be sufficient to recruit and retain employees. To fill CDI vacancies, facilities in such states often rely on contract professionals, many of whom work remotely.

Cash Flow Issues

Given the current healthcare environment, in which costs are increasing, patient volumes are falling, and the use of risk-based payer models is on the rise, healthcare organizations may be challenged to find funding for new programs. Rather than making long-term commitments to hire specialized staff to manage and implement a new outpatient CDI project, the organization may decide to use contractors or outsource the program, at least in the beginning. For example, use of consultants for project management may be more economical than hiring a full-time project manager (PM) (Alexander 2015). Because creative financing is typically a requirement for any broad-based program such as outpatient CDI, the CFO will play an integral role in the program's governance structure.

Physician Leaders

As in other professions, healthcare providers may be more comfortable discussing important business matters with their colleagues than those outside of their profession. Therefore, they may be receptive to CDI proposals presented by physician advisors other than those coming from a project manager or CDS.

Physician advisors with recent medical practice experience can lend a sympathetic ear to colleagues in the current "difficult" healthcare environment, advocate for CDI, and help their peers recognize how program adoption can improve patient care, their personal quality scores, and the accuracy of reimbursement (Provident 2014). With new healthcare legislation always around the corner, healthcare providers struggle to keep abreast of the regulations affecting the financial viability of their practices. Advisors can help them efficiently integrate new policies within the existing practice workflow and operations. The physician advisor can also help physician "extenders," such as physician assistants, nurse practitioners, and clinical nurse specialists, to comply with the clinical documentation requirements associated with claims submission and risk-based payer programs.

The availability of qualified physician leaders to serve as advisors will affect the program's staffing model. Physician advisors may be part time or full time, volunteers, or salaried. In some organizations, a primary physician leader along with several specialty-specific physician advisors may be needed to collaborate, educate, and support the new outpatient CDI program.

The key components of the physician advisor's role in CDI may include the following (Provident 2014):

- Educating staff on ICD-10-CM, CPT/HCPCS, and HCC documentation requirements
- Educating medical staff on the importance of complying with hospital policies and regulations, and explaining specific policy or regulatory changes
- Providing CDI training for physicians individually or in group settings
- Aiding hospital or clinic administrative and CDI staff in preparing documentation for a Medicare compliance audit
- Educating medical staff on coding changes or other procedural shifts
- Bridging the gap between providing quality care and a clinical practice that is focused only on data and reimbursement metrics
- Assisting in the drafting of responses to payer denials (see chapters 5, 6, 7, 10, 12, 14, and 16 for more information on the denials process)
- Mediating clinical documentation–related disagreements between coding, CDI, and physicians

Clearly, physician advisors must understand the guiding principles of accurate and complete clinical documentation. They can learn these principles through mentoring by an experienced CDI physician advisor or manager.

Physician leaders must also be capable of working well with their peers and negotiating changes in clinical documentation processes and workflows. For example, the physician advisor may explain to the medical staff the monitor, evaluate, assess/address, or treat (MEAT) criteria for documenting chronic illnesses in each outpatient visit progress note (refer to chapters 3 and 6 for more information on MEAT). Physician advisors with experience in auditing, denials and appeals, and teaching offer an added level of value to the outpatient CDI program (Hess 2015).

Ideally, physician advisors for the new outpatient CDI program are already well-respected leaders (formal or informal) within the existing medical staff organizational structure. Leaders who have connections to or a position at the pilot CDI implementation site may be good candidates for the physician advisor position because they can share positive insights about the pilot site redesign process with their colleagues.

In situations where physician leaders are willing to lead the new program but lack the knowledge base they would need to be effective advisors, organizations may wish to engage a contractor physician advisor to shadow the facility physician leader and help him or her learn to be an advisor. This process could take a week or longer, depending on the facility leader's existing knowledge base.

The facility physician CDI leader may also benefit from attending a CDI boot camp, such as those sponsored by the American Health Information Management Association (AHIMA) or the Association of Clinical Documentation Improvement Specialists, which is a professional association for CDSs. These boot camps are intensive training programs, usually lasting one to three days. During the program, attendees learn concepts related to CDI and will be provided case scenarios to further define the program educational material.

The facility CDI physician advisor is expected to have difficult conversations with physicians who are noncompliant with the program. When the entire outpatient CDI program is outsourced, the CDI program manager should request that the outsourced implementation team include a physician advisor. This arrangement will ensure that the program is designed to consider the perspectives of physicians and other provider-related issues specific to the facility.

Outsourcing and Employed Staff Options

Options such as apprenticeship, contract-to-hire, and outsourcing are alternatives to staffing the new outpatient CDI program by hiring employees or transferring staff. **Outsourcing** is defined as "assignment of core services or operations of the organization to a provider [vendor] that focuses in that area of service or operation" (Roberts et al. 2013). There are a variety of CDI outsourcing vendors in the healthcare marketplace. They run the gamut from large professional services consulting firms with a broad base of subject matter and project management expertise to small consulting practices where the owners provide most of the consulting support. Often, the smaller firms have owners and subject matter experts who were previously employed by the larger consulting firms. When choosing a company that offers outsourcing options for CDI, healthcare entities should carefully assess the level of expertise of the principals and the depth of subject matter expertise the firm can provide.

When considering a proposal to outsource CDI, the program leaders "must consider (a) reasons why to outsource, (b) obstacles to outsourcing, (c) best practices of outsourcing, and (d) implications to hospital management" (Roberts et al. 2013). To select the best outsourcing option for a facility or healthcare system, the organization (CFO and CDI manager or director) should consider the following factors:

- *Quality of services:* Evaluation of quality should be based on customer references. Once the outsource option is in place, the CDI program manager will monitor the quality of the work product (CDS case reviews). Prior to the outsource implementation, the quality of the work produced is best evaluated through discussion with other clients who have outsourced CDI to the vendor being considered.

- *Scope of work (SOW) and price point:* The healthcare organization should carefully negotiate the SOW for the project, and the associated costs, with the vendor. In addition to high-level milestones, each proposal and contract should spell out who will perform the detailed tasks outlined below each milestone (vendor or client). To ensure that the healthcare entity understands the level of commitment and time required by its employees, it should request a detailed workplan prior to signing the contract, and all parties should agree to who is responsible for each major task (see chapter 10 for additional information about workplans). After identifying internal resources for each task, the CDI program leaders can calculate the entire project cost (internal and external fees) and compare multiple vendor proposals. The outpatient CDI leader should not hesitate to negotiate for lower prices. A larger firm may have the flexibility to negotiate lower prices for large projects that include multiple sites. Smaller firms usually have lower overhead, which may allow them to charge less than larger firms.

- *Experience and expertise of the principals and project manager:* Compared with smaller firms, larger firms may have more experience and expertise overall; however, that does not guarantee that a larger firm will assign an experienced PM to a CDI program.
- *Program targets and metrics:* Before a contract is signed, the vendor should specify the typical metrics used to determine program success and provide examples of the analytics and reports that the CDI steering committee and taskforce will use to monitor the program's progress.

Healthcare organizations should discuss each possible outsourcing option in detail with the vendors. In addition, the outpatient CDI leadership should ask company representatives if the vendor has developed solutions for other clients that may not have been previously discussed. Companies can be very creative in their efforts to encourage potential customers to use their services. Figure 11.3 illustrates the items to consider if outsourcing is an option.

Figure 11.3. Evaluating a scope of work

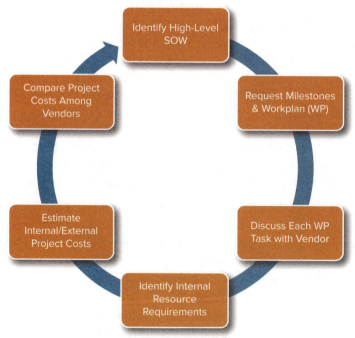

Source: ©AHIMA

Organizations can use a vendor questionnaire during initial discussions with vendors about outsourcing the outpatient CDI program. The questionnaire in figure 11.4 will help assess whether the vendor can address the healthcare entity's requirements; it may be customized to include additional considerations and requirements. The following sections briefly review some typical outsourcing models.

Figure 11.4. Sample questionnaire for CDI service vendors

1.	Have you conducted outpatient CDI program implementations in the past?
2.	Please provide three references for organizations of a similar size and scope to our organization that recently used your program.
3.	Are the proposal prices fixed, or is there room for negotiation?
4.	Do you customize CDI programs, or does your program include only standard project tasks?
5.	If your program is standard and not customizable, what are the program components?
6.	What CDI program metrics does your program track?
7.	For organizations like ours, what are the average program metrics for the following key performance indicators? a. Increase in query rate b. Increase in query response rate c. Increase in query agreement rate d. Average query response turnaround rate (days) e. Average number of CDSs per annual visits/clinics included in the proposed program f. Average number of weeks of training before CDSs are ready to work on their own
8.	Do you offer CDS contractors to cover staff attrition, paid time off, and program expansion?
9.	Will a contract CDI manager and/or PMs be available to our organization during and after program implementation? (The outsourced project may include a CDI manager and/or a PM for the duration of the implementation and possibly beyond, depending on the facility's need for this level of support.)
10.	Can you provide contract physician advisors to be available during and after the project for physician education and to train our physician advisors?
11.	Can you provide contract physician advisors for on-site physician education sessions?
12.	What are the skill sets and experience categories of your CDI program PMs, CDSs, CDI trainers, and physician advisors? Relevant categories could include classification systems, clinic or professional fee operations, and CDI setting (inpatient, outpatient, or professional fee).
13.	Do you have contractors for a prebilling or second-level case review process during and after CDI implementation? If so, what are the skill sets of these contractors?
14.	Do you have a policy and procedure manual for your program implementation?
15.	Do you have educational program materials for CDS, coder, and physician education sessions?
16.	In addition to outpatient CDI program implementation, do you also offer complete outsourcing of the outpatient CDI program?

Source: ©AHIMA

Permanent Outsourcing Solutions

If a healthcare organization decides that a permanent outsourced arrangement is the best solution for the outpatient CDI program, several vendors should be considered. The steering committee, taskforce, and manager or director overseeing the CDI program should review available types of vendors and determine whether the vendor will be a large professional services consulting firm, such as Deloitte, PwC, Accenture, or Huron Consulting Group; revenue cycle firm, such as R1 RCM, Parallon, Vizient, or Navigant Cymetrix; technology firm, such as Nuance Communications or M*Modal; or HIM services firm, such as Himagine Solutions or Optum.

Contract-to-Employed Staff

If the healthcare entity wants to outsource the initial CDI assessment and implementation phase but ultimately bring the outpatient CDI program in-house, the healthcare organization and vendor may agree that the organization will use a vendor's employees as contractors for a period (usually six months) and subsequently allow the organization to hire the consultants. Before an organization makes this type of agreement with the contracting firm, the following points should be settled and the associated cost estimates analyzed:

- Are the contractors going to work remotely or on site? If they are remote, will the healthcare organization be able to hire those who are located out of state? Out-of-state employees can increase the complexity of human resources management from a regulatory, legal, and tax perspective.
- Will the contractors be willing to convert to salaried employees of the healthcare organization? (Contractors may be paid more than staff or prefer contracting for other reasons.)
- Will the contracting vendor agree to provide backup support to the healthcare organization as needed for illness, holiday, and vacation coverage?
- Will the vendor assist with training new staff if attrition of employed staff occurs?

Preceptorship

Some vendors offer a preceptorship option to train inexperienced CDSs. During the **preceptorship**, an experienced CDS mentors and trains the inexperienced CDS in the guiding principles of CDI and the case review process. The trainee may be an employee of the contracting company until the completion of training, or the trainee may be an employee of the healthcare entity from the start of training. Either way, the contracting company agrees to fully train the CDS preceptor, using classroom sessions, online modules, and auditing for quality until the trainee has a quality rating of 95 percent, which is the industry standard for accuracy in the HIM and CDI space (AHIMA 2008). If considering a preceptorship, the healthcare organization should gather proposals from several companies and compare their pricing, training program duration, materials to be covered, levels and percentages of cases audited, training methodologies (classroom, on-site, one-on-one shadowing, webinars, online, and so on), and assistance in identifying candidate trainees.

HIM Apprenticeships

In addition to vendor preceptorships, the **AHIMA Registered HIM Apprenticeship Program** is available through AHIMA and is a good source of staff for a CDI program. The apprenticeship program is certified by the US Department of Labor (DOL) and includes a paid position that students can use as a transition into an HIM career (AHIMA 2016). Roles that are available in the program include hospital coder, CDI specialist, business analyst, and data analyst (AHIMA 2016). Students who are interested in the program and choose to apply must hold an HIM credential such as certified coding associate (CCA), RHIT, or RHIA. The exact credential required depends on the role. The program lasts for one to two years, during which the applicant learns real-world skills through on-the-job training that can lead to a permanent HIM career. The HIM apprentice is a hospital employee, and the salary is determined by the employer.

> The AHIMA Foundation, American Hospital Association, American Medical Informatics Association, and National Center for Healthcare Leadership have joined together to form the Healthcare Workforce Consortium (HWC), which

received notification in 2016 of a $7.1 million award from the US Department of Labor's Employment and Training Administration that positions the HWC as the Healthcare Sector Intermediary for apprenticeships. The US Department of Labor has awarded more than $20.4 million in contract awards to 14 national industry intermediaries and national equity partners to expand apprenticeship opportunities across the US, as part of a historic investment in apprenticeship. The contracts will support the growth of apprenticeship programs in various industries, including health informatics, health information management, health information technology and other healthcare professions, construction, transportation and logistics, manufacturing, and communications technology, and they will support increasing demographic diversity and inclusion in apprenticeship among traditionally underrepresented populations. Changes in technology, social constructs and values, and legislation and regulatory factors in the US have redefined what health professionals do, where they work, and how they work. The Healthcare Sector Intermediary initiative will help address the growing gap between academic training and competencies and the skills needed to ensure workforce readiness. Apprenticeship is a way for employers to build the talent they need to compete and grow and for workers to gain the skills and credentials that put them on the path to successful careers (AHIMA 2016).

Planned Outsourced to Internal Project Management Model

As noted earlier, the healthcare organization may plan to outsource the CDI project until the program assessment and implementation phases are complete and then choose to shift program management and CDS positions to its own employees. When using this model, it is recommended that an in-house CDI leader or manager shadow the consultant PM from the start of the program. The consultant PM will train the client organization's CDI program manager in the tasks required to manage the program on an ongoing basis, such as the following:

- Coordinating the steering committee and taskforce activities
- Managing the quality and productivity of the CDS staff
- Effective medical staff and provider communication
- CDS, coding professional, and provider education activities
- Creating a workplan for expanding the program to new clinics and medical practices
- Analytics, metrics, and reporting for the ongoing program
- Communication of metrics and program successes to stakeholders

Consultant CDSs may be used during the initial implementation to perform case reviews and train in-house CDSs, who may have a portion or all of the skills needed to perform the day-to-day CDI operations.

Because many healthcare organizations today have evolved into complex integrated health systems, one size does not fit all as related to staffing and project management of an ambulatory CDI program. The organizational structure of the program should be discussed with key stakeholders before decisions are made about how to staff the program. Solutions such as complete outsourcing, outsource conversion to an internal program, outsourced CDI staff, preceptorship, and internal staffing models are all options for quickly starting an outpatient CDI program. Careful consideration should be given to the skill requirements for the physician advisor(s), PM, and CDS staff for an efficient and effective outpatient CDI program.

Chapter 11 Review Exercises

1. Which of the following factors should be considered when planning an effective and timely staffing model for the new outpatient CDI program?
   a. Plans for expansion of service lines
   b. The organization's recruiting abilities
   c. Market competition in key service lines
   d. Average RAF score for each specialty clinic

2. Which of the following factors is *most likely* to affect the availability of qualified CDI program staff?
   a. Volume of patients
   b. Age of the program
   c. Location of the facility
   d. Availability of physician leaders

3. An outpatient CDI program covering the outpatient clinic and physician practice organizations could be rolled into the existing inpatient program or could be managed _____.
   a. By a physician specialty leader
   b. Under a separate organizational structure
   c. As part of the specialty clinic manager's responsibilities
   d. As part of the new health information system implementation

4. When selecting an appropriate staffing model for the new outpatient CDI program, options include outsourcing and hiring full-time staff. Which of the following would be a financial reason to outsource at the beginning of the program?
   a. Cash flow issues
   b. Federal tax breaks
   c. Discounted EHR technology
   d. Contractors are usually paid less than employees

5. Quality of services is among the factors to consider when determining the best outsourcing option for a facility or healthcare system. Which of following will be most useful when evaluating the quality of services provided by a prospective CDI outsourcing vendor?
   a. Price point
   b. Customer references
   c. Overall experience or expertise
   d. Metrics showing program success

6. When selecting the best outsourcing option for a facility or healthcare system, which of the following addresses who will perform the detailed tasks outlined by each milestone?
   a. Quality of services
   b. Program targets and metrics
   c. Scope of work and price point
   d. Experiences and expertise of the principals and PM

7. The skill set of the outpatient CDS should include ICD-10-CM and CPT/HCPCS coding skills, and _____.
   a. Auditing experience
   b. Teaching experience
   c. HCC code assignment
   d. Physician practice billing system software development

8. A certified program introducing paid positions that students can use to transition into an HIM career is a _____.
   a. Preceptorship model
   b. HIM apprenticeship model
   c. Contract-to-employed staff model
   d. Planned outsourced to internal project management model

9. Which of the following is *most likely* to be a disadvantage of an integrated inpatient and outpatient CDI program?
   a. It consolidates the CDI program under a single manager.
   b. It expands the authorization of program leadership to allocate required resources.
   c. It leads to higher-level visibility of the HIM director, revenue cycle VP, and CFO within the organization.
   d. It creates a need for the CDI program manager to develop new relationships with leaders in the outpatient setting.

10. A healthcare organization contracts a vendor to train an inexperienced CDS. The trainee, who is employed by the vendor, regularly attends classroom sessions on the guiding principles of CDI as well as the case review process. After several months of training, the vendor certifies that the trainee has achieved a quality rating of 95 percent, and the trainee joins the contracting healthcare organization as a full-time CDS. Which of the following *best* describes the nature of this arrangement?
    a. Preceptorship
    b. HIM apprenticeship
    c. Permanent outsourcing
    d. Contract-to-employed staff

References

Alexander, M. 2015 (June 1). Should you outsource your project management? CIO from IDG. http://www.cio.com/article/2929023/project-management/should-you-outsource-your-project-management.html.

American Health Information Management Association (AHIMA). 2016 (Oct. 7). $7 million award to create new career opportunities through apprenticeships (press release). Chicago, IL: AHIMA.

American Health Information Management Association (AHIMA). 2008. Benchmarking coding quality (audio seminar July 24, 2008). campus.ahima.org/audio/2008/RB072408.pdf.

Hess, P.C. 2015. *Clinical Documentation Improvement: Principles and Practice.* Chicago: AHIMA.

Provident Management Consulting LLC. 2014. The value of a physician advisor. http://www.providentedge.com/the-value-of-a-physician-advisor.

Roberts, J.G., J.G. Henderson, L.A. Olive, and D. Obaka. 2013. A review of outsourcing of services in health care organizations. *Journal of Outsourcing and Organizational Information Management* 2013(2013):985197. doi: 10.5171/2013.985197.

Training the Outpatient Clinical Documentation Specialist

12

Learning Objectives

- Identify the value of the self-evaluation and assessment process for the outpatient clinical documentation specialist (CDS).
- Describe the topics to include in the outpatient CDS training program.
- Discuss the importance of metrics and trending for CDI program sustainability.
- Demonstrate how to maintain the visibility of the clinical documentation improvement (CDI) program.
- Explain the need for critical thinking to enhance the outpatient CDI program.
- Describe examples of critical thinking in the outpatient setting.
- Identify the steps to the critical thinking process.
- Illustrate how to use critical thinking for effective communication.

Key Terms

Bloom's taxonomy
Certified clinical documentation specialist (CCDS)
Certified coding associate (CCA)
Certified coding specialist (CCS)
Certified coding specialist–physician-based (CCS-P)
Certified outpatient coder (COC)
Certified professional coder (CPC)
Clinical documentation improvement practitioner (CDIP)
Critical thinking

This chapter identifies the skills required of an outpatient clinical documentation specialist (CDS). There are a variety of ways to train a CDS in these skills, including online training, on-site classroom training, and college- or graduate-level courses. For example, if the CDS has most of the required skills to work in outpatient clinical documentation but has a gap in *International Classification of Diseases, Tenth Revision, Clinical Modification* (ICD-10-CM), Current Procedural Terminology (CPT), or Healthcare Common Procedure Coding System (HCPCS) coding in the outpatient setting, a college course in ICD-10-CM and CPT/HCPCS might be the best training option. In the example presented in table 12.1, the CDS has all the required credentials and experience to work in the clinical documentation improvement (CDI) program except for an in-depth understanding of Outpatient Prospective Payment System (OPPS) guidelines. This gap can be addressed through an online or college course in CPT/HCPCS and ambulatory payment classification (APC) coding. A combination of training methodologies can also be used as needed. This chapter explains how to assess the knowledge and skills of the outpatient CDS and recommends the most efficient ways to provide training.

Table 12.1. Outpatient CDS skills requirement checklist

Skill Set	Years of Experience or Credential Held
Coding/CDI Credential:	
CCS	
CCS-P	✓
CPC	
CRC	✓
Other Coding	
CDIP	✓
CCDS	
Other CDI	
Coding Experience:	
ICD-10-CM	3
CPT/HCPCS	2
APC	2
HCC	2
OPPS Guidelines	Gap
Hospital charge master and physician fee schedule functionality	1
Ambulatory claims submission, claims scrubber edits, and claims processing work queue functionality	1
Ambulatory denials and appeals process	1
Project management and workflow redesign	1

CDS Skills in the Outpatient Setting

The CDS skills required in the outpatient setting are distinctive, and mastering them is an excellent opportunity for CDI professionals to expand their skill sets and career opportunities (refer to chapters 1–3 of this text for more information on coding and clinical documentation guidelines). At a minimum, the qualifications of the outpatient CDS should include the following:

- *Expertise in ICD-10-CM as it applies to the coding of diagnoses in the outpatient and physician practice settings:* A coding credential, such as the **certified coding specialist (CCS)**, **certified coding associate (CCA)**, **certified professional coder (CPC)**, or **certified outpatient coder (COC)**, is highly recommended. CCS is an AHIMA credential awarded to individuals who have demonstrated skill in classifying medical data from patient records, generally in the hospital setting, by passing a certification examination. CCA is an AHIMA credential awarded to entry-level coding professionals who have demonstrated skill in classifying medical data by passing a certification exam. CPC is a credential sponsored by the American Academy of Professional Coders (AAPC) that certifies the coder has a proven mastery of all code sets (CPT, ICD-10-CM, HCPCS Level II), evaluation and management (E/M) principles, surgical coding, and adherence to documentation and coding guidelines (AAPC 2017). COC, formerly known as *certified professional coder–hospital outpatient*, is a credential sponsored by AAPC that certifies a coder's knowledge of specialized payments related to ambulatory surgery centers or hospital outpatient billing as well as his or her proficiency in accurate medical codes for diagnoses, procedures, and services performed in the outpatient settings (AAPC 2017).

- *Expertise in CPT/HCPCS coding regulations, guidelines, and corresponding clinical documentation requirements:* Because the outpatient CDS will review clinical documentation as it supports procedure, supply, and medication coding on outpatient claims, this person needs knowledge of the guidelines for E/M coding in the outpatient, emergency department, and physician practice settings. A coding credential, such as **certified coding specialist–physician-based (CCS-P)**, CPC, or COC, is recommended. CCS-P is an AHIMA credential awarded to individuals who have demonstrated coding expertise in physician-based settings, such as group practices, by passing a certification examination.

- *CDS credential:* A CDS-related credential can demonstrate that the CDS has mastered the basic tenets of CDI and has experience in that field related to query guidelines, case review, and provider communication in the outpatient setting. Either the AHIMA **clinical documentation improvement practitioner (CDIP)** credential or the Association of Clinical Documentation Improvement Specialists (ACDIS) **certified clinical documentation specialist (CCDS)** credential is recommended. AHIMA awards the CDIP credential to individuals who have achieved specialized skills in CDI. The CCDS credential elevates the professional standing of those who are specialists in the clinical documentation

(ACDIS 2018). Both CDIP and CCDS reflect education in anatomy, physiology, pathophysiology, and pharmacology, as well as an understanding of official medical coding guidelines and reimbursement regulations. Individuals with these credentials have the ability to analyze, interpret, and benchmark clinical data and collaborate with providers to further specify the clinical record.

- *Expertise in HCC code assignment:* The certified risk adjustment coder (CRC) credential from AAPC is a recommended way to demonstrate competency in the risk-based payer methodologies used in the outpatient setting.
- Expertise in claims submission procedures in the outpatient facility and physician practice settings, including how to use the UB-04 and CMS-1500 claim forms.
- Knowledge of hospital chargemaster and physician fee schedule updates and guidelines.
- *Expertise in claims scrubber/claims edit issues within the outpatient facility and physician practice setting:* The CDS must be able to analyze the root causes of such issues and identify workflow challenges related to technology and the coding and claims-processing work queue.
- *Expertise in clinical editor issues identified within the outpatient facility and physician practice setting:* Clinical editors used to determine missing diagnoses and procedures using natural language processing or other software solutions assist the CDS to identify charge capture gaps (see chapter 7).
- Expertise in the denials and appeals process as well as national coverage determinations (NCDs) and local coverage determinations (LCDs).
- *Project management skills:* Project management skills and experience are recommended to facilitate the redesign of clinical documentation workflows in clinics and physician practices and coordinate the educational activities of providers, CDSs, and coding professionals.
- *Healthcare consulting experience:* This experience can facilitate project management activities.
- *Public speaking and communication skills:* These skills are relevant to the CDI program's educational activities, governance committee coordination, and other aspects of program leadership.

Pretraining CDS Assessment

The first step in the outpatient CDS training process is the pretraining assessment. The outpatient CDS skills requirement checklist (table 12.1) can be used to identify a person's basic experience and credentials. Next, the CDI program candidate should complete the pretraining CDS assessment test that can be found in appendix 12A of this text. Figure 12.1 offers a sample of the questions included in the assessment test. A score of 80 percent or higher reflects adequate working knowledge of the key areas needed for the CDS position. A score below 80 percent may reflect areas that require additional training.

Figure 12.1. Sample pretraining CDS assessment questions

1. Progress note states "Chest pain due to gastroesophageal reflux versus esophageal spasm." What is the correct principal diagnosis?
   a. Chest pain
   b. Gastroesophageal reflux
   c. Esophageal spasm
   d. Either gastroesophageal reflux or the esophageal spasm can be the principal diagnosis.
   (Answer: D)
2. Which of the following is characterized by dilated, weak heart, thin ventricular wall, decreased outflow of blood from the heart, and a low ejection fraction?
   a. Congestive heart failure (CHF)
   b. Acute CHF
   c. Diastolic heart failure
   d. Systolic heart failure
   (Answer: D)
3. Which of the following statements related to the term *risk adjustment* is true?
   a. Risk-adjustment data are pulled from procedure code data reported from claims data and health record documentation from physician offices and hospital inpatient and outpatient settings.
   b. Risk adjustment is the process by which the Centers for Medicare and Medicaid Services (CMS) reimburse Medicare Advantage plans based on the health status of their members.
   c. Implemented to pay commercial insurance long-term care plans more accurately for the predicted health cost expenditures of members under the age of 65 by adjusting payments based on demographics (such as age and gender) as well as health status.
   d. Risk adjustment is the use of APC codes in the physician practice setting to reimburse for claims related to primary care.
   (Answer: B)

Source: ©AHIMA

Job Description for the Outpatient CDS

The outpatient CDS job description in figure 12.2 can be used as a starting point to establish the customized, facility-specific description of the position. Each CDI program is distinctive, and the combination of resources used within the program may vary.

Figure 12.2. Example of an outpatient CDS position description

Clinical Documentation Improvement Specialist			
Job Description			
Job/Position Title:	Ambulatory Clinical Documentation Improvement Specialist	**Reports to:**	Health Information Management Director
Dept:	Ambulatory CDI	**Review Date:**	12/15/2017
Job/Position Code:	CDI-0453	**Status:**	Exempt

Purpose: Under minimal direction, the Ambulatory Clinical Documentation Improvement Specialist will provide active concurrent and retrospective review, provide feedback, and educate clinical care providers to improve the documentation of all conditions, treatments, and care plans within the health record to accurately reflect the condition of the patient and promote patient care. In addition, documentation should reflect documentation associated with APC and HCC assignment, severity of illness, risk of mortality, physician profiling, hospital profiling, quality measures, and reimbursement rules.

Figure 12.2. Example of an outpatient CDS position description (*Continued*)

Coordinates and maintains the elements and requirements of the Clinical Documentation Improvement Program, including staff and physician education, to ensure the highest quality of documentation in support of compliance and accurate representation of the care provided to the patient.

Education/Experience		
Healthcare Degree	Bachelor's degree in healthcare field (e.g., health information management or nursing) OR equivalent combination of education and experience required.	
Work Experience	Minimum of 1-3 years experience in health information management, coding, clinical quality, utilization management, case management, nursing, or a related field. Minimum of 1 year experience in ambulatory coding (ICD-10-CM, CPT/HCPCS, APC, HCC).	Prefer 2-3 years of experience in a Clinical Documentation Improvement Program with previous experience in health information management, coding, clinical quality, utilization management, case management, nursing, or a related field.
Credentials	CDIP or CCDS Preferred. CCS or CPC required.	
Skills/Knowledge	Successful leadership skills with the use of critical thinking, problem solving, and deductive reasoning required. Successfully manages multiple priorities required. Successful completion of specialized training in organizational, analytical, writing, and interpersonal skills required. Specialized training in advanced computer skills with proficiency in Microsoft Word, Excel, PowerPoint, and Outlook required. Additional training in Access database management; Medicare Part A, B and C programs; APC and HCC assignment; and knowledge of SOI/ROM preferred.	
Essential Job Functions	1. Coordinate and maintain all elements of the outpatient clinical documentation improvement program to meet the goals and objectives of the organization and its stakeholders. 2. Meet CDI program objectives, goals, and balance scorecard metrics. 3. Ensure timely, accurate, and complete documentation of clinical information used for measuring and reporting physician and hospital outcomes. 4. Ensure effective communications with physicians and other key stakeholders. 5. Conduct compelling physician educational sessions. 6. Revise clinical documentation workflows to meet program goals and objectives. 7. Collaborate with denials management to identify root cause and provide training on related clinical documentation improvement. 8. Analyze data and create reports to meet desired outcomes. 9. Identify trends and opportunities for improvement in clinical documentation. 10. Meet program quality and productivity guidelines and standards. 11. Collaborate with coding professionals to fully support the needs of clinical code assignment; communicate proficiently with coding professionals to resolve identified discrepancies. 12. Work effectively with CDI team members to accomplish departmental goals. 13. Demonstrate continued advancement in professional growth.	
Key Success Indicators and Attributes	1. Ability to prioritize and multitask in a multifaceted environment. 2. Demonstrate strong organizational skills and be detail oriented. 3. Demonstrate ability to self-motivate, set goals, and meet deadlines.	

Source: AHIMA 2016a.

CDS Self-Evaluation

After the CDS candidate has completed the pretraining CDS assessment, the candidate should review the position description and complete a CDS self-evaluation, such as the one in figure 12.3. By using this tool, the candidate can identify the areas where he or she needs additional training to become a CDS. The CDI manager and candidate can then discuss the most efficient ways to address any gaps in experience or knowledge that the candidate may have. After the training program is complete, the CDS can retake the self-evaluation, using the last column in figure 12.3. This process provides feedback on the quality of the training program for the manager as well as feedback for the CDS about areas where he or she needs additional training and mentoring.

Figure 12.3. Outpatient CDS self-evaluation

OUTPATIENT CDS SELF-EVALUATION

Directions: Please complete the following statements by indicating your level of knowledge and familiarity with the concepts addressed BEFORE the start of the clinical documentation improvement program as well as your knowledge of the same concepts AFTER completion of the training program. Circle the number that best represents your level of knowledge and familiarity both before and after training. "1" signifies no knowledge, and "5" represents a strong knowledge of the concept.

	My knowledge of:	Before Training					After Training				
		Weak				Strong	Weak				Strong
1	The relationship between documentation and coding	1	2	3	4	5	1	2	3	4	5
2	The relationship between coding and reimbursement	1	2	3	4	5	1	2	3	4	5
3	APC assignment and the OPPS system	1	2	3	4	5	1	2	3	4	5
4	Risk-based payment methodology	1	2	3	4	5	1	2	3	4	5
5	HCC assignment and payment methodology	1	2	3	4	5	1	2	3	4	5
6	Outpatient quality measures including those under the MIPS program	1	2	3	4	5	1	2	3	4	5
7	Coding and reimbursement in the outpatient facility setting	1	2	3	4	5	1	2	3	4	5
8	Coding and reimbursement in the professional practice setting	1	2	3	4	5	1	2	3	4	5
9	ICD-10-CM coding	1	2	3	4	5	1	2	3	4	5
10	CPT and HCPCS coding	1	2	3	4	5	1	2	3	4	5
11	Physician documentation requirements in the outpatient clinic setting	1	2	3	4	5	1	2	3	4	5
12	Physician documentation requirements in the professional practice setting	1	2	3	4	5	1	2	3	4	5
13	How to review medications, diagnostic test results, and other clinical indicators for query opportunity	1	2	3	4	5	1	2	3	4	5
14	The impact that secondary diagnoses and chronic illnesses have on reimbursement in the outpatient clinic and professional practice setting	1	2	3	4	5	1	2	3	4	5
15	The importance of identifying etiology for symptoms (if known)	1	2	3	4	5	1	2	3	4	5

Figure 12.3. Outpatient CDS self-evaluation (*Continued*)

16	The importance of documenting differential diagnoses for symptoms with uncertain etiology	1	2	3	4	5	1	2	3	4	5
17	The relationship between physician documentation and healthcare report cards such as Healthgrades	1	2	3	4	5	1	2	3	4	5
18	The relationship between physician documentation and Medicare quality indicators	1	2	3	4	5	1	2	3	4	5
19	The physician query process in the outpatient setting	1	2	3	4	5	1	2	3	4	5
20	The denials and appeals process in the outpatient setting	1	2	3	4	5	1	2	3	4	5
21	The workflow around claims processing in the outpatient setting	1	2	3	4	5	1	2	3	4	5
22	The typical claims scrubber edits and their root causes	1	2	3	4	5	1	2	3	4	5
23	The hospital chargemaster and physician fee schedule functionality	1	2	3	4	5	1	2	3	4	5
24	Metrics and trending used in the outpatient CDI setting	1	2	3	4	5	1	2	3	4	5

I would like to know more about:

Source: ©AHIMA

Training Topics and Resources

In the inpatient setting, a basic six-week program in fundamentals of clinical documentation and diagnosis-related group (DRG) assignment for the inpatient provides the skills that an inpatient CDS needs to begin inpatient concurrent case review. If the inpatient CDS is not proficient in coding, he or she can learn inpatient coding guidelines and skills over time through ongoing collaboration with the inpatient coding staff. However, an effective training program for the outpatient CDS requires more extensive use of outside resources to teach skills related to ICD-10-CM, CPT, HCPCS, APC, and HCC code assignment, as well as the clinical documentation requirements to support the codes and prevent denials based on code errors and medical necessity issues. The following sections of this chapter present topics that should be covered during outpatient CDS training, as well as resources that can be used to provide the training. Some of the resources are available through professional organizations, and others are taught in college- and graduate-level courses in health information management (HIM) programs.

CDI Program Process and Design

The CDS needs a clear understanding of the CDI program's purpose, process, and design to develop and implement of an effective CDI program. According to AHIMA,

> The purpose of a CDI program is to initiate concurrent and, as appropriate, retrospective reviews of health records for conflicting, incomplete, or nonspecific provider documentation. These reviews usually occur on patient care units, in outpatient

clinics, [or] the professional practice or they can be conducted remotely via the electronic health record (EHR). The diagnoses and procedures documented in the record need to be clearly supported by clinical indicators so that the ICD-10-CM/PCS codes assigned are accurate and correctly assigned. The method of clarification used by the CDI professional is often written queries in the health record. Verbal and electronic communications are also methods used to make contact with providers. These efforts result in improved accuracy and completeness in documentation, coding, reimbursement, and severity of illness (SOI) and risk of mortality (ROM) classifications. Often, CDI programs begin with focused concurrent review of a specific payer type (such as Medicare) or specific payment types (such as HCC coding for the Medicare Advantage patient), but this is not a requirement and the focus will depend on the individual organization. Although CDI programs are traditionally found in the acute inpatient setting, they also exist in other healthcare settings such as provider offices, ambulatory care, acute rehabilitation hospitals, and skilled nursing facilities (AHIMA 2016a).

Clarification of these key terms may be helpful to understand the purpose of the CDI program discussed above:

- Severity of illness (SI or SOI): A type of supportive documentation reflecting objective clinical indicators of a patient's illness (essentially the patient is sick enough to be at an identified level of care) and referring to the extent of physiologic decompensation or organ system loss of function
- Risk of mortality (ROM): The likelihood of an inpatient death for a patient
- Medicare Advantage Plan: A program that provides Medicare recipients with more choices among health plans; formerly called Medicare + Choice Plans (CMS 2017)

This excerpt from AHIMA's Clinical Documentation Toolkit (2016 Version) provides an overview of CDI as a concept and methodology for improving clinical documentation in the inpatient, outpatient clinic, and professional practice settings.

CDS Training Programs and Topics

A variety of CDS training programs are available. The basic skills needed for assessing clinical documentation to support the quality of care and claims submission are the same in all settings. They include the use of clinical indicators to identify query opportunities, knowledge of requirements for high-quality clinical documentation, communication skills for collaboration with providers, writing skills for clear and concise written query communication, and organizational skills to quickly but accurately review a clinical record for specificity and clinical documentation gaps. Therefore, basic CDS training programs can benefit the outpatient CDS who has not previously had that level of in-depth training. In addition to this text, the following resources can be used to augment the training of the outpatient CDS on CDI theory and application:

- AHIMA's Clinical Documentation Toolkit (2016 Version)
- AHIMA online courses (AHIMA 2017a): AHIMA offers four self-paced courses that focus on documentation assessment and improvement as they support code assignment. The courses are not designed to teach how to code. All materials are online, and there is no requirement to purchase textbooks. The student can begin any time after payment is received and can continue the courses for a period of one year after enrollment.

In addition to CDI theory and practice, the outpatient CDS will benefit from basic and advanced skill sets in ICD-10-CM and CPT/HCPCS coding. AHIMA offers online courses that may be purchased and completed at the learner's own pace (AHIMA 2017b). If the outpatient CDS candidate is not skilled in ICD-10-CM and CPT/HCPCS coding, these courses are highly recommended.

Data Review Training

As part of the CDS training process, the CDI manager should discuss with the CDS the methodology in place for identifying targets for case review. The CDI manager will explain how to identify cases using the EHR and other data analytics reports. For example, in the case of the Medicare Advantage patient targeted for HCC review, EHR reports should be available to identify Medicare Advantage patients scheduled for the following day or week. For quality metrics, the CDS will consider the patient population being monitored for each metric. In many cases, the entire patient population may be monitored. For other metrics, the target may be patients with a specific diagnosis or procedure group. The denials department or software tool should provide denials trend reports with a "drill down" to the patient account level for those denials groups that are being monitored by the outpatient CDS. For example, if a denials trend is identified for patients with a magnetic resonance imaging (MRI) of the spine, the NCDs and LCDs should be reviewed for the required ICD-10-CM codes supporting medical necessity. Insurance companies publish NLDs and LCDs on their websites and include a list of ICD-10-CM codes that indicate medical necessity for specific CPT procedures performed. If the CDS is planning to review the medical necessity for MRI of the spine, the NCD will provide the list of acceptable ICD-10-CM codes. The CDS would then identify patients scheduled for MRI of the spine and would conduct case review prior to the procedure to ensure that the clinical records reflect specificity for an approved ICD-10-CM code.

ICD-10-CM, CPT, HCPCS, APC, and HCC Training

As discussed earlier, AHIMA has excellent tools for training in ICD-10-CM, CPT, HCPCS, APC, and HCC. Outpatient CDSs need to understand the various disease and procedure classification systems (ICD-10-CM, CPT, and HCPCS) and reimbursement systems (OPPS/APC, and so on), used in outpatient documentation (refer to chapter 3 for additional information on ICD-10, CPT, and HCPCS classification systems).

If an outpatient CDS lacks a coding background, the recommended training is college-level course in ICD-10-CM and CPT/HCPCS coding. These courses are offered online as well as in classrooms. After training, it is recommended that the CDS attain one of the coding credentials offered by AHIMA (CCS) or AAPC (CPC, CPC-P, and COC).

Other training options include Medicare Learning Network web-based training modules, which are offered for free by CMS and include courses in Medicare program basics, Medicare billing, ICD-10-CM and CPT coding, the Quality Payment Program, and provider compliance (CMS 2018).

Outpatient Clinical Documentation Case Review

Training in outpatient case review is best taught by a trainer with CDS and coding credentials. The trainer may be a CDI manager or an experienced CDS on the

CDI team. Case reviews for CDI can be conducted for a variety of reasons, such as the following (refer to chapter 6 for additional detail on the case review process):

- Accuracy of HCC assignment based on supporting clinical documentation
- Charge capture issues related to clinical documentation gaps, charge capture workflow, CPT/HCPCS code description and code mismatch, or coding errors
- Root causes of claims denials, such as coding or claims submission errors or documentation that does not show medical necessity
- CPT/HCPCS code accuracy and APC grouping accuracy
- CMS quality measures, including those related to Merit-based Incentive Payment System (MIPS) and value-based purchasing
- Clinical documentation to support E/M code assignment

The timing of the case review is based on the workflow established when the outpatient CDI program is initiated in each clinic or professional practice. At minimum, the cases should be reviewed prior to the patient visit (on the day before the day of the visit), if possible. Then, a concurrent or postvisit review should be done to evaluate whether queries submitted during the previsit review were answered and the requested documentation was present; if feasible, a case review concurrent with the visit is preferable to next-day review. These reviews can be performed remotely or on site. At the start of the outpatient CDI program at each clinic, it is best to have the case review performed on site so that the process can be streamlined. Training for this case review process should be continued until the CDS achieves a 95 percent accuracy rate for the query documentation and communication process.

Query Process

The query process and workflow for a particular facility are determined by the CDI program manager during the initial pilot phase of the program (refer to chapter 15 for further detail on the query process). The use of EHR templates, notes, alerts, and tasks is recommended for provider communication. After the workflow is streamlined, the CDI manager or CDS trainer can explain the process, show the CDS how to submit the query, and then watch the CDS perform the task.

The standards for writing an inpatient query are also used in the outpatient setting. All queries should be AHIMA compliant (see chapter 15) and meet the guidelines established by AHIMA (2016b).

The generation of a query should be considered when the health record documentation

- Is conflicting, imprecise, incomplete, illegible, ambiguous, or inconsistent,
- Describes or is associated with clinical indicators without a definitive relationship to an underlying diagnosis,
- Includes clinical indicators, diagnostic evaluation, and/or treatment not related to a specific condition or procedure
- Provides a diagnosis without underlying clinical validation (AHIMA 2016b).

Training of the outpatient CDS in the AHIMA-approved query process should include the following:

- Review of all previous and most recent AHIMA practice briefs on the query process. These practice briefs can be found in the appendix 12B of this text. The AHIMA Query Toolkit is also a helpful reference (AHIMA 2017c).
- Discussion of any query templates or standard query formats used by the facility. Inpatient query formats should be revised as appropriate for the outpatient setting.
- Discussion of the query process and workflow to include use of EHR templates, alerts, notes, tasks, and other automated EHR features to streamline the query process for the provider.
- Trainer shadowing of the trainee during query preparation, delivery, and responses.

Further education of the outpatient CDS should be conducted by the trainer when the response rate for the trainee's queries is lower than expected. Low response rates may indicate that the queries are ineffectively worded. Effective queries should be clear and concise and include a brief synopsis of the clinical scenario.

Role of Physician Advisor

The outpatient CDS in training should learn about the role of the physician advisor(s) in the outpatient setting (see chapter 11). The CDS should be introduced to the physician advisor in person, if possible, or via a conference call. The physician advisor can explain the best ways for the CDS to communicate with providers and the reasons behind the communications. The outpatient CDS should be encouraged to work closely with the physician advisor to determine the best way to communicate and build working relationships with the medical staff.

Typical reasons for the CDS to contact the physician advisor are as follows:

- Implementation of a new CDI process (for example, data capture for MIPS measures)
- A staff physician does not respond to queries
- Need for physician CDI education, such as a group presentation by the physician advisor or a one-on-one discussion between the physician advisor and a staff physician
- A question related to a clinical documentation issue or case

Metrics and Trending

Each outpatient CDS should understand the metrics that are captured as part of the outpatient CDI program. These metrics not only keep the individual CDS informed of his or her progress and ongoing performance, but they also assist the stakeholders in program monitoring and offer information to clarify the return on investment (ROI) of the program. The CDI manager should meet with the new outpatient CDS and go over the reports that are used to track each CDS, each physician, and the program. This meeting will provide an opportunity for the CDS to ask questions and understand how the data are captured. The CDS should be able to use critical thinking skills to review the data each month, determine whether the data seem reasonable, and, as appropriate, participate in further investigation of how the data should be collected.

Program data and reports are used on an ongoing basis to share the program successes and provide feedback to stakeholders on areas that need improvement. The CDI targets will change as issues are resolved and new issues are identified. The outpatient CDS with an in-depth knowledge of program analytics, data-gathering methods, and program targets can help the CDI manager identify root causes of issues, resolve them, and identify new focused targets for improvement.

During the CDS training process, the AHIMA Clinical Documentation Toolkit (AHIMA 2016a) can be used to demonstrate the use of metrics to support the outpatient CDI program. The toolkit can be used as a teaching aid and provides examples of reporting that can be adapted to outpatient settings. Figure 12.4 is an example of a report that could be created for the physician practice HCC capture process. The report shows the number of queries, answers, and response rates by quarter for HCCs related to diabetes mellitus (DM) for the physician practice in a single year. In the first quarter, the response rate was from 61 percent to 72 percent. The response rate was similar for the second quarter (from 61 percent to 77 percent). In the third and fourth quarters, the response rates trended upward (from 66 percent to 79 percent), except in October (54 percent). This type of report can be used to demonstrate improvement in physician response, which in turn reflects improved collaboration and adoption by the provider of the outpatient CDI program. The root causes of the notable changes in responses would be further investigated; for example, the October dip noted in figure 12.4 might be attributed to the arrival of a new group of residents in the internal medicine and family practice groups.

This type of report can also be used to track changes in query rates by the outpatient CDS. For example, according to the report in figure 12.4, 150 and 180 DM queries were made in the first and second quarters, respectively. The number of DM queries dropped to 172 in the third quarter and 99 in the fourth quarter. Root cause analysis attributes the increase in queries in the first half of the year to the CDS's increasing proficiency in the query process; the drop in queries in the second half of the year is explained by the physicians learning what documentation is required and consistently providing the necessary information. The data from figure 12.4 can also be depicted in a graph (figure 12.5), which can be used during a one-on-one or specialty-group discussion with providers or in a presentation to the outpatient CDI steering committee or taskforce.

Figure 12.4. Diabetes monthly physician response to query process report

| Diabetes (DM) Monthly Physician Response to Query Process Report ||||||||
| 1st quarter |||| 2nd quarter ||||
Mo.	# DM Queries	# Answers	% Response	Mo.	# DM Queries	# Answers	% Response
JAN	150	92	61%	APR	180	110	61%
FEB	89	61	69%	MAY	160	104	65%
MAR	110	79	72%	JUN	98	75	77%
3rd quarter				4th quarter			
Mo.	# DM Queries	# Answers	% Response	Mo.	# DM Queries	# Answers	% Response
JUL	172	133	77%	OCT	99	53	54%
AUG	132	87	66%	NOV	186	141	76%
SEP	169	115	68%	DEC	201	159	79%

Source: ©AHIMA

Figure 12.5. Diabetes monthly physician response to query process trend report

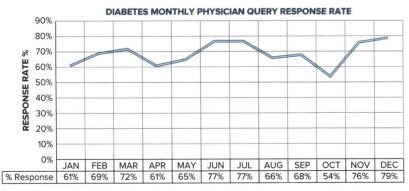

	JAN	FEB	MAR	APR	MAY	JUN	JUL	AUG	SEP	OCT	NOV	DEC
% Response	61%	69%	72%	61%	65%	77%	77%	66%	68%	54%	76%	79%

Source: ©AHIMA

Figure 12.6 reports on the average risk adjustment factor (RAF) for a professional practice group's HCCs for a four-year period (refer to chapter 3 for further discussion on RAF scores). For example, the report reflects the increase (improvement) in RAF score from 1.6342 for the first quarter 2014 to 1.8301 in the fourth quarter of 2017. This report can be used to highlight the ROI for the program during the four-year period.

Figure 12.6. Four-year average risk adjustment factor—HCCs

Risk Adjustment Factor—HCCs Quarterly Report

Year	1st QTR HCCs	2nd QTR HCCs	3rd QTR HCCs	4th QTR HCCs
2014	1.6342	1.6471	1.7539	1.8004
2015	1.7681	1.7734	1.7384	1.7621
2016	1.7762	1.7526	1.8189	1.8345
2017	1.8011	1.8101	1.8112	1.8301

Quarterly Risk Adjustment Factor—HCCs Quarterly Report

	1	2	3	4
1st QTR HCCs	1.6342	1.7681	1.7762	1.8011
2nd QTR HCCs	1.6471	1.7734	1.7526	1.8101
3rd QTR HCCs	1.7539	1.7384	1.8189	1.8112
4th QTR HCCs	1.8004	1.7621	1.8345	1.8301

Number of Patients per Quarter

Year	1st quarter	2nd quarter	3rd quarter	4th quarter
2014	8245	8007	8116	8351
2015	8349	7998	8205	8391
2016	8298	8016	8377	8432
2017	8460	8127	8423	8501

Source: ©AHIMA

The report in figure 12.7 provides a snapshot of the HCC-capture activity for patients during a four-year period. The assumption for this scenario is that the outpatient CDI program started in 2014. The report is like the one in figure 12.6, except figure 12.7 reflects the number of patients, number of HCCs, and average number of HCCs per patient during the four-year period. For example, the average number of HCCs per patient in the fourth quarter of 2014 was 13.95. In the fourth quarter of 2017, the average number of HCCs per patient was 14.93. The program metrics show the improvement in HCC capture over the four-year period since the start of the program in 2014. Training in the use of metrics reports is an important part of the CDS knowledge base and assists the CDS in determining future areas of focus for the program.

Figure 12.7. Quarterly HCC diagnoses report

Quarterly HCC Diagnoses Report

	1st quarter			2nd quarter		
Year	# Patients	# HCCs	Avg # HCCs/Pt	# Patients	# HCCs	Avg # HCCs/Pt
2014	1521	21085	13.86	1601	22368	13.97
2015	1796	25231	14.05	1802	25231	14.00
2016	2123	30625	14.43	1963	28652	14.60
2017	2475	36432	14.72	2179	32380	14.86
	3rd quarter			4th quarter		
Year	# Patients	# HCCs	Avg # HCCs/Pt	# Patients	# HCCs	Avg # HCCs/Pt
2014	1681	23500	13.98	1605	22390	13.95
2015	1801	25664	14.25	1736	24790	14.28
2016	1916	27782	14.50	1873	27140	14.49
2017	1920	28435	14.81	1898	28337	14.93

Source: ©AHIMA

Maintaining Program Visibility

Program sustainability is the primary target once the CDI program implementation phase is complete. A sustainable program is one that does the following:

- Develops solutions for improved clinical documentation and accurate coding to support quality metrics and medical necessity
- Continually addresses new issues and identifies new targets for case review and monitoring and develops corresponding solutions

- Maintains a solid ROI through strategic planning and management of resources
- Maintains a high-level customer (physician) satisfaction rate, and validates this rate through surveys and in-person discussions

To ensure a sustainable program, each CDS must be trained in case review, the query process, the role of the physician advisor, and the use of metrics and data analytics. Metrics with positive trend lines, improved quality scores, decreased denials rates, improved RAF scores, and coding accuracy rates of at least 95 percent are indicators of a sustainable clinical documentation program. The CDI manager should discuss the details of this process and encourage the outpatient CDS to be aware of program metrics and offer suggestions for CDI as root causes and solutions are identified.

Posttraining Evaluation

After the new outpatient CDS has been in place for 90 days, he or she is evaluated by the CDI manager. The 90-day evaluation can include a score for each of the functions listed in figure 12.8 or others selected by the CDI manager. Comments are used to provide positive feedback as well as recommendations for improvement. In addition, the outpatient CDS can take a posttraining test

Figure 12.8. 90-day evaluation form for a CDS

Clinical Documentation Improvement Specialist 90-Day Evaluation

Purpose: The purpose of the 90-day evaluation is to identify CDI development opportunities. The value of the review lies in the communication between manager and specialist.

Employee Name: _____ Hire date: _____
Evaluation date: _____

1 = Poor (Unable to complete basic job functions) *requires action plan*
2 = Less than satisfactory (Lacks knowledge in basic job functions)
3 = Satisfactory (Adequate grasp of job functions)
4 = Very good (Understands all phases of functions)
5 = Superior (Has completely mastered all functions) *requires comments*
** scores of 1 or 5 require comments

Function	1	2	3	4	5	Comments
Job Knowledge (Test Score)						
Quality of Work (Query Validation Score)						
Quantity of Work (Query Rate)						
Responsibility						
Attendance (less than 3 absences)						
Communication						
Initiative						

Performance Strengths: _____
_____
_____
_____
_____

Source: ©AHIMA

similar to the pretraining assessment to provide feedback for the CDI manager about any additional areas of study and training the CDS might need. A posttraining assessment test is included in appendix 12C this text.

The AHIMA Foundation has established professional competencies for the HIM profession. These competencies include CDI practice. Part of the process to establish new curricula for college and university HIM programs throughout the United States is to consider new methods for teaching students (Tyczkowski 2015). For example, as HIM programs move to the next level, educators can use "unfolding" case studies. This type of case study "fosters a learner-centered classroom, where the student is actively engaged in the learning process. In this format, information is presented in several stages. At each stage, the student engages in critical thinking and problem solving" (Tyczkowski 2015).

Critical Thinking Defined

Critical thinking involves the following key tasks (Hess 2015):

- Validating information
- Identifying exceptions
- Analyzing trends
- Considering what is not there
- Thinking "outside the box"
- Being creative

To accomplish these tasks, the critical thinker must be open to new information and alternative explanations as well as an unbiased consideration of what one presumes to be true about a given situation or problem before a conclusion is reached. "The primary difference between thinking and thinking critically is the added dynamic of having a purpose and control for the thought process" (Alfaro-LeFevre 2014).

Thinking critically requires more than criticism of the current state of affairs. Rather than a negative activity, it is a positive process developed to identify effective solutions to complex issues. Steps for critically considering a positive solution to a complex problem might be as follows:

- Gather and analyze information.
- Develop a set of assumptions that will be a basis for the thought process.
- Use scientific methods to develop conclusions.
- Discern the validity of knowledge sources using questions and judgment.
- Apply a creative thought process to develop possible solutions.
- Analyze the feasibility, advantages, and disadvantages of possible solutions.
- Determine necessary action.
- Positively communicate a proposal to stakeholders.
- Implement best-practice solutions.

The use of critical thinking allows for confidence through success, independent action, collaboration when needed, and effective and creative solutions that improve job satisfaction (Hess 2015; Alfaro-LeFevre 2014).

Why Is Critical Thinking Necessary in Healthcare?

Critical thinking skills are necessary in today's healthcare environment because of the complexity of the industry today. Healthcare professionals must apply analytic skills to complex decisions for high-quality patient care delivery. The intricacies of the EHR and associated interoperability issues have added a layer of complexity for the provider and healthcare workers. The Internet has exponentially increased the amount of available information on any subject. The large amount of information available to professionals today has resulted in specialization and subspecialization by providers as well as other clinicians and nonclinicians. Historically, there may have been one type of professional performing a combination of functions such as HIM management, quality assurance, utilization review, and CDI activities; today, however, each of these functions is typically performed by someone who specialize in that area.

Critical thinking skills are an area of focus for many healthcare managers as they encourage their staff to think through problem-solving at a higher level. CDSs may have been selected for their CDI positions based on their clinical expertise. Today's CDI team members must be competent in many other areas. CDI managers are calling for more highly skilled thought leaders who not only learn their specific area of expertise but also keep abreast of current research in interrelated areas to tie together a bigger picture of issues they face on a daily basis. The outpatient CDS should therefore learn about the organizational goals and objectives, budget issues, staffing constraints, key performance indicators, and strategic plans that affect the outpatient CDI areas during the day-to-day problem-solving process.

Critical thinking skills allow the CDS to become a transformational leader and someone who can do the following:

- *Challenge preliminary solutions.* Example: The outpatient CDS has been the key CDI staff member on the new outpatient CDI pilot clinic implementation. She understands that the hospital has been closely monitoring budgets because of a downturn in revenue related to the increase in risk-based payer plans. The initial plan for the CDI program rollout to additional clinics involved adding one outpatient CDS to each site. After working on the initial clinic implementation, the outpatient CDS streamlines some of the workflows to decrease time requirements and allow for remote CDSs to cover multiple clinics. The outpatient CDS presents this new process to the CDI taskforce. The CDI manager compliments the outpatient CDS for her critical thinking skills and for saving money for the health system.

- *Expand root cause analysis.* Example: The outpatient CDS reviews the response and agreement rates for all her clinics on a weekly basis. She notices that the response and agreement rates for Dr. Smith are much lower than those for the other providers in the internal medicine clinic. After collaboratively discussing the issue with Dr. Smith, the CDS learns that he travels to several of the outlying clinics because his subspecialty is endocrinology. Because of his travel schedule, he misses out on a benefit of providing patient care at the internal medicine clinic: At the clinic, a nonprovider clinician helps during the query process by notifying a physician just before the patient encounter if there are outstanding queries for the case. To ensure that Dr. Smith also gets previsit notification of queries, the outpatient CDS and Dr. Smith agree to a revised workflow for him that would include the use of an EHR alert on the patient's record. This alert will allow Dr. Smith to see the query prior to the patient encounter or as he is opening the case while in the patient room. The new process results in a significant increase in query responses and agreements by Dr. Smith.

- *Use critical thinking to identify more streamlined solutions and workflows.* Example: The outpatient CDS notices that the MIPS measure that includes diabetic eye exam is not being captured by the primary care providers. Provider education has been conducted on several occasions, but the capture rate has not improved. During a recent meeting with the new EHR vendor, the outpatient CDS learns of enhancements to the system that include in-line documentation prompts that could be used to query providers about the need for a diabetic eye exam on diabetic patients. The outpatient CDS creates the wording for the prompt and the exact point in the documentation process where the prompt should occur. She then sets up a meeting with the CDI manager and EHR vendor to discuss the possibility of including this prompt during the new system implementation.

The outpatient CDS should always be on the lookout for opportunities to use critical thinking skills to improve the workflow, provider communication process, and stakeholder collaboration. The issue at hand is not always obvious after a high-level investigation. A more in-depth root cause analysis, although more time-consuming, may lead to more cost-effective processes, improved key performance indicators (KPIs), and better collaboration among stakeholders.

Critical Thinking and the Learning Process

To improve one's critical thinking skills, one must focus on learning and be open to new ways of doing things. Research has shown that traditional learning approaches in which the student reads a textbook and listens to lectures are focused on the instructor rather than the student (Tyczkowski 2015). This method of learning is *passive*. An example of passive learning is requiring the student to read specific chapters and research articles to prepare for a quiz. In contrast, using the assigned materials as the starting point for a research project is an *active* form of learning that helps to solidify the information studied. As discussed in chapter 13, active learning methods are more successful than passive methods. Learning environments in all disciplines, including medical education, are moving toward active learning models (Frieden 2015).

Bloom's taxonomy (figure 12.9) categorizes levels of learning from low to high. The active learning model aims to move learning from recall, understanding, and application (lower-order thinking) to analysis, evaluation, and creation (higher-order thinking). The typical CDI trainee may begin practicing at the knowledge level, learning and recalling the basic concepts of CDI as they are introduced by managers and during training. The trainee may enter the job from a college or university program or from another healthcare job within the current facility. The next step, understanding, occurs as the CDI trainee begins the case review process while being shadowed by the trainer. The CDI trainee moves to the application level as he or she applies the knowledge of CDI and the case review process to identify opportunities for queries based on clinical indicators, knowledge, or medical necessity guidelines and quality measures. The analysis step occurs when the CDI trainee reviews metrics on query, response, and agreement rates to determine gaps for specific providers. Evaluation is demonstrated when the CDI trainee reviews the clinical documentation process for providers with response and agreement gaps. During this root cause analysis, the CDI trainee determines the reason why the provider has not responded or agreed at the expected rate. During the evaluation stage, the CDI trainee must collaborate with the providers and staff to develop a new workflow that corrects the problem. The highest level of thinking, the creation state, occurs when the CDI practitioner, who is no longer a trainee, has become a subject matter expert and presents findings and solutions to the CDI manager and taskforce. These solutions can typically be used to assist other practitioners to improve KPI metrics, provider adoption, and provider collaboration.

Figure 12.9. Bloom's taxonomy

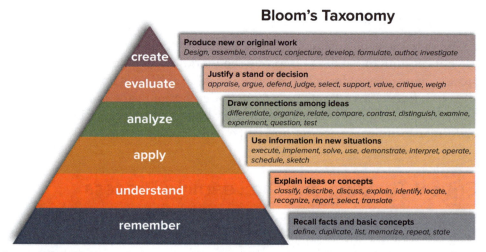

Source: Vanderbilt University Center for Teaching. 2018 (January). "29428436431_170dc675d7_o.png." Digital Image. Flickr.

The following case example applies Bloom's taxonomy to categorize an outpatient's levels of thinking when approaching the issue of accurate HCC capture for diabetes-related conditions.

Case Example

While conducting an audit of primary care cases, the outpatient CDS notices that many of the physicians in the primary care clinics throughout the health system document type 1 or type 2 diabetes in their progress notes during most encounters with diabetic patients. The physicians also frequently document a condition that may be a complication of diabetes, such as retinopathy. The CDS may question whether additional documentation including the word "with" is required to code these two diagnoses documented as (1) type 1 diabetes and (2) retinopathy. Section I.A.15 of the *ICD-10-CM Official Guidelines for Coding and Reporting* states the following about the use of the word "with:

> The word "with" should be interpreted to mean "associated with" or "due to" when it appears in a code title, the Alphabetic Index, or an instructional note in the Tabular List (NCHS, 2018). The word "with" in the Alphabetic Index is sequenced immediately following the main term, not in alphabetical order. To clarify guidance, for example, to accurately assign the E11.319, Type 2 diabetes mellitus with retinopathy, the physician documentation does not need to provide a link between the diagnoses of diabetes and retinopathy; this can be assumed since the retinopathy is listed under the subterm "with" (NCHS 2017).

Problem Resolution without Critical Thinking

Knowledge
The outpatient CDS learns from a recent HCC seminar that diabetes is one of the primary HCC documentation gaps. She uses her knowledge of HCC capture to identify that the primary care physicians are not documenting secondary and associated diabetic complications, such as peripheral neuropathy, peripheral vascular disease, and diabetic retinopathy. If the patient's additional comorbid conditions associated with diabetes are not documented, the clinical record is incomplete.

Comprehension
The outpatient CDS completes an audit of the primary care practices and compiles a report that includes the total cases reviewed, total cases with documentation gaps, and percentage of documentation gaps.

Application
The outpatient CDS presents the information to the CDI manager, and they discuss a corrective plan of action. The action plan is to present the findings at the monthly primary care provider meeting.

The lower-order thinking process is outlined in the flowchart in figure 12.10.

Figure 12.10. CDS uses lower-order thinking process to address a clinical documentation gap

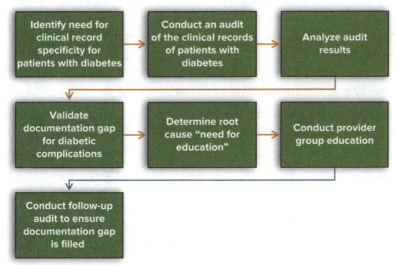

Source: ©AHIMA

Problem Resolution with Critical Thinking

Analysis

The outpatient CDS has recently attended a lecture on using critical thinking skills in the healthcare operations setting. She reconsiders the data and her original conclusion that the problem was that the physicians were not educated about the need to document diabetic complications in the progress note for each encounter in which the monitor, evaluate, assess/address, or treat (MEAT) requirements were met. (Refer to chapters 3 and 6 for more information on MEAT.) She decides to further evaluate the data and clinical documentation workflow by scheduling a shadowing session with one of the providers who has the highest gap in diabetic complication documentation.

At the clinic, the outpatient CDS describes the audit process and her initial analysis. She then explains that she wants to better understand the clinical documentation workflow and perform a more in-depth root cause analysis. The provider agrees to allow the outpatient CDS to observe during a four-hour period, while patients are being seen in the clinic. The outpatient CDS follows these steps during the four-hour shadowing session:

1. Reviews the patient's record, including historical clinical records in the inpatient, outpatient, and professional practice and provider settings, before the visit;
2. Observes the provider to determine whether he reviews clinical records before entering the examination room to see a patient;
3. Observes the provider as he interviews the patient and documents in the clinical record; and
4. Reviews the clinical record for the concurrent encounter to determine any documentation gaps.

Evaluation

The outpatient CDS observes the clinical documentation workflow for 10 patients with diabetes during the four-hour period. She notes that the provider

- Does not review the clinical record before entering the examination room;
- Opens the clinical record for the first time during the patient's examination and discussion;
- Conducts only a cursory review of the problem list (which, the CDS also notes, does not contain all diabetic complications);
- Does not ask the patient about possible diabetic complications during the history-taking part of the encounter;
- Documents "diabetic exam" as the reason for the encounter; and
- Submits the claim with only one ICD-10-CM code for type 1 or type 2 diabetes.

After the shadowing period is complete, the outpatient CDS considers the gaps in the clinical documentation process to be as follows:

- The provider did not have the information on the patient's diabetic complications at the time of the visit. The provider needs quick access to this information at the time of the visit.
- The problem list was inaccurate and had not been updated for several years. A new workflow for problem list update is needed.
- The EHR did not provide prompts, alerts, or templates that would help the provider include additional specificity about the patient's diabetic condition.

Creation

The outpatient CDS determines that a new workflow is needed to ensure provider access of historical patient information related to diabetic complications. In a redesigned workflow, an outpatient CDS could review the patient's records before the encounter and use a query to alert the physician about potential diabetic complications in the patient's historical record. An updated problem list and an automated solution using in-line documentation templates, alerts, or prompts could be incorporated in the EHR to help the physician create the encounter progress note. The outpatient CDS develops the following task list reflecting the root cause analysis and recommendations for resolution:

- Present the findings to the CDI manager with detailed root cause analysis and recommended solution and implementation steps. Collaborate with the manager on a proposal about the best way to move forward.
- Present the new solutions to the CDI taskforce for further discussion and approval.
- Establish and implement a process for a CDS to shadow providers before, during, and after patient encounters.
- Meet with the primary care physicians individually to discuss a streamlined approach and adoption of the process.
- Develop an in-line documentation template for encounters with patients with diabetes, and meet with the primary care physicians to discuss proposed content and functionality.
- Meet with the information technology (IT) team to discuss an EHR technology solution for in-line documentation to include prompts, alerts, and templates.
- Develop a timetable for implementation of new solutions.
- Present the new solutions to the CDI manager and gain approval.
- Present the findings and proposed solutions to the CDI steering committee.
- Ensure that the IT team implements the solution.
- Monitor the progress using metrics, and communicate metrics to the providers, CDI taskforce, and CDI steering committee.

The higher-order thinking process is outlined in figure 12.11.

Figure 12.11. CDS uses higher-order thinking process to address a clinical documentation gap

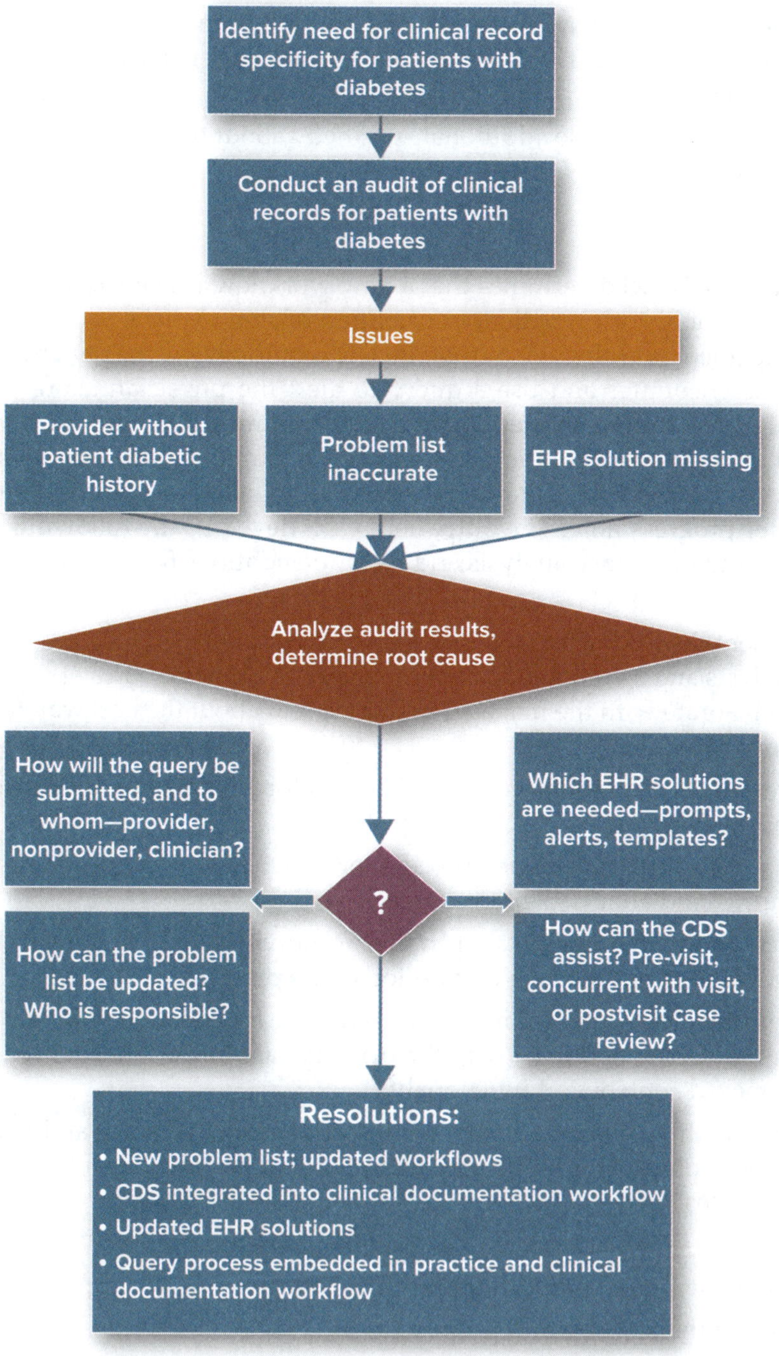

```
            Identify need for clinical record
            specificity for patients with
                     diabetes
                         ↓
             Conduct an audit of clinical
             records for patients with
                     diabetes
                         ↓
                      Issues
                         ↓
   ┌─────────────────┬──────────────────┬────────────────────┐
   Provider without    Problem list       EHR solution missing
   patient diabetic    inaccurate
   history
   └─────────────────┴──────────────────┴────────────────────┘
                         ↓
             Analyze audit results,
             determine root cause
                         ↓
                         ?
```

- How will the query be submitted, and to whom—provider, nonprovider, clinician?
- Which EHR solutions are needed—prompts, alerts, templates?
- How can the problem list be updated? Who is responsible?
- How can the CDS assist? Pre-visit, concurrent with visit, or postvisit case review?

Resolutions:
- New problem list; updated workflows
- CDS integrated into clinical documentation workflow
- Updated EHR solutions
- Query process embedded in practice and clinical documentation workflow

Source: ©AHIMA

Using Critical Thinking to Surmount Barriers to Success

In any process, barriers to success must be overcome. Table 12.2 lists the barriers identified in the previous case study, along with the critical thinking skills used to surmount them.

Table 12.2. Critical thinking to address barriers to success

Barrier	Critical Thinking Skills
Lack of historical patient data available to provider at the time of the visit	Creative approach to utilizing EHR functionality to provide historical patient information. Technology skills for communicating with physician using multiple system functionality
Lack of CDS interaction to assist in diagnostic specificity in the clinical record	Creative analysis of workflow design and redesign process
Ineffective or absent query communication process	Effective communication skills and workflow redesign techniques for collaborating and developing new query process
Absent EHR in-line documentation process	Analytic and technology skills required to create new technology workflow and collaborate with IT developers in new system functionality design

First Barrier: Historical Patient Data Unavailable to the Provider at the Time of the Visit

The first potential barrier to the capture of diabetic complications in the clinical record is a lack of historical patient data available to the provider at the time of the visit. The following questions can help identify whether this is a barrier and then address the root cause of the problem:

- Under the current workflow, how can the provider review a patient's historical clinical data?
- Are multiple systems involved, and is interoperability an issue?
- Does the provider have time to review patient history information in multiple EHR systems prior to the patient visit?
- Is there a technology or CDS workflow solution that can streamline the process of reviewing patient histories? For example, if the provider is currently required to review a patient's historical data from multiple EHRs, can the problem list be used as an alternative to validate current and historical diagnoses within the continuum of care?

The CDS must investigate the various EHR systems that include historical clinical information and determine whether providers can access them easily and efficiently before the patient visits. Assuming that the provider does not have time to review multiple EHR systems, the CDS must also assess the use of the problem list as an alternative and determine whether the problem list is periodically updated and accurate. If the CDS must create a streamlined solution for the provider, he or she must look for the most cost-effective solution. For example, should technology functionality be changed, should the CDS shadow the provider, or should both of these steps be implemented?

Second Barrier: Lack of CDS Interaction with Providers to Help Ensure Diagnostic Specificity in the Clinical Record

The second potential barrier to the capture of diabetic complications in the clinical record is a lack of CDS interaction with providers to help ensure diagnostic specificity in the clinical record. If this is a barrier, a shadowing process could be integrated into the provider practice workflow so that the CDS could review the historical records and query the provider, if necessary, to include the diabetic complication documentation that fit the MEAT criteria. The following questions should be considered:

- Does the CDS understand the current workflow and the best way to communicate query information to the provider?
- Does the CDS understand the EHR system functionality required for query communication?
- Is the provider open to working with the CDS during the previsit, concurrent, or postvisit query process?

The CDS must investigate the various options for communication with the provider and determine which is most efficient and streamlined so that the day-to-day patient interactions and provider workflow are not impaired. This investigation occurs through observation of the workflow and collaborative discussion of communication options (verbal, electronic) and timing (pre-encounter, concurrent with the visit, or postencounter). The CDS must have in-depth knowledge of EHR functionality and options, which may require learning from the IT department about the current process and options for enhancements. The CDS staff should also be kept abreast of the latest changes in ICD-10-CM coding guidelines (such as the coding of diabetes and diabetes comorbidities).

Third Barrier: Ineffective or Absent Query Communication Process

The third potential barrier to the capture of diabetic complications in the clinical record is an ineffective or absent query communication process. The CDS must determine whether an effective query process is currently in place. The following questions should be considered:

- Is there a query process in place? If so, how many queries are submitted, and what are the response and agreement rates?
- If response and agreement rates are low, what are the reasons?
- What is the provider preference for query communication? Alerts, prompts, templates?
- Should the query be submitted to the provider or a nonprovider clinician?
- What is the most efficient and compliant way to notify the provider of a patient's history of chronic illnesses that might affect HCC capture?

The answers to these questions may be found by reviewing chapter 16.

Fourth Barrier: Absence of an EHR In-line Documentation Process

The fourth potential barrier to the capture of diabetic complications in the clinical record is the absence of an EHR in-line documentation process. If queries only come to the provider via e-mail, the provider may not be aware of them while documenting a patient encounter. In contrast, in-line documentation allows the provider to respond to prompts and queries shown within the EHR during the clinical documentation process (see chapter 7). The CDS must determine whether an in-line process is in place and not being used or if there is no process available. The following questions should be considered:

- Does the EHR system have in-line documentation functionality?
- If it does, why is the process not being used by the physicians?
- If it does not, is the physician open to using in-line documentation instead of e-mail queries or EHR alerts, prompts, and templates?
- Does the CDS have adequate knowledge of EHR functionality to assist the provider in the use of current functionality?
- Are IT resources available to develop in-line documentation functionality (internally or through the IT vendor)?

The CDS must possess sufficient knowledge of EHR functionality to assess the current system or assist in the development of new EHR functionality. Therefore, the CDS may need to study the existing EHR functionality and possible enhancements. If the functionality is in place, or if new functionality is installed, the CDS will educate the provider on its use. The CDS should also follow up to see whether the provider is using the functionality as designed.

Integrating Effective Communication

Implementing or changing a process such as the clinical documentation workflow is never just a mechanical or technical challenge. It also involves human factors, such as the many personalities of the participants and the political environment of the setting, and, for that reason, it requires effective communication. Effective communication is part of the critical thinking process. By adopting the following habits, the CDS can enhance his or her critical thinking skills and become a more effective communicator:

- Demonstrate open-mindedness through open communication with other departments and leaders. Collaborate with others using critical thinking techniques to identify root causes and comprehensive solutions to problems.
- Communicate with stakeholders in person whenever possible, either one-on-one or collaboratively in a group setting. E-mails, memos, and instant messages do not work as well as in-person communication when people must cooperate to resolve operational issues, and no one appreciates hearing about a problem secondhand. In-person discussions allow stakeholders to be part of the solution.
- Collaborate with stakeholders to find out details of the workflow and historical roadblocks to problem-solving. This saves time during root cause analysis and avoids repeat trials of proposed resolutions that previously failed.
- Share your insights about case scenarios with colleagues and mentors. They might benefit from what you have learned in their own professional practice, and they can also provide feedback on your ideas.

Chapter 12 Review Exercises

1. The leaders of a CDI program are in the process of onboarding a new outpatient CDS and want to gain a better understanding of her baseline credentials and experience. Which of the following tools would be *best* utilized for this task?
   a. Pretraining assessment
   b. Posttraining assessment
   c. Skills requirement checklist
   d. Résumé and college transcripts

2. A recently hired outpatient CDS lacks a coding background and decides to pursue professional development opportunities to advance his career. As part of this initiative, he completes an online course in ICD-10-CM and CPT/HCPCS coding. After training, he decides to pursue a coding credential to supplement the training and bolster his professional standing. Which of the following credentials would be *most appropriate* to pursue, given his background and needs?
   a. CCA
   b. CCS
   c. CDIP
   d. CCDS

3. Which topic covered during outpatient CDI specialist training involves reviewing all previous and most recent AHIMA practice briefs; discussion of templates, standard formats, and workflow; and trainer shadowing?
   a. Data review training
   b. Query process training
   c. Program process and design training
   d. Clinical documentation case review training

4. Which of the following functions is assessed as part of the 90-day CDS evaluation?
   a. HCC RAF score
   b. Query Validation Score
   c. Provider-specific case mix index
   d. Physician group participation score

5. A sustainable CDI program is one that develops solutions for improved clinical documentation and accurate coding to support quality metrics and medical necessity. Which of the following *best* describes a characteristic of a sustainable CDI program?
   a. Maintains a 90 percent HCC capture rate
   b. Ensures a 50 percent bonus-sharing plan with Medicare Advantage
   c. Demonstrates an upward case mix index trend for all specialty clinics
   d. Provides a solid ROI through strategic planning and management of resources

6. A CDS may contact a physician advisor for various reasons, including to seek advice when implementing a new CDI process. For which of the following reasons would a CDS be *most likely* to contact a physician advisor?
   a. Need for physician education
   b. Decreased historical RAF score average
   c. Marketing strategy for the oncology clinic
   d. New physician assistant in the cardiology clinic

7. Which of the following learning methods is *most likely* to improve critical thinking skills?
   a. Active learning
   b. Passive learning
   c. Traditional learning
   d. Lower-order learning

8. Which of the following barriers to success would be *best* addressed through a workflow redesign that aims to improve collaboration?
   a. Absence of an EHR in-line documentation process
   b. Ineffective or absent query communication process
   c. Limited availability of historical patient data to the provider at the time of the visit
   d. Lack of CDS interaction with providers to help ensure diagnostic specificity in the clinical record

9. Which of the following describes a likely use of a query process report?
   a. Demonstrating improvement in physician response
   b. Highlighting ROI for the CDI program
   c. Measuring improvement in HCC capture during a given period
   d. Identifying Medicare Advantage patients scheduled for a particular day or week

10. Critical thinking is an important part of the CDS skillset and vital to the CDI problem-solving process. Which of the following is *least likely* to support critical thinking among CDI staff?
    a. Strong purpose behind the thought process
    b. Ability to criticize the current state of affairs
    c. Willingness to entertain alternative explanations
    d. Lack of bias in characterizing the facts surrounding a problem

References

Alfaro-LeFevre, R. 2014. What are critical thinking, clinical reasoning, and clinical judgment? In: *Critical Thinking, Clinical Reasoning, and Clinical Judgment: A Practical Approach*, 5th ed. St. Louis, MO: Elsevier: 1–22.

American Academy of Professional Coders (AAPC). 2017. http://www.aapc.org.

American Health Information Management Association (AHIMA). 2017a. AHIMA online education. http://www.ahima.org/education/onlineed/Programs/cdi.

American Health Information Management Association (AHIMA). 2017b. AHIMA online coding courses. http://www.ahima.org/education/onlineed/Programs/cb.

American Health Information Management Association (AHIMA). 2017c. AHIMA query toolkit. http://bok.ahima.org/PdfView?oid=302140.

American Health Information Management Association (AHIMA). 2016a. Clinical documentation toolkit (2016 version). http://bok.ahima.org/Toolkit/CDI#.WSHwEoWcG3A.

American Health Information Management Association (AHIMA). 2016b. AHIMA practice brief: Guidelines for achieving a compliant query practice (2016 update). http://bok.ahima.org/PB/QueryCompliance#.WhDAX0qnE2w.

Association of Clinical Documentation Specialists (ACDIS). 2018. https://acdis.org/certification/about.

Centers for Medicare and Medicaid Services (CMS). 2018. Medicare Learning Network. MLN Web-Based Training. https://www.cms.gov/Outreach-and-Education/Medicare-Learning-Network-MLN/MLNProducts/WebBasedTraining.html.

Centers for Medicare and Medicaid Services (CMS) Glossary. 2017. https://www.cms.gov/apps/glossary/default.asp?Letter=ALL&Language=English.

Frieden, J. 2015 (August 7). Changing face of medical education: it's all about the system. Medpage Today. https://www.medpagetoday.com/PublicHealthPolicy/MedicalEducation/52990.

Hess, P.C. 2015. *Clinical Documentation Improvement: Principles and Practice*. Chicago: AHIMA Press.

National Center for Health Statistics (NCHS). 2017. ICD-10-CM Official Guidelines for Coding and Reporting FY 2018. https://www.cms.gov/Medicare/Coding/ICD10/Downloads/2018-ICD-10-CM-Coding-Guidelines.pdf.

Tyczkowski, B. 2015. New health information management (HIM) competencies? Teaching critical thinking using an unfolding case study. *Educational Perspectives in Health Information Management*. http://eduperspectives.ahima.org/new-health-information-management-him-competencies-teaching-critical-thinking-using-an-unfolding-case-study.

Vanderbilt University Center for Teaching. 2018. Bloom's Taxonomy. https://cft.vanderbilt.edu/guides-sub-pages/blooms-taxonomy.

Provider and Clinical Staff CDI Education in the Outpatient Setting

13

Learning Objectives

- Explain effective methods to teach physicians and clinical staff about clinical documentation improvement (CDI).
- Identify the different types of providers and clinicians who can benefit from CDI training.
- Describe the content for educational sessions about CDI for physicians, nonphysician providers, and clinical staff.
- Describe the steps included in an outpatient CDS clinical documentation workflow supported by clinical staff.
- Explain how to encourage attendance and participation in CDI educational sessions.
- Understand how to structure a slide presentation for a CDI educational session.

Key Terms

Audit and feedback
Certified medical assistants (CMAs)
Clinical nurse specialists (CNSs)
Computerized decision support system data

Continuing medical education (CME)
Nonphysician providers (NPPs)
Passive dissemination
Real-time computerized reminders

The learning methods used in provider training about clinical documentation improvement (CDI) should reflect evolving worldviews in medicine and complement and support the efforts of the healthcare industry to re-create itself and shift from volume-based to outcome-based payment models. Provider education in CDI can help mitigate the challenges associated with multitasking, time management, and physician adoption of technology-based solutions. Physician educators, including those teaching providers about CDI, should "start with the end in mind, figuring out what doctors need to be able to do and know" (Frieden 2015a). In the context of the outpatient CDI program, the instructor should be well versed in the program content, understand physician attitudes and how each physician learns best, and be able to apply measurable goals and objectives that validate the physician trainee's success. Using the new approaches in medical education discussed in this text, the outpatient CDI manager can evaluate the target physician groups or individuals and develop programs based on the providers' understanding of the healthcare delivery system.

Trends in Physician Education

> "As medicine becomes more of a patient-centered, team-provided service, medical education must adapt to adequately prepare medical students. New information delivery methods are necessary to help students themselves adapt to a changing professional environment" *(Lefler 2013)*.

Compared with more experienced providers, physicians who have recently entered the workforce may be more open to workplace training in CDI because of recent shifts in medical school curricula. Whereas medical education has historically involved two years of coursework in basic science followed by two years of clinical training, newer programs are incorporating training in soft skills such as compassion and team orientation. In at least some medical schools, small-group, team-based learning that focuses on the collective success of the group, rather than the individual's success, is considered the future of medical education (Lefler 2013). US medical schools are also developing curricula focused on healthcare delivery issues, such as courses in "health policy, health economics, the role of community agencies, the importance of electronic health information, the importance of teamwork, leadership, evidence-based care, and healthcare financing, including about the Affordable Care Act and how it affects patients" (Frieden 2015b). These types of courses familiarize new physicians with issues related to CDI, such as value-based purchasing and risk-based payment, the relationship of clinical documentation to accuracy in reimbursement, quality measures, and provider-to-provider collaboration. Additionally, innovative options for learning and training, such as online courses, are being used as part of medical school education (Lefler 2013).

Like medical school curriculum, **continuing medical education (CME)** is also evolving in directions that can support CDI training for providers. CME refers to an educational activity for physicians that is conducted for the purpose of increasing their professional practice knowledge and skills. The content of these activities is typically in the areas of medical science and public health, and physicians must complete CME hours to maintain licensures, certifications, and credentials (ACCME, 2017). Organizations offering CME can submit the outline of the CME activity to the Accreditation Council for Continuing Medical Education to receive prior approval for the number of CME hours that physicians can earn by participating (ACCME 2017).

In CME, there is a trend toward more active forms of learning, such as programs that facilitate physician discussion with the use of clinical case reviews, and away from passive methodologies, such as simply disseminating printed educational materials and the formal, didactic classroom approach. In a systematic review of 14 reviews of interventions designed to get physicians to implement guidelines in clinical practice, "active forms of continuing medical education and multifaceted interventions were found to be the most effective methods for implementing guidelines into general practice. Additionally, active approaches to changing physician performance were shown to improve practice to a greater extent than traditional passive methods" (Mostofian et al. 2015). Table 13.1 provides an overview of the types of interventions included in the systematic review and indicates whether each is a passive or active approach. Most of the studies included in three of the reviews (71 percent) in this study showed "positive change in physician behavior when [physicians were] exposed to active educational methods and multifaceted interventions" (Mostofian et al. 2015). The use of multiple educational methods (multifaceted interventions such as audit, feedback, reminders, and CME) was most effective in changing physician behavior, even though some of the interventions were passive (Mostofian et al. 2015).

Table 13.1. Passive versus active forms of interventions to encourage implementation of guidelines by physicians

Type of Intervention	Passive vs Active
Audit and feedback	Passive
Computerized decision support systems	Active
Didactic lecture–based CME	Passive
Interactive CME facilitating physician discussion and clinical case review	Active
Influence of local opinion leaders	Passive
Marketing	Passive
Passive dissemination of information	Passive
Real-time computerized reminders	Active
Manual reminders (paper-based reminders)	Active

Source: Mostofian et al. 2015.

Recommended Approaches to Physician Education about CDI

Extrapolating from the current research on effective learning methodologies, we can conclude that the outpatient CDI physician education program should be a multifaceted combination of active and passive interventions (Frieden 2015a; Frieden 2015b; Frieden 2015c; Mostofian et al. 2015; Lefler 2013). Recommended educational interventions include the following:

- *Audits and feedbacks:* An **audit and feedback** intervention summarizes "clinical performance on patient care over a specified period based on medical records, computerized databases, patient surveys, or observation" (Mostofian et al. 2015). Research indicates that audit and feedback interventions are most effective when the feedback is provided at the time of decision making (Mostofian et al. 2015); therefore, feedback on case audit results should be provided to each physician separately. After removing case-identifying information, trainers can also use the initial audit of the focus area as a case study to discuss during CME presentations.

- *Analysis of **computerized decision support system data***: Metrics, trends, and other data used by computerized decision support systems to improve to clinical decision making can be discussed during CME presentations and provided as part of a monthly or quarterly report for individual physicians in the form of a scorecard that includes peer benchmarking information.

- *Interactive CME that facilitates physician discussion and clinical case review*: During the CME presentation, the presenter should engage participants using polling questions; interactive, small group sessions and case study discussions; and rapid redesign sessions for identifying streamlined workflows for new CDI processes.

- *Annual compliance training*: Consider adding a module that includes outpatient CDI to the annual compliance assessment.

- *Online training modules*: In some healthcare organizations, the education department may have sophisticated learning platforms for online training. If that technology is not available, slide decks and the related audio from live CME presentations on CDI can be recorded and then used as part of a work-at-your-own-pace online module that includes exercises or questions to measure understanding.

- *Passive dissemination of information*: **Passive dissemination** refers to activities such as providing reading materials rather than having an interactive discussion. Prior to and during CME programs, trainers can provide take-home information that includes data and information providers will need in the future to accomplish the objectives outlined during the program. The information may be distributed as printed material or an electronic file or via a link to an online training module.

- *Real-time computerized reminders*: **Real-time computerized reminders** are electronic health record (EHR) alerts and prompts that can be used to help the physician during the clinical documentation process. For example, EHRs can offer information and prompts to guide the provider as he or she documents clinical indicators, signs, symptoms, and medications that may be related to specific disease processes or procedures (see chapter 7).

Nonphysician Providers

The number of physicians globally and in the United States is decreasing, causing a physician shortage (Weldon 2014). The Global Health Workforce Alliance (GHWA), whose secretariat is the World Health Organization, was established in 2006 as a partnership of governments that will address crisis situations and advocate for solutions (GHWA 2013). The GHWA estimates that by 2035 the global shortage of healthcare providers will be 12.9 million (GHWA 2013). This shortage is applicable not only to physicians but also to other healthcare providers. To mitigate this broad-reaching healthcare issue, nonphysician clinicians are delivering healthcare to patients in a variety of settings. The year-over-year growth for **nonphysician providers (NPPs)**, also called mid-level providers, is roughly 160 percent, which is significantly higher than the 10 percent to 20 percent increase for other healthcare positions (MGMA 2016).

NPPs work under the supervision of an attending physician in both the inpatient and ambulatory settings in a variety of inpatient and outpatient settings. Types of NPPs include physician assistants (PAs), nurse practitioners (NPs), optometrists, physical therapists, and certified registered nurse anesthetists (CRNAs). The most common types of NPPs are the PA and NP. PAs and NPs typically work with teams of physicians and allow the physicians to provide services to a broader patient base in a timelier manner, with higher quality of care at a lower cost.

"Nurse practitioners are well suited to careers in primary care" (Dark 2011). They diagnose, manage and treat illness, disease, and impairments, as well as engage in preventive and promotive care (Brown et al. 2011). An NPP will have a master's or doctorate degree with two or more years of additional postbaccalaureate studies. These requirements can be condensed into the criteria shown in figure 13.1.

Figure 13.1. Mid-level providers

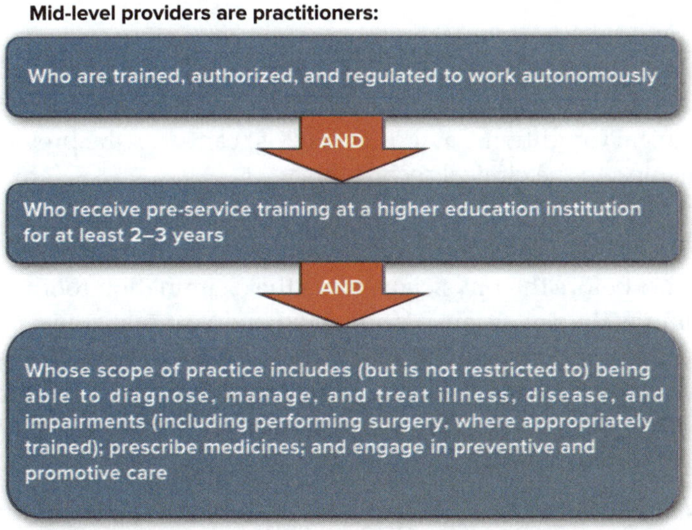

Mid-level providers are practitioners:

- Who are trained, authorized, and regulated to work autonomously

AND

- Who receive pre-service training at a higher education institution for at least 2–3 years

AND

- Whose scope of practice includes (but is not restricted to) being able to diagnose, manage, and treat illness, disease, and impairments (including performing surgery, where appropriately trained); prescribe medicines; and engage in preventive and promotive care

Source: Brown et al. 2011.

Clinical nurse specialists (CNSs) may also be categorized as NPPs. A CNS is a nurse with a bachelor's degree in nursing as well as a master's or doctorate degree from a clinical nurse specialist program (NACNS 2017). CNSs specialize in and focus their practice on a specialty area of disease management.

Medicare and state laws regulate the scope of practice for all types of NPPs, including CNSs. If allowed under their state's regulations, NPPs can provide and be reimbursed for selected Medicare services. NPPs often work independently in private practice, and Medicare will assign their unique Medicare provider numbers. However, reimbursement of NPPs by Medicare is capped at 85 percent of the Medicare Physician Fee Schedule (Wier 2013).

An understanding of the roles, education, and degrees of autonomy of NPPs is essential to the understanding of their clinical documentation workflow. NPPs document most of the clinical information in the patient's record. Their documentation may be used to report *International Classification of Diseases, Tenth Revision, Clinical Modification* (ICD-10-CM), Current Procedural Terminology (CPT), and Healthcare Common Procedure Coding System (HCPCS) codes on the claim. If NPPs practice in the facility, it is essential to include them in provider education sessions. The NPP role is vital in achieving best-practice clinical documentation and coding.

Nonprovider Clinicians

In addition to the NPPs, nonprovider clinicians contribute to the care and treatment of patients in the outpatient setting and can provide supporting clinical documentation. Types of nonprovider clinicians include registered nurses (RNs), licensed practical nurses (LPNs), and **certified medical assistants (CMAs)**. CMAs are trained in medical assistance through an accredited postsecondary program (AAMA 2017).

Nonprovider clinicians can greatly contribute to the success of the new outpatient CDI program by doing the following:

- *Identifying and monitoring the focus area in cases for review by the outpatient clinical documentation specialist (CDS).* Example: The CMA performs a case review of all cases scheduled for the following day to determine whether Hierarchical Condition Categories (HCCs) captured the previous year are documented in the clinical record this year.

- *Ensuring that the provider reviews and responds to the CDS query.* Example: The RN reviews an electronic query for a patient scheduled today. Just before the physician enters the examination room, the RN reminds the physician to review the query so that clinical documentation can be added where appropriate to support the coding of chronic conditions affecting treatment or medical decision making.

- *Reminding the physician or other provider to include additional clinical documentation as needed to support medical necessity, quality measures, and coding/billing guidelines.* Example: The LPN notes an electronic query submitted by the outpatient CDS yesterday. The query requests that the physician review the problem list stating the patient is immunocompromised. This chronic condition will alter the capture of Merit-Based Incentive Payment System (MIPS) measures and exclude the patient from the denominator group, therefore improving the MIPS score on acute sinusitis patients with computed tomography scan ordered unnecessarily.

- *Assessing the quality of the clinical documentation postvisit and prompting the provider to add additional information as needed.* Example: the RN reviews the patient's record immediately after a visit to ensure that "immunocompromised" was entered into the clinical record on today's visit.

Establishing Group Educational Sessions

The outpatient CDI program manager must decide who (NPPs or nonprovider clinicians) will be included in the educational sessions. In general, NPPs should be included in the education sessions for physicians. Physicians and NPPs work closely together in teams, and the NPPs often support the physician by completing the clinical documentation for the visit progress note, consultation report, or surgical procedure report. If both physicians and NPPs are included in the same session, they will be able to discuss the clinical documentation workflow process and streamline the implementation of the outpatient CDS shadowing, case review, and query process.

Before educating physicians and NPPs, it may be beneficial to have a separate educational session for the nonprovider clinician group so that the nonprovider clinicians can openly discuss strategies for physician–NPP engagement and adoption of the process. In this session, the details of the workflow for each individual physician can be reviewed, and suggested modifications can be made to the process, so that the presentation of the new workflow to the provider group is well thought out.

Figure 13.2 depicts the outpatient CDS workflow using nonphysician clinicians to support the process. This process should be discussed during the training sessions for the nonphysician clinician groups.

Figure 13.2. Outpatient CDS clinical documentation workflow

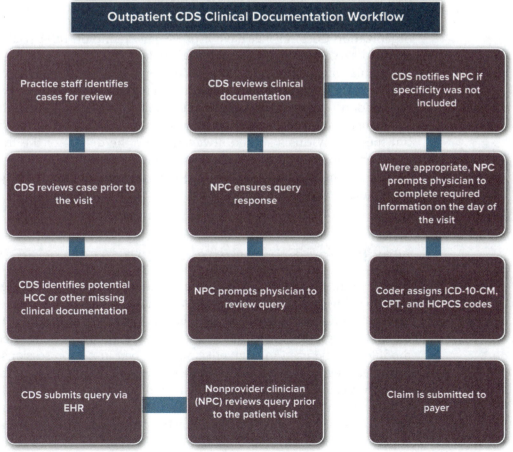

Source: ©AHIMA

Selecting Instructors for Nonprovider Clinician CDI Educational Programs

Professionals tend to learn best from a peer whom they trust and respect (Hess 2015). The instructor(s) for the nonprovider clinician session should include the outpatient CDI program manager or CDS as well as a nonprovider clinician leader. This leader may be a clinic or practice nurse manager. Buy-in and support from the leadership of the group are essential for successfully revising the existing workflow.

In addition to the slide presentation in figure 13.3, interactive workflow redesign discussions are important so that each staff member can express concerns and present ideas for a streamlined process that will be different in each practice and for each provider.

Selecting Instructors for Physician CDI Educational Programs

A CDI program physician advisor is an excellent candidate for the position of peer instructor for physician education about CDI. In addition to the peer instructor, it is also recommended that a CDI subject matter expert participate in the instruction. This instructor may be an outpatient CDS or the outpatient CDI manager or director. Involving both the peer instructor and the CDI expert in the training program will increase the likelihood of program success. If the organization does not yet have a physician champion or specialty leader in place to serve as a peer instructor, an outside consultant can be retained to function as the peer trainer. The outside consultant should have experience in CDI physician training and collaboration and be well versed in current industry standards and guidelines related to clinical documentation. Either the outside consultant or the CDI program leader can develop the training materials, but these individuals should always review the details of the training plan together before to the training begins. This discussion will ensure that both parties are sharing the same message with providers about the organization's policy and practices.

Maximizing Educational Program Attendance

If feasible, all physicians who practice in a setting where an outpatient CDI program is being implemented or is in place should receive training in some form. In-person presentations are recommended because they are effective for the team-building and buy-in processes. However, online or self-paced recorded modules can be used to augment training when in-person sessions are not an option for some or all providers. After training, instructors should follow up with physician participants to ensure that all of their questions are answered.

When training physicians in private practice, a group training session on the practice premises during breakfast, lunch, or dinner may encourage attendance. A personal call to the office manager and physician leader of the practice from the physician advisor or CDI manager is essential to gain buy-in and attendance at the training session. The CDI manager should ask whether physicians have specific clinical documentation issues and concerns that they will likely want to discuss during the session and then help the physician peer trainer prepare to address their questions. Understanding the practice organization, market issues, reimbursement landscape, and physician personalities is also beneficial when preparing an effective training session.

Where possible, having an educational session away from the clinic or practice is suggested. At a minimum, the session should be held in a separate conference room away from the patient care area. Having the discussions in the hallway will not allow for the attention to detail by the participants.

CME Presentation Content

CME presentations on CDI should reflect the specialties, personalities, and quality and reimbursement issues of the participants. The following presentation, which may be modified for each specialty group, is included in appendix 13A. The presenter can use the slide deck in the appendix to practice the presentation, add to the slide notes, and modify the slide content as needed to reflect the makeup of the group attending the presentation (for example, their specialties, preferences, practice patterns and time constraints).

A typical time frame for the presentation is 30 to 60 minutes. The presentation may be shortened if it is given during a physician department meeting. The presenter should incorporate group discussion during the presentation, if possible, and allow time for questions and answers at the end. Organizations can apply for CME credit for the physician attendees with the ACCME (ACCME 2017). In most healthcare entities, the education department is familiar with the steps to obtain CME and can assist in this process (AMA 2017).

Educational Session Content

Each educational session for nonprovider clinicians should reflect the specialty and makeup of the group. Small group sessions are preferable for effective workflow redesign discussions. A small group could include a specialty practice or group of informal leaders who are being asked to support and encourage other providers in the CDI process.

How to Use the Sample Presentation

The outpatient CDI team (manager and CDS team) can use the sample presentation to customize a program for the nonprovider clinical staff. Each slide in the presentation can be modified to fit the organization's culture, policies and procedures, and workflows. Prior to the nonclinician provider presentation, the outpatient CDI team should review each slide and discuss as a group any changes needed to the content. As part of this review, the CDI team should anticipate questions from the group and determine how the presentation content may be modified to aid the group's understanding of challenging topics. Wherever possible, examples from the CDI staff's experiences should be used in the presentation to illustrate points made in the slides.

Suggested Slide Presentation

Figure 13.3. Example of a CDI presentation title slide

Continuing Medical Education for the Physician Practice

Presented by:

CDI Physician Advisor

The presentation begins with a title slide (figure 13.3), which introduces the purpose of the program and the presenters. At this point in the presentation, the educator may:

- Provide information regarding the CDI process and establish a forum for collaboration and knowledge transfer related to guidelines for high-quality clinical documentation
- Discuss CDI issues of concern to the audience, such as HCC capture for risk-based payers, increasing payer denials because of coding and medical necessity gaps, and quality scorecards for MIPS and the Centers for Medicare and Medicaid Services Quality Payment Program.

Figure 13.4. Example of a slide outlining a team-based approach to CDI

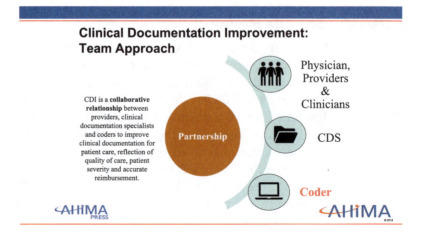

Figure 13.4 focuses on the team approach to CDI. The presenter may use this slide to This slide can be used to launch a larger discussion. While showing the slide the educator may do the following:

- Introduce the outpatient CDI program.
  - What are the primary tasks of the program? For example, the presenter might emphasize case review for clinical documentation gaps, streamlined query process for communication with providers, metrics and reporting to showcase the program progress, provider query support, and provider education on clinical documentation gaps.
  - How is the program organized within the health system and medical practice plan?
  - Who is the leader of the program, and what is that person's reporting relationship to the executive leadership?
- Explain the pilot program for the initial CDI program rollout, if one has been established. For example, the presenter could note the pilot locations and the number of outpatient CDSs assigned to them.
- Discuss the collaborative relationships and team approach needed for successful implementation of the program.
- Stress the benefits of CDI for the providers, including accurate reflection of the quality of care; data on patient severity levels and observed versus expected mortality rates; and improved reimbursement through value-based and risk-adjusted incentive payments.

Figure 13.5. Example of a slide defining CDI in the ambulatory setting

What is Clinical Documentation Improvement in the Ambulatory Setting?

- Change in the "quality" not necessarily the quantity of physician documentation
- Physician training that identifies problematic diagnoses and corresponding key words using a streamlined process not disruptive to the physician practice
- Use of templates by physicians that include prompts or reference to essential information based on the patient's diagnosis
- Documentation that supports the continuity of patient care among clinicians
- Documentation that supports medical necessity for the treatment and services provided – decreased payer denials for your practice
- Clinical record that supports the quality of patient care provided at your facility

Figure 13.5 defines CDI in the outpatient setting and identifies the following details about high-quality clinical documentation in the outpatient setting that the educator will emphasize:

- The goal of CDI is to improve the quality of clinical documentation, not increase the quantity.
- EHR templates can be used to prompt providers for more specific clinical documentation.

- Continuity of documentation across the continuum of care can eliminate inconsistent or inaccurate documentation, as well as the need to revise documentation.
- Improved supporting documentation will demonstrate the medical necessity of the services rendered.
- CDI can lead to fewer payer denials.
- Clinical documentation can reflect the high quality of care and severity level of patients treated at the facility.

Figure 13.6. Example of a slide summarizing the physician query process

Physician Query Process

- Simply put – a physician query is a question that is asked of the physician to clarify clinical details of the diagnoses and treatment provided – same process and purpose as in the inpatient setting
- Queries are electronic using (in EHR communication such as alerts, notes or tasks, email, phone texts
- The query and response is not maintained as part of the permanent record and an addendum to the record must be made
- The query is also part of the HIM record completion process and a deficiency notice may be sent to the physician via email
- The AHIMA practice brief, "Guidelines for Achieving a Compliant Query Practice" is used as a guideline for provider queries. Leading queries are not permitted.

The slide in figure 13.6 explains the physician query process and may be supplemented with additional discussion as follows:

- Like inpatient queries, outpatient queries ask the physician to clarify clinical diagnoses and treatments or procedures. The content of the query may not be as extensive in the outpatient setting and may relate more about diagnostic specificity than clinical indicators or clinical validation.
- The query method will depend on the EHRs used in the outpatient and professional practice setting and the interoperability of EHRs across the continuum of care. Taking into account the EHR functionality and interoperability issues within the health system, the presenter can explain how and why the CDS may intervene in the query process.
- Some facilities keep the query and response in the permanent record; others do not. therefore, the presenter should describe the facility's process and guidelines for the clinical record addendum process. If the query is not maintained as part of the legal record, the presenter should describe the facility-approved process for adding the query response to the clinical record. In most cases, the provider will open the EHR progress note or report and add an addendum to the clinical record.
- A query may also be part of the health information management record completion process as a deficiency notice may be sent to the physician

via e-mail. The presenter can explain how the provider will be notified of pending or delayed responses.
- The AHIMA practice brief "Guidelines for Achieving a Compliant Query Practice" (AHIMA 2016) is a great resource for participants in outpatient CDI. Portions of practice brief, such as the prohibition on leading queries (questions with an obvious answer), may be discussed during the presentation. However, the presentation should be short. Therefore, detailed query guidance may be better delivered in a newsletter or handout for the attendees to review later.

Figure 13.7. Example of a slide describing how to determine when to query

When to Query

- The generation of a query should be considered when the health record documentation:
  - Is conflicting, imprecise, incomplete, illegible, ambiguous, or inconsistent
  - Describes or is associated with clinical indicators without a definitive relationship to an underlying diagnosis
  - Includes clinical indicators, diagnostic evaluation, and/or treatment not related to a specific condition or procedure
  - Provides a diagnosis without underlying clinical validation
  - Is unclear for present on admission indicator assignment
  - Is required to further specify the details of chronic illnesses identified in the clinical documentation in other settings (inpatient, emergency department, observation, outpatient clinic/surgery) or for previous visits in the provider practice

- Figure 13.7 lists reasons why a query might be needed. When discussing this slide, the presenter may wish to provide illustrative examples of documentation gaps, such as those related to HCC capture and the use of clinical records from other settings or during previous encounters to document chronic illnesses.

Figure 13.8. Example of a slide explaining how to determine who to query

Who to Query

- Which physician should be queried?
  - The treating physician whose documentation in unclear or requires further clarification should be queried
  - If there is conflicting information, the attending physician's documentation will be used for coding purposes - query to the physician whose documentation is in question

The slide in figure 13.8 summarizes who should be queried when the clinical documentation from two treating physicians is conflicting. CDI students and practitioners often struggle with this topic, and the slide can be used to initiate a discussion about why a query is sent to one treating physician versus the other.

Figure 13.9. Example of a slide making a case for outpatient CDI

Making a Case for Outpatient CDI

- Emerging CDI opportunities beyond reviewing for MS-DRG based major complications and comorbidities (MCCs) and complications and comorbidities (CCs).
- CDI programs are expanding the scope of work to include support of risk based payer methodologies and quality reporting metrics.
- CDS skills sets are expanding to include not only clinical, coding, and communication skills, but also the ability to manage work flow redesign, quality, compliance, and regulatory initiatives.
- CDI programs are moving outside the walls of the traditional inpatient acute-care setting into other settings, such as hospital outpatient and physician offices.

Citation: Endicott, M. (2016). CDI: Beyond Acute Care Reimbursement. ICD10Montior. Retrieved from https://www.icd10monitor.com/cdi-beyond-acute-care-and-reimbursement

Figure 13.9 makes a case for outpatient CDI. It explains why CDI is evolving into the ambulatory sector of healthcare and identifies the need for new skills sets for the outpatient CDS vs the inpatient CDS.

Figure 13.10. Example of a slide outlining components of the outpatient facility and professional practice

Outpatient Facility & Professional Practice Components

- Governance structure
- Data analytics for focus areas
- HCC capture
- CDS Collaboration (inpatient, outpatient & provider practice CDS)
- System interoperability, EHR templates, consistent data (problem list)
- CDS physician shadowing
- Staffing
- Education
- Repeat the process

Figure 13.10 defines the components of the CDI program in the outpatient facility and professional practice. In the presentation, the featured topics may be covered at a cursory level and brisk pace; providers will be less interested in the granular details of the program components than in the broader component topics themselves. However, the presenter should encourage questions from participants about specific topics on the list. Individual topics may be addressed as follows:

- *Governance structure:* Explain the structure established by the organization, which may be part of an overarching CDI program or may be separate for the ambulatory setting.
- *Data analytics for focus areas:* Explain the technology and resources used to identify areas of focus for root cause analysis, such as the chargemaster, claims scrubber, HCC capture audits, outpatient CPT/HCPCS audit, evaluation and management code audits, ICD-10-CM audits, quality metrics, MIPS measures, or denials trends
- *HCC capture:* Explain the review process for all settings (inpatient, outpatient, and professional practice)
- *CDS collaboration:* Explain the organization's inpatient, outpatient, or provider practice CDS staff and how they will collaborate and work together to improve the clinical documentation workflow.
- *System interoperability, EHR templates, consistent data (problem list):* Discuss disparate systems and how the CDS will review each to resolve clinical documentation gaps, such as inaccurate HCC capture.
- *CDS physician shadowing:* Discuss the rationale for having a CDS shadow physicians and how to establish an efficient shadowing process that minimizes disruptions to the facility's workflow and patient care.
- *Staffing:* Describe the CDS support that will be provided to physicians and others involved in clinical documentation.
- *Education:* Describe the ongoing educational process, such as follow-up information, additional group sessions, and one-on-one meetings.
- *Repeat the process:* Explain that the CDI process is an ongoing effort, in which new focus areas will be targeted as current issues are resolved.

Figure 13.11. Example of a slide analyzing a sample risk score

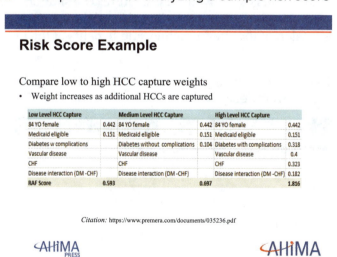

Figure 13.11 is an example of a risk score (Premera 2015). In this example, the added clinical documentation related to diabetes mellitus (DM) and corresponding complication of vascular disease resulted in the addition of two HCCs with weights of 0.318 and 0.40. The addition of congestive heart failure (CHF) resulted in assignment of the disease-interaction HCC related to diabetes

and CHF, with a resulting HCC weight of 0.182. Refer to chapter 3 of this text for more information on HCC weights and risk-adjustment factor (RAF) score calculation. The presenter can use this slide when discussing the following:

- The methodology of HCC capture and how clinical documentation specificity affects the risk-adjusted weight
- Similarities and differences between HCCs and the diagnosis-related groups (DRGs) assigned in the inpatient setting
- Similarities and differences between the RAF score and the case-mix index (CMI) in the inpatient setting.

Figure 13.12. Example of a slide describing the HCC redesign process

Redesigned Clinical Documentation Process

HCC Redesign Begins in the Professional Practice
- Clinical Data requirements
- HCC audit
- Socializing the concept
- Redesign work flow
- Pilot site(s)
- Improve HCC capture and improved clinical documentation

Figure 13.12 presents an outline of the redesigned clinical documentation process for a program whose goal is improved HCC capture. The slide should be edited to reflect the goals, objectives, and workplan tasks of the specific CDI program and support discussion of the sites, timeline, and benefits of the initiative.

Figure 13.13. Example of a slide providing additional discussion on workflow redesign

More on Work Flow Redesign

In-line documentation for HCC data capture
- In-line documentation refers to the process of allowing the provider to document measure related information within the body of a progress note template.
- Example: Diabetic Patient
  - The provider is prompted to document information about the patient's most recent diabetic eye examination.
  - The provider is given a series of menu choices that will be mapped to the requirements for this measure.
  - The provider may also be prompted to:
    - Generate an ophthalmology referral
    - Document that the patient has declined the dilated eye examination, because the most recent examination took place within the specified timeframe and was normal. Documentation of a diabetic eye exam is part of MIPS Measure #117.

Citation: Marron-Stearns, Michael. "How MACRA Changes HIM" Journal of AHIMA 88, no.3 (March 2017): 22-25.

Figure 13.13 explains workflow design for a CDI program focused on compliance with MIPS (Marron-Stearns 2017). This slide lists prompts that might be shown to the provider related to eye care for a patient with diabetes. If this slide is used, the presenter should be prepared to explain MIPS measure 117, which requires that a retinal or dilated eye exam is performed annually for patients with diabetes, and how the measure affects Medicare reimbursement. The presenter may also emphasize that in-line documentation technology can be used to enhance the capture of chronic illness diagnoses for HCC risk-based payment programs.

Chapter 13 Review Exercises

1. Which of the following is *not* a current trend in physician education identified in this chapter?
    a. Soft skills training
    b. Curricula focused on healthcare delivery issues
    c. Use of educational technology such as online coursework
    d. Customized teaching models to promote individual student success

2. Based on current research, which of the following approaches is most recommended to instill positive changes in physician behavior?
    a. Classroom lectures
    b. Multifaceted intervention
    c. Small-group collaboration
    d. Single-method intervention

3. Which of the following teaching interventions would *best* facilitate physician discussion and case review?
    a. Interactive CME
    b. Online training modules
    c. Annual compliance training
    d. Passive dissemination of information

4. Which of the following would be *least* important to consider when developing slide content for CME presentations on CDI topics?
    a. Specialties of the participants
    b. Personalities of the participants
    c. Long-term goals of participants
    d. Time constraints of the participants

5. The leadership of an outpatient facility has recently decided to initiate group CDI educational sessions for its physician staff. The leaders spent considerable time debating whether the program should be instructed by a well-regarded outside consultant or in-house CDS. Ultimately, they decided the sessions would be more effective if instructed by the staff CDS. Which of the following provides the *most likely* explanation for the facility leadership's decision?
    a. They wish to avoid the expense of hiring an outside consultant.
    b. They believe the trainees will learn better from an instructor they know and trust.

c. They are skeptical about the subject matter expertise of the outside consultant.
d. They are unsure if the outside consultant understands the facility's policies and practices.

6. When introducing the outpatient CDI program during a continuing education presentation, the instructor should discuss which of the following?
   a. The history of CDI
   b. Any questions the attendees may have
   c. The backgrounds and experience levels of attendees
   d. How the program is organized within the health system or medical practice plan

7. In the context of staff CDI educational programs, which of the following is *most likely* to be a difference between experienced providers and physicians who have recently entered the workforce?
   a. Openness to workforce education
   b. Necessity for workforce education
   c. Effectiveness of workforce education
   d. Preferred learning methods during workforce education

8. A private practice is implementing an outpatient CDI educational program and has scheduled the sessions to coincide with staff meal periods. Which of the following is *most likely* a primary benefit of timing the educational sessions in this way?
   a. Maximized attendance
   b. Minimized distractions
   c. Improved focus of attendees
   d. Reduced overtime wage expense

9. Which of the following factors would be *most likely* to improve the effectiveness of workflow redesign discussions during nonprovider CDI educational sessions?
   a. Casual environment
   b. Small-group structure
   c. Staff-wide participation
   d. Regular (quarterly, annual) occurence

10. Which of the following *best* accounts for the recent year-over-year growth of NPPs in the workforce?
    a. Relaxed licensure requirements for NPPs has made it easier to enter the profession.
    b. Increasing salaries across all categories of NPP have made the profession more attractive.
    c. A declining number of physicians in the workforce has led to a shortage of providers worldwide.
    d. Falling costs of postbaccalaureate programs has made medical education more accessible than ever.

References

Accreditation Council for Continuing Medical Education (ACCME). 2017. CME content: definition and examples. http://www.accme.org/requirements/accreditation-requirements-cme-providers/policies-and-definitions/cme-content-definition-and-examples.

American Association of Medical Assistants (AAMA). 2017. What is a CMA (AAMA)? http://www.aama-ntl.org/medical-assisting/what-is-a-cma#.WkFgyt_tzIU.

American Health Information Management Association (AHIMA). 2016. Practice brief: Guidelines for achieving a compliant query practice (2016 update). http://bok.ahima.org/PB/QueryCompliance#.WtYyo4jwY2w.

American Medical Association (AMA). 2017. Continuing Medical Education. https://www.ama-assn.org/education/continuing-medical-education.

Brown, A., G. Cometto, A. Cumbi, H. de Pinho, F. Kamwendo, U. Lehmann, W. McCourt, B. McPake, G. Pariyo, and D. Sanders. 2011. Mid-level health providers: A promising resource. *Peruvian Journal of Experimental Medicine and Public Health* 28(2): 308–315.

Dark, C. 2011 (April 4). Non-physician clinicians. Policy Prescriptions. http://www.policyprescriptions.org/non-physician-clinicians/.

Frieden, J. 2015a (August 6). Changing face of medical education: Big data, self-paced learning. MedPage Today. http://www.medpagetoday.com/publichealthpolicy/medicaleducation/52973?pop=0&ba=1&xid=tmd-md&hr=trendMD.

Frieden, J. 2015b (August 7). Changing face of medical education: It's all about the system. MedPage Today. https://www.medpagetoday.com/PublicHealthPolicy/MedicalEducation/52990.

Frieden, J. 2015c (August 10). Changing face of medical education: Integrating basic science. MedPage Today. http://www.medpagetoday.com/PublicHealthPolicy/MedicalEducation/53016.

Global Health Workforce Alliance (GHWA). The Global Health Workforce Alliance 2013 Annual Report: Rising to the grand challenge of human resources for health. Geneva, Switzerland: World Health Organization. 2013.

Hess, P. 2015. *Clinical Documentation Improvement: Principles and Practice*. Chicago, IL: AHIMA.

Lefler, D. 2013. New and future approaches to medical education. In-Training. http://in-training.org/new-and-future-approaches-to-medical-education-3725.

Marron-Stearns, M. 2017. How MACRA changes HIM. *Journal of AHIMA* 88(3): 22–25.

Medical Group Management Association (MGMA). *The Rising Trend of Nonphysician Provider Utilization in Healthcare: A follow-up to the MGMA 2014 Research & Analysis Report*. 2016.

Mostofian, F., C. Ruban, N. Simunovic, and M. Bhandari. 2015. Changing physician behavior: what works. *American Journal of Managed Care* 21(1):75–84.

National Association of Clinical Nurse Specialists (NACNS). 2017. What is a CNS? http://nacns.org/about-us/what-is-a-cns.

Premera Blue Cross. 2015. Medicare Advantage risk adjustment coding. https://www.premera.com/documents/035236.pdf.

Weldon, D. 2014 (May 28). Non-physician providers: An unexpected route to revenue increases. Healthcare Finance. http://www.healthcarefinancenews.com/news/non-physician-providers-unexpected-route-revenue-increases.

Wier, R.R., Jr. 2013. Billing Medicare for non-physician providers. *HBMA Billing* 18(3): 24–25.

Educational Programs for Outpatient Coders

14

Learning Objectives

- Describe the recommended attendees for the educational program on outpatient clinical documentation improvement (CDI) for medical coders.
- Illustrate methodologies to engage the medical coder in the CDI program.
- Describe the content of a comprehensive CDI educational program focused on the interaction between the clinical documentation specialist and the coder.
- Identify the best instructors for the outpatient CDI educational session for medical coders.
- Discuss the challenges in promoting and delivering an effective outpatient CDI educational program for medical coders.

Medicare uses a risk-based model to reimburse providers who care for patients enrolled in Medicare Advantage (MA) plans. Under this model, the severity of a patient's condition affects the annual risk-adjusted payment to the provider for services to treat that patient. In other words, "higher payments are made to providers who care for 'sicker' patients" (AHIMA 2017). This reimbursement model established a relationship between the ICD-10-CM code assigned to an outpatient clinical record and payment. Thus, MA plans, as well as other changes in the requirements for documenting and reporting patient care in the outpatient setting, have expanded the scope of work and required skill sets for outpatient coding professionals. This chapter reviews the skill sets that outpatient coders need to succeed and the educational training that will help them acquire those skills.

Medical Coding Professionals in the Outpatient Setting

The medical coding professionals working in outpatient settings are a diverse group, and their required competencies and job descriptions will vary depending on the setting, the health system's organization, and other factors.

Required Competencies

Risk-adjustment coding requires a detailed understanding of the Hierarchical Condition Category (HCC) model. Outpatient coding professionals should also be competent in the use of Current Procedural Terminology (CPT), Healthcare Common Procedure Coding System (HCPCS), and *International Classification of Diseases, Tenth Revision, Clinical Modification* (ICD-10-CM) codes in the clinic and professional practice settings. The *ICD-10-CM Official Guidelines for Coding and Reporting* include a section on ambulatory ICD-10-CM coding (Section IV; Diagnostic Coding and Reporting Guidelines for Outpatient Surgery) (CDC 2018). CPT guidelines are published by the American Medical Association (AMA 2018), and the CPT code set can be purchased from a variety of companies, including the AMA. The AMA also publishes *CPT Assistant*, a periodical that offers in-depth guidance in the coding of procedures and services. The Centers for Medicare and Medicaid Services (CMS) offer guidance on HCPCS on the CMS website (CMS 2018).

Additionally, the outpatient coding professional must understand the following:

- *CMS quality programs:* For example, the Merit-Based Incentive Payment System (MIPS) program was established by CMS for quality measurement in the physician practice.
- *Denials management:* Coders should be familiar with the process of tracking and trending denials. They also should know how to analyze root causes of clinical documentation improvement (CDI) gaps and find solutions for these gaps.
- *Claims editor functionality:* Hospital and professional practice billing systems include claims editors that scrub the data for errors prior to the bill drop. There are also stand-alone clinical claims editors that provide

deeper insight into claims issues related to quality scores, coding, and medical necessity (see chapter 7).
- *Hospital chargemaster:* The hospital chargemaster is a system file that includes the line items used for claims reporting. The file includes CPT and HCPCS codes, which should be matched correctly with line-item services; mismatched codes and line items may be a root cause of coding errors.
- *Fee schedules:* The fee schedule file is used in the physician practice for the same purpose as a chargemaster in a hospital. CPT and HCPCS code errors in the file could result in an inaccurate reimbursement or denied claims.
- *Clinical documentation guidelines and methodologies:* The guidelines and methodologies discussed in this textbook are essential for the success of the outpatient CDI program.

Each of these areas is important, and all affect the accurate payment and quality scores in the outpatient setting.

Educational and Training Background

Before a CDI program is implemented, the medical coding professional working in the outpatient setting may have proficiency in several, but not necessarily all, of the following skill sets:

- CPT
- HCPCS
- Ambulatory payment classification (APC) assignment
- Outpatient Prospective Payment System (OPPS) guidelines
- ICD-10-CM
- HCC assignment
- Physician practice coding
- Outpatient facility coding
- Observation patient coding
- Emergency department coding

The CDI manager should assess the existing skill set of each outpatient coding professional to determine his or her educational needs. The staff may have a broad range of experience and formal education. Some coding professionals have had no training other than what they received on the job. Others have two-year associate degrees in health information management (HIM), four-year HIM baccalaureate degrees, or graduate degrees in HIM, informatics, business, public health, hospital administration, healthcare administration, or another healthcare-related discipline. Their university-level coursework may or may not have included CDI, management, data analytics, health information management, revenue cycle and coding consulting, HIM operations, health informatics, information technology (IT) support, health data security and privacy, information governance, physician practice management, or clinic operations.

Job Responsibilities

The role of an outpatient coding professional may vary depending on the setting but typically includes the following responsibilities:

- Review clinical information, including charges, to ensure accurate charge capture and diagnostic code assignment.
- Query the attending physician to clarify unclear, inconsistent, or incomplete clinical information and to ensure that the clinical documentation supports the diagnosis and treatment provided.
- Use coding manuals, encoders, or computer-assisted coding software, assign ICD-10-CM, CPT, and HCPCS codes for diagnoses and services provided.
- Collaborate with CDS staff to learn more about the clinical indicators for specific disease processes.
- Resolve claims edits such as those related to the National Correct Coding Initiative (NCCI), coder or modifier edits, and national coverage determination (NCD) or local coverage determination (LCD) medical necessity issues.
- Submit the claim.
- Assist with denials resolution and prevention.
- Support continuous quality improvement processes through special projects, education, and training.
- Audit claims and coding accuracy and provide on-the-job mentoring of new staff.
- Assist with chargemaster or fee schedule CPT and HCPCS code updates.

Each ambulatory coding task should be reviewed by the CDI team to ensure that it fits within the current workflow of the CDI program. Tasks may be added or revised as needed to customize the ambulatory coding professionals' workflow.

Preparing for and Running CDI Educational Sessions

Educational sessions for coding professionals should be planned for specialty-specific groups if possible. For example, coding professionals working in surgical specialty clinics could be invited to attend a presentation that will address their issues with coding and clinical documentation. The presentation slides provided in online appendix 14A may be modified to meet the needs of the specific group. The instructor should add case scenarios to provide real-life examples of challenging or problematic coding and clinical documentation issues.

The program should focus on how the coder can best function as part of the clinical documentation team. The sessions should include a discussion of ongoing collaboration between CDSs and coders as well as strategies for effective communication between the groups. For example, the groups may hold weekly meetings, participate in lunch-and-learn sessions, and openly discuss problematic cases and provider adoption issues.

The initial training session can review the CDI workflow so that the coding professional understand where their tasks fit into the outpatient CDI program.

Refer to figure 13.2 in chapter 13, which depicts an outpatient CDI workflow. The graphic can be used during the training session discussion. The workflow begins when the practice staff identifies the cases that will be the focus of CDI review and shows how the nonphysician provider (NPP) and CDS work together to ensure that the physician or other provider enters complete and specific clinical documentation into the record. Types of NPPs include physician assistants, nurse practitioners, clinical nurse specialists, and certified nurse midwives. See chapter 13 for additional discussion about NPPs.

The instructors for the medical coder educational sessions should include the outpatient CDI program manager or CDS as well as the HIM coding manager or director. Buy-in and support from the leadership of the coder group is essential to encourage collaboration and teamwork between coders and CDSs.

In addition to giving a slide presentation (such as the one in online appendix 14A), the instructors should lead interactive discussions of ways that CDSs and coders can streamline their collaborative efforts during the query and coding process. Each staff member should be encouraged to express concerns and present ideas for a streamlined workflow, which may be tailored to each practice and each provider.

If coders and CDSs work in the clinic or physician practice setting, an educational session away from the clinic or practice may be more productive than one held in the workplace. At a minimum, the session should be held in a separate conference room away from the patient care area, so participants can pay close attention to the presentation and discussion.

Small group sessions are preferable when discussing effective workflow redesign. The information discussed during the redesign portion of the session may focus on individual provider preferences, time constraints, and practice patterns.

Educational Session Content

When customizing a presentation for the coding staff, the outpatient CDI team (manager and CDS team) should use slides that fit the organizational culture, policies and procedures, and workflows, and address any specialty-specific issues (such as coding related to obstetric or surgical care). Before the presentation, the outpatient CDI team should review each slide and discuss as a group how to customize the content for the attendees. Whenever possible, the presentation should include relevant examples from the CDI staff's experience. During this preparatory discussion, the team should also anticipate questions that participants are likely to ask.

The rest of this chapter outlines presentation topics appropriate for CDI educational sessions for coding professionals. Appendix 14A provides PowerPoint slides for these topics, which the instructor can edit to create custom presentations.

Introduction (Title Slide)

Each presentation should begin with a title slide. At this point, the lead instructor can introduce the topics to be covered, other presenters, and executive sponsors for the CDI program. The presenter can also explain briefly why the program has been developed and implemented.

Clinical Documentation Improvement: Team Approach

An initial presentation on CDI may focus on team building and collaboration throughout the continuum of care. Objectives may include the following:

- Discuss the collaborative relationships among all providers, clinicians, CDS and coding staff as well as the team approach needed for a successful implementation of the CDI program.
- Stress the importance of collaboration between coding professionals and CDSs to support the mission, goals, and objectives of the health system. This collaboration can
  - Improve the accuracy and specificity of clinical documentation by providers and clinicians, thereby supporting the delivery of high-quality patient care
  - Help generate coded data used in publicly available forums such as Healthgrades and other websites to measure the quality of care provided at the facility
  - Ensure accurate data on patient severity levels and accurate observed versus expected mortality rates
  - Support accurate reimbursement through fee-for-service, value-based, and risk-adjusted incentive payments

Outpatient CDI Defined

Objectives related to this topic may include the following:

- Explain why CDI is evolving in outpatient healthcare.
- Introduce the rationales for clinical documentation requirements for value-based purchasing and risk-adjustment payment methodologies.
- Compare the skills sets for the outpatient CDS versus the inpatient CDS. The outpatient CDS must understand
  - CPT/HCPCS Coding
  - APC grouping and OPPS guidelines
  - HCC for risk-adjustment payments
  - ICD-10-CM specificity for quality measure scores and medical necessity
- Emphasize the need for improved clinical documentation in all settings, including hospital outpatient clinics, the emergency department, physician offices, long-term care facilities, and home healthcare.

CDI in the Outpatient Setting

This topic focuses on how outpatient CDI can enhance high-quality clinical documentation in the outpatient setting. For example, the outpatient CDI program can accomplish the following:

- Improve the quality, not quantity, of documentation.
- Facilitate use of EHR templates to prompt providers for more specific clinical documentation.
- Improve the continuity of documentation across the continuum of care, eliminate inconsistent or inaccurate documentation, and reduce the frequency of revisions.

- Ensure that providers enter support documentation to substantiate the medical necessity of the services rendered.
- Reduce payer denials caused by problems with clinical record specificity to support accurate ICD-10-CM coding and accurate claims submission, including the physician order to determine the patient status (inpatient, observation, or outpatient).
- Ensure that the content of the clinical record accurately reflects the quality of care and severity levels of patients treated at the facility. Accuracy in these data will improve the quality scores of the physicians well as the healthcare facility or practice.

Outpatient Facility and Professional Practice Components

This topic leads participants through the following components of the outpatient CDI program:

- *Governance structure:* Explain the program's governance structure, as established by the organization. For example, the program may be included as part of a comprehensive inpatient-outpatient CDI program, or there may be a separate program for the outpatient setting.
- *Data analytics for focus areas:* Explain the technologies and methodologies used to identify areas of CDI focus, such as the chargemaster, claims scrubber, HCC capture audits, CPT and HCPCS audits, evaluation and management (E/M) audits, ICD-10-CM audits, quality metrics, MIPS measures, denials trends, and root cause analyses.
- *HCC capture:* Explain the case review process for all settings (inpatient, outpatient, and ambulatory) used to ensure accurate capture of HCC codes for a patient encounter.
- *CDS collaboration (inpatient, outpatient, and provider practice):* Describe the roles of the organization's CDS staff, and explain how they will collaborate and work together to improve clinical documentation workflow.
- *System interoperability, EHR templates, consistent data (problem list):* Discuss the interoperability challenges posed when outpatient clinical documentation is found in disparate EHR systems, and how CDI can resolve them (for example, the CDS could review documentation from each EHR for HCC capture).
- *CDS physician shadowing:* Briefly discuss the query process and why the CDS will shadow physicians to observe their clinical documentation workflow. Emphasize that the CDS will collaborate with physicians and staff to design an efficient shadowing process that does not disrupt patient care or other work.
- *Staffing:* Describe the CDS support that will be provided for each individual physician or physician group.
- *Education:* Describe the educational objectives for this meeting as well as the process for sharing follow-up information and plans for additional group and one-on-one meetings.
- *Repeat the process:* Explain that the CDI process will be an ongoing endeavor. As high-risk, high-dollar issues are identified and resolved, a new set of issues will become the focus of the CDI program.

HCC Shadowing Process

If HCC capture is an area of focus for the CDI program, the educator can explain the CDI process that will occur in the clinic or practice:

- *Clinical data requirements:* Explain that the outpatient CDS's first task is to determine the best way to identify the patients whose cases will be reviewed. For example, the health information system may be able to provide a schedule of MA patients who will be seen in the following week.
- *HCC audit:* Describe the preliminary audit that will be done by the outpatient CDS to determine how HCCs are captured currently.
- *Socializing the concept:* Explain that the outpatient CDS will meet individually with the physicians in the practice setting to determine the best way to submit and receive a query as needed for HCC capture.
- *Redesign workflow:* Explain that the clinical documentation workflow will be revised if needed to incorporate the CDS shadowing and query process (the previsit, concurrent visit, and post-visit case review process).
- *Pilot site(s):* Discuss the process used to select pilot sites for implementing the CDI program (for example, large primary care practices may be the first sites because they treat the greatest number of MA patients). Also discuss the schedule to roll out the CDI program to the remaining practices.
- *Improve HCC capture and improve clinical documentation:* Emphasize the benefits of this CDI initiative.

HCC Shadowing Process Drill-Down

If HCC capture is an area of focus for the CDI program, the educator may wish to walk coding professionals through the details of the CDS shadowing process.

- *Previous clinical record review for scheduled patients:* Explain how the CDS will review a patient's records before the visit, looking for previously identified chronic illnesses that could be assigned an HCC code.
- *HCC identification:* Explain how the CDS will identify whether an HCC code was assigned, or might have been assigned, to a chronic condition during a previous visit.
- *Query provider for potential HCCs and update problem list with current HCCs:* Explain the predetermined method for querying the provider when a historical HCC is identified in the clinical record.
- *All queries must meet the American Health Information Management Association (AHIMA) guidelines for query submission:* Discuss compliance with the AHIMA query guidelines, including the guideline against the use of leading queries (AHIMA 2016).
- *Provider and/or nonprovider clinician reviews query:* Further discuss the query workflow, such as whether nurses or other nonprovider clinicians will initially review queries and, if so, how the provider will subsequently view the query.

- *Provider determines if the query is valid and, if it is, enters additional more specific documentation according to MEAT guidelines:* Explain the monitor, evaluate, assess/address, or treat (MEAT) guidelines, emphasizing that the condition must be monitored, evaluated, assessed/addressed, or treated to be coded on the claim for the current visit.
- *CDI performs postencounter case review.* Explain that the CDS will review the clinical record after the visit to determine whether all necessary documentation is present to support accurate coding. The CDS will notify the physician immediately if there is a documentation gap that needs to be addressed.
- *CDS tracks HCC capture in automated tool or spreadsheet:* Explain how the CDS will track identification of new HCCs to highlight the program's progress and success.

Physician Query Process in the Outpatient Setting

The following fundamental aspects of the outpatient query process may be topics for discussion:

- How to transmit queries electronically, using communication such as EHR alerts, notes, or tasks, as well as e-mail and text messages.
- The organization's current process for submitting queries, such as via EHR alerts or templates, in-person conversations with on-site providers, or phone calls to providers who are off site.
- The legal aspects of queries. Some facilities keep the query and response in the permanent record; others do not. Describe your facility's policy regarding addenda to clinical records. The decision whether to keep the query as part of the clinical record is typically decided by the facility's or clinic's legal counsel.
- The current process used when queries are part of the HIM record completion process, such as when a deficiency notice may be sent to the physician via e-mail.
- The AHIMA practice brief "Guidelines for Achieving a Compliant Query Practice (2016 Update)" provides guidance for provider queries (AHIMA 2016). When discussing the guidelines, use examples from the CDI team to illustrate the differences between compliant and noncompliant queries.

When to Query

When discussing the reasons why a coding professional might query the provider, the instructor can illustrate the rationales for queries by providing examples from the CDI team. These examples should describe cases where clinical indicators are not definitively associated with an underlying diagnosis in the documentation.

For example, if the CDS or coding professional finds that a patient's record documents above-normal blood glucose levels and insulin therapy but does not include a diabetes diagnosis, the CDS or coder should submit a compliant query to the provider about the test results and treatment information. Similarly, if the CDS identifies that a chronic illness was documented during previous visits or in a patient's records from other settings, the CDS should query the provider to consider whether the previous diagnosis is relevant to the current visit. These types of queries can ensure that documentation reflects the medical necessity of treatments and improve HCC capture.

When discussing the timing of queries, the instructor can explain that the outpatient CDS will submit the query before or during the encounter. As in the inpatient setting, the outpatient coder may identify a query opportunity after the visit. If records are coded soon after the encounter, there may be time for the query to be submitted and answered prior to bill drop.

Who to Query

Coding professionals must know what to do situations in which they identify potentially conflicting information in documentation from different providers and need to query for clarification. The instructor can illustrate this presentation with examples specific to the areas of focus for the outpatient CDI program.

For example, two physicians within the practice document two different visits in same year. The clinical record for the first visit includes a diagnosis of diabetes. Documentation for the second (current) visit records low blood sugar but does not include a diabetes diagnosis. The patient also has a history of peripheral vascular disease related to the diabetes, which was documented in a visit note from the previous year. The outpatient CDS reviewing the clinical documentation after the most recent visit submits a query to the physician who saw the patient in that encounter. The query notes that diabetic peripheral vascular disease was mentioned last year and asks which diagnoses are applicable for the current visit. The physician's response will allow for accurate coding of diagnoses for HCC capture.

Growing Demand for CDI to Support Risk Adjustment

As noted earlier in this chapter, coding professionals need to be aware of how risk-adjustment payment models are driving the need for outpatient CDI programs. Learning objectives for this topic may include the following:

- Explain the basic concepts of risk adjustment, including the use of risk scores for negotiating payer contracts.
- Explain that risk-adjustment calculations include diagnoses related to chronic illness as well as demographics such as age, sex, disability, and Medicaid status.
- Explain that scores are predictive in nature and that the information collected this year will be used two years later to determine risk scores and the corresponding impact on reimbursement.

Common HCCs

If HCC capture is an area of focus for the outpatient CDI program, the instructor may wish to accomplish the following objectives:

- Discuss the most frequently identified HCCs at the facility or clinic. Diabetes, chronic kidney disease, congestive heart failure (CHF), chronic obstructive pulmonary disease (COPD), malignant neoplasms, acute myocardial infarction, cerebrovascular accident, and hip fractures are some of the most frequently identified HCCs.
- Explain that there are 9000 ICD-10-CM codes with corresponding HCCs, and the CDS will use an encoder or other electronic HCC list to determine which ICD-10-CM codes in clinical documentation have a corresponding HCC.

Risk Score Example

When discussing HCC capture, the instructor may wish to achieve the following objectives, particularly if trainees are familiar with inpatient coding:

- Explain the methodology of HCC capture and how specificity in clinical documentation affects the risk-adjusted weight. Note that this methodology is similar to the use of DRGs in the inpatient setting.
- Explain how the risk-adjustment factor (RAF) used with HCCs is similar to the case-mix index in the inpatient setting.
- Present an example that explains how to calculate the RAF score. The example in the slide for this topic in appendix 14A shows how HCC capture and the RAF score change when vascular disease (a diabetes complication) and CHF (a disease interaction with diabetes) are documented.

Return on Investment for the MA Plan

To measure the benefits of a CDI program, coding professionals can apply the formula to calculate the return on investment (ROI) for providers participating in the plan.

- The following steps are used to determine the payment for care provided to an MA patient:
    1. All unique HCC weights for the patient during a one-year period are added together. In this example, the sum of the weights equals 1.223.
    2. Multiply the sum of the HCC weights by the per-patient-per-month (PPPM) contract rate. The PPPM contract rate can be found on the CMS website. It is unique to the specific county where the facility is located. The PPPM rate in this example is $897.90.
    3. Multiply the result from step 3 by 12, because there are 12 months in the year.
    4. The annual payment for this patient to the MA Plan is $13,178 (1.223 × 897.90 × 12).
- If the facility and MA plans are separate, each MA plan contract must be reviewed to calculate the ROI for the facility. It is determined by the shared-savings bonus agreement between the MA plan and the facility (see chapter 3 for further information).

OIG Risk-Adjustment Data Validation Audit

MA risk-adjusted data may be audited by the Office of Inspector General (OIG) of the US Department of Health and Human Services. The following learning objectives can prepare coding professionals for this possibility:

- Discuss why OIG reviews risk-adjusted data submitted to the Medicare Advantage plan.
- Review some of the errors identified by the OIG.
- Discuss that the highest error rate identified was for "unsupported diagnosis coding," which results from lack of specificity in the clinical documentation to support the ICD-10-CM code.

- Explain that coders play an important part in the accuracy of the coded data. Only diagnoses that are well supported in the clinical data should be submitted on the claim. The coder should query the physician for further specificity and clarification if needed to report an accurate code.
- Explain that CMS also conducts ongoing risk adjustment data validation audits of risk-adjusted coding submitted by the MA plan to CMS for payment.

Clinical Data Requirements

The following are some educational objectives related to clinical data requirements for HCC capture:

- Explain that payers of MA plans have a stake in accurate HCC assignment. The payers may be able to provide reports that show HCCs submitted on historical claims. Some of these plans offer summary-level data, and others provide specific HCC code assignment by patient. The payer's HCC reports can be helpful for identifying those patients with historical HCC submission on past claims. Identifying HCCs claims from past years can alert the provider that the chronic condition may still be present.
- Describe the process of HCC case review. The CDS must access all clinical records in the inpatient, outpatient, and professional fee settings to determine accurate HCC identification for a calendar year. A specific HCC can be reimbursed for only once during a calendar year, and the CDS must verify that all HCCs were identified during the period of the review.

Conduct an HCC Audit

When HCC capture is an area of focus for the outpatient CDI program, outpatient coders will likely conduct a sample audit of providers most affected by HCC reimbursement, such as physicians in primary care and internal medicine. Instructors should therefore explain the following HCC audit process steps:

- *Select accounts from the MA patient list to audit:* If a report from the MA plan include HCCs submitted at a claim level, that report can be used to select a random sample of patients to audit. If this type of report is not available, the facility can review a random sample of claims and screen for HCC capture gaps. Twenty-five records per provider is a sufficient sample size for the initial review.
- Review the clinical record and corresponding ICD-10-CM codes on each claim, and then identify the HCCs for each claim. Review the patient's clinical records from the inpatient, outpatient, and professional fee settings for the current and previous years.
- Add each HCC to the audit spreadsheet used for RAF score calculation. An example of the spreadsheet is provided to show the group what is used for data capture.
- Validate each HCC submitted on the claim and add HCCs not submitted.
- Identify HCCs that are newly reported for the current year.
- Share the results of the audit with the provider.

Example Scenario: HCC Case Review

Discussion of an example of HCC case review can help coding professionals understand how HCCs are identified and captured. A sample case review is provided in the slide for this topic in appendix 14A. The review was conducted over a three-year period. HCCs identified in previous years are probably relevant and should be documented in the current year. In the example, four patient encounters were reviewed. The CDS identified six HCCs, but only two were submitted. Four HCCs were identified as being missed on the claim. Only one HCC in the example is reimbursable in the current year. New HCCs identified and not captured on the original claim were COPD, chronic viral hepatitis C, and recurrent manic depressive disorder.

Incorporate Other Focus Areas

Many facilities focus their outpatient CDI program solely on HCC capture, but some also choose other areas of focus. Learning objectives for this topic include the following:

- Identify possible focus areas to be included in the outpatient CDS's case review and shadowing process, such as MIPS measures, medical necessity–based denials, coding error trends and missing charges.
- Explain that the ambulatory CDI program manager can start the process of choosing areas of focus by identifying up to 10 high-volume, high-dollar issues. The Hospital Outpatient Quality Reporting (OQR) measure OP-8: MRI Lumbar Spine for Low Back Pain is one possible focus area.
- Discuss who selects the areas of focus and the selection criteria. The selection of areas of focus should be based on the resources available and the potential ROI if the issue identified is corrected.

Example 1: Outpatient CDI Focus Area

A case example can illustrate how an outpatient facility selects CDI areas of focus. A sample case related to the new comprehensive APCs is provided in the slide for this topic in appendix 14A. Using this example, the instructor can explain that an associated add-on secondary procedure code is required to receive the higher-level payment in the APC group.

Example 2: Outpatient CDI Focus Area

Another example of a focus area for outpatient CDI is the OQR measure OP-8: MRI Lumbar Spine for Low Back Pain, which is used to screen for unnecessary magnetic resonance imaging (MRI) scans performed on patients with low back pain. While discussing this measure, key objectives are as follows:

- Explain that when specified secondary diagnoses codes are reported, the MRI is not counted for OP-8. The case is excluded from the OP-8 measure, and an unnecessary MRI is not reported.
- Review CMS guidance for OP-8, which provides a listing of diagnosis code exceptions. Some examples are history of lumbar spine surgery, infectious condition, treatment fields for radiation therapy, trauma, unspecified immune deficiencies, and cancer.

Provider Program Adoption

Among the biggest challenges to the success of the outpatient CDI program are providers who do not engage in CDI implementation because they do not recognize its benefits. The instructor can help coding professionals explain benefits to providers, such as the following:

- Improved clinical record for quality patient care and provider collaboration
- Improved observed and expected mortality scores
- Improved physician scorecards on Healthgrades and other public reporting forums
- Improved reimbursement in risk-based, fee-based, and value-based payment systems

In addition, the following are steps that coding professionals can take to increase awareness and interest in the program by the providers:

- Select executive sponsors to include the medical staff leaders and specialty physician.
- Meet with small groups of specialty-specific providers.
- Present a high-level overview of the HCC audit performed for their specialty.
- Discuss a couple of case examples for their specialty and explain the impact on the RAF score.
- Explain that a pilot site(s) will be selected so that the methodology and ROI can be validated prior to rolling the program out to other practices.
- Discuss best ways to present the concept to the general medical staff and to encourage buy-in for the program.

Technology for Outpatient CDI

Coding professionals should understand the sources for data used in analysis and identification of focused review targets. Data can be found by reviewing

- The hospital chargemaster or physician fee schedules including volume data
- Claims scrubber edit reports
- Quality measure capture reports
- Denials software reports, including trends in medical necessity denials due to lack of a patient status order
- Clinical editors using a natural language processing (NLP) engine to flag suspect diagnoses based on clinical indicators, diagnostic test results, and medication administration records
- Coding audit information about error trends related to clinical documentation gaps

Technology for HCC Capture

Coding professionals should also understand what technology is available at the facility to identify clinical documentation gaps that affect HCC capture. Examples include the following:

- NLP engines to identify missing diagnoses and procedures. Applications include computer-assisted coding (CAC), CDI modules, HCC forecasting, suspecting, and score calculation. The CDI manager should identify available applications and provide further detail about their use.
- EHR functionality, such as templates for in-line clinical documentation; templates and drop-down lists for ICD-10 specificity; and alerts, tasks, and notes for physician query communication.
- Encoders that can identify and assign HCC codes to ICD-10-CM coded data. This functionality is helpful to the CDS and coder during the HCC capture process.

The concept of system interoperability as it relates to HCC capture is another important topic for educational sessions on CDI technology. Key points for discussion include the following:

- Interoperable systems help the CDS and coder to efficiently perform a complete HCC historical and concurrent case review. However, when there are multiple systems used by the hospital, clinic, and physician practice, it is easy to miss clinical documentation related to specific HCCs, especially information related to "history of" a condition.
- If there are interoperability issues, further analysis of the existing functionality should be conducted by the CDI manager with subsequent training provided to the CDS and coding staff.
- Maintaining up-to-date problem lists is a challenging process when multiple EHR systems are in use. These issues require further investigation and workflow redesign to ensure sharing of accurate and current problem lists information between the CDI sites (inpatient, outpatient, and physician practice).

More on Workflow Redesign

If in-line documentation is available to providers, or is an option being considered, coding professionals should be familiar with its functionality and benefits. Appendix 14A includes a case study related to compliance with the MIPS measure for eye examinations for patients with diabetes. In this example, the inline documentation tool prompts the provider to document the following information related to the MIPS measure:

- Date of most recent eye exam
- Ophthalmology referral
- Patient declining eye exam because of recent exam elsewhere

While discussing this case study, the instructor can emphasize the benefits of the in-line documentation capture process:

- It includes built-in templates or prompts that ask the questions during the documentation process.
- The physician is not required to exit the EHR to record the measured information.
- The streamlined process saves time for the provider.

Outpatient CDI Mastery for Coders

This topic explains the requirements for coding and auditing in outpatient settings. It should be noted that, depending on their job descriptions, coders may not be required to have experience in each competency.

- Outpatient coders who work primarily on observation cases must be familiar with all relevant requirements, including HCC assignment.
- A coder who is working primarily in the facility cardiology clinic setting may be required to have experience in the following:
  - CPT and HCPCS
  - ICD-10-CM
  - Value-based purchasing, risk adjustment, and HCC assignment
  - OPPS/APC guidelines
  - E/M coding

Credentials for Outpatient Coders

Coding professionals should understand the need for certified coders and the coding credentials available for professionals working in the outpatient setting. Appendix 14A provides four slides on these credentials, which are reviewed in chapter 12 of this textbook.

Outpatient Coding and CDI Resources

In addition to attending educational sessions, coding professionals should be encouraged to study on their own those areas where they need additional training (for example, risk-adjustment coding for both the outpatient facility and physician practice setting).

In addition to this textbook, instructors can identify helpful resources from AHIMA, AAPC, and Association of Clinical Documentation Improvement Specialists, such as practice briefs and position papers; journal articles; books; boot camps; webinars; and online courses. Relevant resources from CMS, such as its website on risk adjustment (CMS 2017a), can also be highlighted.

Knowledge Base for Outpatient Coders

The Knowledge Base slides in appendix 14A can be used to provide instruction to outpatient coders about a range of topics that they may be expected to understand about CDI. These competencies are in addition to ICD-10-CM, CPT, HCPCS, and HCC coding skills.

Knowledge Base for Coders: Making the Case for CDI

Chapter 1 of this textbook offers a high-level introduction to outpatient CDI theory and application. An educational session built around this chapter should offer insight into resources the coders can use as they begin to enhance their skills and understanding of outpatient CDI.

Each chapter of this text includes corresponding PowerPoint presentations, available online, which may be modified to expand the coder group presentation to include outpatient CDI theory and application.

Knowledge Base for Coders: Physician Fee Schedules

Chapter 3 presents a high-level introduction to physician fee schedules. An educational session on this topic could and explain what RVUs are and how they are used to calculate a payment under the payment policies for Medicare Part B Physician Fee Schedules (PFSs).

The calculation is shown in figure 14.1.

Figure 14.1. Medicare PFS payment rates formula

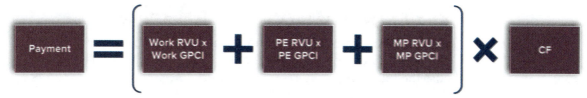

Source: CMS 2017b.

During instruction on this calculation, participants should become familiar with all the variables.

- *RVUs:* Three separate RVUs are associated with calculating a payment under the *Medicare PFS*: The work RVU reflects the relative time and intensity associated with furnishing a Medicare PFS service. The practice expense (PE) RVU reflects the costs of maintaining a practice (such as renting office space, buying supplies and equipment, and staff costs). The malpractice (MP) RVU reflects the costs of malpractice insurance.
- *GPCIs:* Each of the three RVUs is adjusted to account for geographic variations in the costs of practicing medicine in different areas of the United States. These adjustments are called GPCIs, and each kind of RVU component has a corresponding GPCI adjustment.
- *Conversion factor (CF):* To determine the payment rate for a particular service, the sum of the geographically adjusted RVUs is multiplied by a CF in dollars.

Finally, participants in training on PFS should learn that the Physician Fee Schedule final rule is updated annually, with new RVU weights and a new CF.

Knowledge Base for Coders: Hospital Chargemaster

An educational session providing a high-level introduction to the hospital chargemaster can be based on content from chapters 3 and 6 of this textbook. The instructor can emphasize the following points:

- The chargemaster, which is also known as the charge description master (CDM), is a system file within the hospital billing system that includes a list of all items billed.
- Each line item includes the CDM description, department, CDM item code, revenue code, and price.
- In most facilities, the revenue integrity department is responsible for annual updates and revisions to the CDM as new services are added or deleted.
- An annual evaluation of the CDM should be conducted by the revenue integrity department.
- The outpatient CDS or coder may identify issues with CDM accuracy during an outpatient coding and CDI audit.
- These issues should be discussed with the revenue integrity department so that the CDM file can be updated and the charge capture mechanism revised as needed.

Knowledge Base for Coders: Claims Editors

An educational session providing a high-level introduction to claims editors can be based on content from chapter 7 of this textbook. The session may discuss the following:

- The purpose of the clinical editor is to identify coding gaps and quality issues related to coding and clinical documentation and to prevent denials from inaccurate claims based on coding or medical necessity.
- The claims editor system can generate reports that can be reviewed by the CDS and coder. These reports can identify high-volume claims editor issues. Then, those areas the CDI and coding teams can target those issues for root cause analysis and workflow redesign.

To illustrate issues related to claims editors, participants in this session can discuss the case example provided in online appendix 14A.

Knowledge Base for Coders: Denials Management

An educational session providing a high-level introduction to denials management can be based on content from chapters 6 and 7 of this textbook. The instructor can focus on the following primary functions of the denials management department:

- Receiving the denials information, which may be communicated electronically on remittance advice, via denials software, or via letter
- Reviewing the denials detail to determine trends and preliminary root causes such as medical necessity, lack of preauthorization, coding error, technical claim error, or lack of information
- Reviewing the clinical record to validate the root cause

- Communicating with the relevant stakeholder (coder or provider) to verify the cause of a denial and identify additional information that can be added to the clinical record as an addendum and used to prepare the denial letter to respond to the payer
- Monitoring the denials process for trends and collaborating with CDI program to develop solutions such as coder or provider training, EHR template design, EHR enhancements, and CDI workflow redesign

Knowledge Base for Coders: CMS Quality Programs in the Outpatient Setting

An educational session providing a high-level introduction to CMS quality programs for outpatient facilities can be based on chapter 4 of this textbook. Appendix 14A includes two slides on this topic.

This session may accomplish the following objectives:

- Discuss the quality program at the facility and how it supports CMS.
- Provide a brief overview of the OQR.
  - CMS implemented OQR specifically for outpatient facility services. It requires hospitals to submit data related to the quality of services provided in the outpatient setting.
  - These quality measures can be categorized into four types: process, outcome, structure, and efficiency.
  - The program dictates that hospitals that do not meet OQR requirements will receive a decrease in their OPPS annual payment update of 2 percent. The data collected through the OQR program are available for the public to view on the Hospital Compare website (CMS 2017c).
- Provide a brief overview of the Physician Quality Reporting System (PQRS).
  - CMS defines the PQRS "as a quality reporting program that encourages individual eligible professionals (EPs) and group practices to report information on the quality of care to Medicare. PQRS gives participating EPs and group practices the opportunity to assess the quality of care they provide to their patients, helping to ensure that patients get the right care at the right time" (CMS 2017d).
  - The program established a negative payment adjustment for providers who did not meet the quality measure for covered professional services in 2013. Providers who met the requirements for 2016 will avoid the 2018 PQRS negative payment adjustment. CDSs should be familiar with this subject matter so that they can assist the physician practice in establishing streamlined data collection solutions to ensure accurate data capture.
  - *Note:* 2016 was the last program year for PQRS. PQRS transitioned to the Merit-based Incentive Payment System (MIPS) under the Quality Payment Program. The final data submission timeframe for reporting 2016 PQRS quality data to avoid the 2018 PQRS downward payment adjustment was January through March 2017. The first MIPS performance period is January through December 2017. For more information, visit the Quality Payment Program website (CMS 2017d).

- MIPS:
  - MIPS consolidates reporting under three existing Medicare programs: PQRS, Value-Based Modifier (VM), and Meaningful Use of Certified Electronic Health Record Technology (CEHRT).
  - Those programs have been replaced by four performance categories—quality (formerly PQRS), resource use (formerly VM), advancing care information (formerly Meaningful Use of CEHRT)—and clinical practice improvement activities (CPIAs) (a new performance category).
  - Selected providers are included in MIPS (CMS 2017e):
    - Physician
    - Physician assistant
    - Nurse practitioner
    - Clinical nurse specialist
    - Certified registered nurse anesthetist
  - Under the MIPS program, each provider will receive a composite performance score (CPS) that ranges from 0 to 100 points. Each of the performance categories has a corresponding weight.
  - The payment received under the program is dependent on the amount of data submitted as well as the performance results (CMS 2017e).

Knowledge Base for Coders: HCC and Outpatient Code Assignment

Instructors may wish to provide a high-level introduction to HCC, CPT, HCPCS and ICD-10-CM assignment and emphasize the need for in-depth knowledge of these classification systems in the outpatient setting.

- It is important to let the coder know which coding systems they should be familiar with for outpatient coding and CDI coding. They will most likely be familiar with each of these systems.
- Resources such as online and live training are available, as are community and university courses in these classification systems. Coders with credentials such as CCS, CCS-P, CCA, CPC, and COC will already have the basics. Additional study may be needed for specific areas of focus. The CRC credential preparation course prepares the ambulatory coder to work with risk-based coding.

Knowledge Base for Coders: Data Analytics, Metrics, and Trending

A high-level introduction to data analytics and its use for improving clinical documentation, quality score, and reimbursement can be based on chapter 6 of this textbook.

- Discuss the types of data that are used in outpatient CDI programs. The most frequently used data are denials reports, HCC capture reports, claims edit reports, coding audits, quality score trends, the hospital chargemaster or physician fee schedule with volumes, and outpatient research identifiable file or outpatient charge data file.
- Discuss how data analysis can identify CDI gap trends that can become focus of further auditing, root cause analysis, and workflow redesign.

- Explain that it is not practical to audit and resolve issues for all trends identified because of the high volume of clinical documentation in the outpatient setting. Instead, outpatient CDI works to identify those gaps that result in high-dollar revenue loss, high-volume denials, quality score issues, and clinical documentation that is incomplete or lacks the necessary specificity of detail.
- Explain that data analytics can also be used to monitor the progress of CDI implementation, identify successes, and develop solutions to new issues.

Questions

Every session should allow time for a question-and-answer period at the end. Instructors can ask the participants if they have any questions on the material presented, and if there are areas of focus that came to mind during the discussion. As the session ends, the instructors should encourage the participants to keep the program in mind as they do their daily work and to become collaborative members of the CDI team by identifying CDI gaps and being part of the resolution process.

Chapter 14 Review Exercises

1. The move toward risk-based payment has increased the need in both the clinic and professional practice setting for which of the following professionals?
    a. Outpatient coders
    b. Nurse practitioners
    c. Nonprovider clinicians
    d. Nonphysician providers

2. Risk-adjustment coding requires a detailed understanding of which of the following?
    a. HCC codes
    b. Case-mix index
    c. APC assignment
    d. Fee-schedule RVU weights

3. What should be the topic of focus on a presentation to medical coding professionals during an outpatient CDI coding professional education session?
    a. Clinical workflows for a variety of specialty areas
    b. Key differences between inpatient and outpatient CDI
    c. Improving quantity rather than quality of documentation
    d. How the coder can assist in the clinical documentation team process

4. Outpatient CDI leaders should stress the importance of the collaboration between coding professionals and CDSs to support the mission, goals, and objectives of the health system by _____.
    a. Explaining the HCC scores and how they are predictive in nature
    b. Comparing accurate outpatient reimbursement processes to inpatient guidelines

c. Discussing the query workflow and determining whether the nonprovider clinician will initially review queries
d. Improving and ensuring accurate and specific clinical documentation is available for providers and other clinicians to ensure high-quality patient care

5. A coder who is working primarily in the facility's cardiology clinic setting may be required to have experience in which of the following areas?
   a. E/M coding
   b. UB-04 claims submission guidelines
   c. CMS Hospital Acquired Condition guidelines
   d. Inpatient Prospective Payment System guidelines

6. Outpatient CDI can enhance high-quality clinical documentation in which of the following ways?
   a. By increasing the quantity of documentation
   b. By promoting a decrease in documentation that supports medical necessity requirements
   c. By enhancing clinical record specificity to support accurate ICD-10-CM coding and accurate claims submission
   d. By using paper chart templates or handwritten notes to prompt providers to document more specificity in the clinical documentation

7. Providers may not engage in CDI initiatives because they do not think it offers them a direct, individual benefit. Which of the following benefits should therefore be emphasized when discussing CDI with the providers?
   a. Improved physician scorecards on public reporting forums
   b. Opportunities for career advancement for coding professionals
   c. Improved charge capture, chargemaster maintenance, and claims submission
   d. Increased clarity of clinical documentation for clinical and administrative staff

8. Several coders who work at a surgical specialty clinic have been asked to attend a medical coder educational session led by their organization's outpatient CDI program manager. Which of the following locations would be *best* suited for the training session?
   a. A nearby convention center
   b. An on-site conference room
   c. The facility's operating theater
   d. A quiet hallway within the clinic

9. Which of the following factors would be *least* likely to have an impact on the effectiveness of an outpatient CDI educational program?
   a. Buy-in from staff
   b. Size of the trainee group
   c. Gaps in trainees' coding skills
   d. Location of educational sessions

10. Who among the following would be *most* appropriate to lead an educational session on outpatient CDI for medical coding professionals?
    a. Experienced CDS
    b. Specialty physician
    c. Leader of the coder group
    d. CDI program's executive sponsor

References

American Health Information Management Association (AHIMA). 2017. Practice brief: Evolving roles in clinical documentation improvement: Physician practice opportunities. *Journal of AHIMA* 88(5):54–58.

American Health Information Management Association (AHIMA). 2016. Practice brief: Guidelines for achieving a compliant query practice (2016 update). http://library.ahima.org/doc?oid=301357#.WutyyYgvzcs.

American Medical Association (AMA). 2018. *Current Procedural Terminology, Professional Edition 2018*. Chicago: AMA.

Centers for Disease Control and Prevention (CDC). 2017. ICD-10-CM Official Guidelines for Coding and Reporting FY 2018. https://www.cdc.gov/nchs/data/icd/10cmguidelines_fy2018_final.pdf.

Centers for Medicare and Medicaid Services (CMS). 2018. HCPCS general information. https://www.cms.gov/Medicare/Coding/MedHCPCSGenInfo/index.html.

Centers for Medicare and Medicaid Services (CMS). 2017a. Risk adjustment. https://www.cms.gov/Medicare/Health-Plans/MedicareAdvtgSpecRateStats/Risk-Adjustors.html.

Centers for Medicare and Medicaid Services (CMS). 2017b. Medicare Learning Network fact sheet: Medicare Physician Fee Schedule. https://www.cms.gov/Outreach-and-Education/Medicare-Learning-Network-MLN/MLNProducts/downloads/MedcrePhysFeeSchedfctsht.pdf.

Centers for Medicare and Medicaid Services (CMS). 2017c. Hospital Outpatient Quality Reporting Program. https://www.cms.gov/Outreach-and-Education/Medicare-Learning-Network-MLN/MLNProducts/downloads/MedcrePhysFeeSchedfctsht.pdf.

Centers for Medicare and Medicaid Services (CMS). 2017d. Physician Quality Reporting System. https://www.cms.gov/Medicare/Quality-Initiatives-Patient-Assessment-Instruments/PQRS/index.html.

Centers for Medicare and Medicaid Services (CMS). 2017e. MIPS: Advancing Care Information deep dive. https://www.cms.gov/Medicare/Quality-Initiatives-Patient-Assessment-Instruments/Value-Based-Programs/MACRA-MIPS-and-APMs/MIPS-ACI-Deep-Dive-Webinar-Slides.pdf

Physician Queries in the Outpatient Setting

15

Learning Objectives

- Explain the need for physician queries in the outpatient setting.
- Describe the process of physician shadowing and query submission.
- Identify the components of a compliant query.
- Discuss examples of specialty-specific queries.
- Explain how to improve the outpatient query process.

Key Terms

Compliant query
Physician shadowing
Query metrics
Query templates

The query process has become a basic component of the inpatient clinical documentation improvement (CDI) process but is used less frequently in outpatient clinics and physician practice documentation workflows. As in the inpatient setting, the clinical documentation specialist (CDS) or coder primarily submits queries to the provider. However, the outpatient CDI process encourages a team approach in which nonphysician clinicians assist with query responses. Refer to chapter 13 for additional information on nonphysician clinicians. This chapter explores the components of the query process in outpatient settings.

When to Submit a Query

Queries should be submitted when clinical documentation does not meet the criteria for high-quality documentation: legibility, completeness, clarity, consistency, precision, reliability, and timeliness (Hess 2015).

In the outpatient setting, a query may be submitted to the provider prior to, during, or shortly after the visit. Given the sheer volume of outpatient claims, the outpatient CDI program manager must identify areas of focus for the query process. For example, queries may be submitted to clarify the presence of chronic conditions for Hierarchical Condition Category (HCC) capture, to validate or further specify treatments and procedures, and to ask for clarification on signs, symptoms, and clinical indicators. When problematic documentation trends—such as claims denials related to medical necessity, Current Procedural Terminology (CPT) and Healthcare Common Procedure Coding System (HCPCS) procedure code specificity, or *International Classification of Diseases, Tenth Revision, Clinical Modification* (ICD-10-CM) diagnosis code specificity—are identified, queries to address these areas of focus may also be targets of the CDI program.

Criteria for Query Submission

The American Health Information Management Association (AHIMA) Query Toolkit outlines the following reasons for query submission, which may be applied in the outpatient setting (AHIMA 2017):

- Clinical indicators of a diagnosis but no documentation of the condition
- Clinical evidence for a higher degree of specificity or severity
- Uncertainty whether there is a cause-and-effect relationship between two conditions or organisms
- Only the treatment is documented (without a diagnosis documented)
- Clinical validation of a diagnosis

Outpatient records should maintain the same high-quality standards for clinical documentation that are expected in the inpatient setting. Each entry in the outpatient record should meet the following objectives (Hess 2015):

- Address clinical significance of abnormal test results.
- Support the intensity of patient evaluation and treatment, and describe the thought process and complexity of medical decision making.
- Identify all diagnostic and therapeutic procedures, treatments, and tests ordered and performed, in addition to the results.

- Document any changes in the patient's condition, including psychological and physical symptoms.
- Include all conditions that coexist at the time of the encounter or that affect the treatment received.

During the case review process, the outpatient clinical documentation specialist (CDS) should monitor the content of the record as a whole. Trends that indicate documentation does not meet quality standards should lead to provider education and monitoring.

Query Process

The general guidelines for outpatient query process are as follows (AHIMA 2017):

1. Queries may be either verbal or written and may be generated in one or more of the following ways:
   - Previsit (prior to the encounter to clarify chronic conditions that may exist at the time of the visit)
   - Concurrent (during the patient encounter)
   - Retrospective (post-encounter)
2. Queries may be submitted in writing or by e-mail, or via EHR [electronic health record] alert, task, or notes and will be made utilizing compliant query templates.
3. Where query templates are used, they may be edited only as follows:
   - Deletion of any part of the query form not pertinent to the current query
   - Addition of any pertinent clinical findings as documented in the health record
4. Verbal and telephonic queries will follow the same format as written queries.
5. All queries will be:
   - Clear, concise, and nonleading (AHIMA 2017)
   - Simple and direct
   - Itemized to reflect clinical indicators or clues found in the clinical record—for example, those mentioned in the nursing documentation but not in the primary provider's documentation, lab findings, and radiological findings
6. The query should contain all of the patient's identifying information such as account number, name, and date of service, as well as clear, concise itemization of the clinical findings with supporting documentation resulting in a specific question for the provider.
7. Queries may be initiated by either coding professionals or CDI professionals.
8. All queries will be logged for follow-up, to track responses, and to trend for any documentation issues that may indicate additional documentation improvement educational opportunities for providers or overuse of queries by CDI professionals or coding professionals.

Query templates, which are structured forms in which the fields required for query submission are prepopulated, can be used for query development, but the use of templates must follow the policies and procedures of the healthcare entity and adhere to the AHIMA compliant query guidelines (AHIMA 2016). A query that meets the AHIMA industry-standard guidelines outlined the AHIMA Query Toolkit (see appendix 15A of this textbook) can be described as a **compliant query**. Policies and procedures related to the query process should include the key elements mentioned in the eight recommendations outlined previously from the AHIMA Query Toolkit (AHIMA 2017). Established policies and procedures help ensure that the process is effective and that stakeholders understand the industry guidelines; the result is improved clinical documentation in the EHR.

Examples of templates are featured in this chapter. These templates can be customized by the CDI program manager based on clinical indicators in this textbook, the AHIMA Query Toolkit, and each facility's medical staff recommendations. Figure 15.1 presents a generic template recommended by AHIMA (2017) as a format to support the submission of a compliant query. This figure also includes a case scenario to illustrate how case-specific clinical indicators are added to each query. In this example, a query is submitted to clarify the type of diabetes the patient has and to specify the relationship between the two diagnoses documented in the clinical record, peripheral neuropathy and diabetes. The appropriate wording of the query is important; the CDS's query must not lead the provider to a specific diagnosis. Refer to appendix 15B for a detailed reference on query wording and nonleading query documentation.

Figure 15.1. Query template with diabetes complication case scenario

Account Number:
Patient Name:
Date of Service:
Dear (add provider's name):

Diabetes and peripheral neuropathy were documented in the physician progress notes on 12/5. *Example scenario:* This 70-year-old patient has had glucose tests for a chronic type 2 diabetic condition present for 6 years. The progress note today specifies diabetes. The patient is currently on U-100 insulin subcutaneously 3 times per day, 30 minutes prior to the start of a meal. A progress note from a previous encounter last year reveals peripheral neuropathy.

Based on the clinical indicators and your professional judgment, select one of the options below.

- Type 1 diabetes (if so, please specify any associated hypoglycemia or hyperglycemia or any other diabetes complications)
- Type 2 diabetes (if so, please specify any associated hypoglycemia, hyperglycemia, or any other diabetes complications)
- Other explanation of clinical findings (please provide further clarification of diabetes-related complications and or comorbidities) _____
  _____
- Unable to determine
- No further clarification needed

Source: AHIMA 2017.

In a query, demographic information such as account number, patient name, and date of service may be autopopulated, depending on the software used for the query. Portions of the clinical scenario information may also be autopopulated if the software includes natural language processing (NLP) capabilities. (Refer to chapter 7 of this text for more information on NLP.) The AHIMA Query Toolkit includes dropdown menus with options for clinical indicators in the case scenario portion of the template, such as signs, symptoms, risk factors, and treatment.

The template guides the CDS in the development of a compliant query by providing a standardized format for the query. The template then assists the CDS to identify the opportunity. In the example from figure 15.1, the patient's age and history of a type 2 diabetic condition is noted, along with the number of years that the condition has been documented. The patient's treatment (U-100 insulin) is provided, including the dosage, timing, and route. An additional diabetes complication diagnosis (peripheral neuropathy) identified in previous visit notes was added. This information is pertinent to the case because the addition of peripheral neuropathy to the current documentation will result in a higher HCC weight.

The template also clearly presents the question being posed to the provider by listing the options for answering the query: type 1 or type 2 diabetes, other explanation, unable to determine, and no further clarification needed. The query is clear and concise and provides the clinical scenario necessary for the provider to answer the query. After the query is completed by the provider, it can be included as part of the legal clinical record if that is dictated by the health system guidelines. If queries are not included as part of the clinical record per facility guidelines, the provider must addend the clinical record to include the new query response information. Refer to appendix 15C for further discussion of the legal clinical record (AHIMA 2011).

Metrics for Query Submission and Response

Each outpatient CDI program must establish **query metrics** for evaluating the efficiency and effectiveness of clinical documentation queries. These metrics should include the following ratios, which can be calculated for a specific CDS, provider, clinical practice, or the program as a whole.

- *Case review volume:* The number of cases reviewed (in initial and subsequent reviews).
- *Query rate:* The number of queries divided by the number of case reviews.
- *Response rate:* The number of provider responses divided by the number of queries.
- *Agreement rate:* The number of provider agreements divided by the number of provider-specific queries. *Provider agreement* refers to the provider agreeing with the clinical documentation query.
- *Educational sessions held (hours):* The number of CDS hours spent in educational sessions to provider groups.

- *One-on-one provider/coder discussions (hours):* The number of hours spent by coders in one-on-one discussions with providers.
- *Educational material development (hours):* The number of CDS hours spent developing CDI-related provider handouts, newsletter articles, and training materials.

The first four metrics listed here are typically monitored as part of the outpatient CDI program. The remaining three (hours spent in educational sessions, one-on-one discussions, and educational material development) are not typically tracked. However, if the productivity and success of CDSs are measured only by case review volume and query rate, the larger picture of the essential CDS activities will be missed by the CDI program manager or project manager.

As the CDI program evolves, the amount of CDS time spent in each activity will change. A new program requires a relatively large number of queries because providers are learning the concepts and guidelines related to outpatient CDI documentation issues. As providers become more knowledgeable about outpatient CDI, fewer queries will be required (the query rate will drop). As the outpatient CDS becomes more skilled and proficient in the query process, the provider agreement rate should increase. The provider agreement rate will also increase as the program matures and providers become knowledgeable about clinical documentation.

Each CDI program must establish metrics and benchmarks based on the healthcare entity's policies, CDS procedures, and clinical documentation workflow. At the start of a new program, the CDI manager should establish a target weekly amount of time to be spent by the CDS performing each task. Industry standards suggest that 10 new and 15 subsequent case reviews may be completed by the CDS in an 8-hour workday. The actual volume of case reviews performed daily will vary widely based on the amount of time that CDSs spend performing case reviews versus the time allotted for provider education and queries. The level of patient severity will also be a factor in determining the volume of case reviews. For example, fewer case reviews can be conducted per day at an academic medical center than in a community hospital because cases in the academic medical center tend to be more severe. The amount of time spent in educational program development and delivery, as well as newsletter content development, will vary depending on the facility. Many CDI managers do not establish a case review productivity standard for these reasons. Refer to appendix 15D for additional information on CDI productivity standards (Combs 2016).

The AHIMA Clinical Documentation Improvement Toolkit (2016) suggests the following metrics for provider query participation:

- Provider *response* rate: ≥ 80%
- Provider *agreement* rate: ≥ 80%

These standards are prevalent in the CDI industry and have been accepted by many CDI program managers as a CDI metric. The provider response rate reflects the level of cooperation by the provider and also reflects the level of collaboration between the provider and CDS. It is not unusual to see providers with a higher agreement rate for one CDS than another. Similarly, the agreement rate speaks to the clear, concise, and thoughtful query development by the CDS as well as the level of cooperation by the provider. A high response rate and low agreement rate could reflect an issue related to the query content created by the CDS, or it could indicate that the provider lacks understanding of coding guidelines and clinical documentation. To determine the root cause, the CDI manager should review a sample of query disagreements. The process should include a review of the clinical record, the query submitted, and the provider response. For each case, the reason why the provider disagreed should be determined. The CDI manager may also benefit from a conversation with the provider to get feedback on the query process and determine the reason for a high disagreement rate.

Improving the Physician Query Process

To develop an efficient and effective query process, the provider's clinical documentation process must be modified. The typical clinical documentation steps for an outpatient encounter without a query process are as follows:

1. The patient is placed in the examination room.
2. The provider enters the room and reviews the EHR for historical information and current vital signs and laboratory findings.
3. The provider asks the patient about his or her chief complaint and reason for the visit.
4. The provider examines the patient.
5. The provider discusses the prognosis and treatment plans with the patient.
6. The provider documents the discussion and exam in the EHR (during or immediately after the visit).
7. The patient visit ends.
8. The coder codes the record from the EHR and drops the bill.

In this scenario, the provider has no interaction with the CDS or coder.

In the revised clinical documentation process, the outpatient CDS is an active participant who interacts with the physician through written or verbal queries. The clinical documentation process steps, including CDS query process, are as follows:

1. **REVISED**—The CDS reviews the patient history information, including problem lists, for focused issues such as HCC capture, charge capture gaps, or medical necessity gaps. The CDS submits any appropriate provider queries via e-mail or through EHR alerts, notes, or tasks, using the AHIMA compliant query template. This step can be performed the day or week prior to the visit or on the same day just prior to the visit.
2. The patient is placed in the examination room.

3. The provider enters the room and reviews the EHR for historical information, current vital signs, and laboratory findings.
4. **REVISED**—The provider reviews the CDS query communication regarding CDI-focused issues such as HCC capture, charge capture gaps, or medical necessity gaps. This provider may perform this step just before entering the room or, if the note or prompt is brief, during the visit.
5. The provider asks the patient about his or her chief complaint or reason for the visit.
6. The provider examines the patient.
7. The provider discusses the prognosis and treatment plans with the patient.
8. **REVISED**—The provider considers the CDS query information and makes a clinical determination about whether the query includes diagnoses pertinent to today's visit based on MEAT criteria (monitor, evaluate, assess/address, or treat). Refer to chapter 6 for more information on MEAT criteria.
9. The provider documents the discussion and exam in the EHR (during or immediately after the visit).
10. The patient visit ends.
11. **REVISED**—The CDS reviews documentation of the visit in the EHR immediately or as soon as possible after the visit.
12. **REVISED**—The CDS queries the provider immediately, or as soon as possible, after the visit, if an original query was not addressed in the note or if a new query is needed.
13. **REVISED**—The provider responds to queries and updates the visit documentation as soon as possible after the CDS response.
14. **REVISED**—The CDS reviews the clinical record to evaluate the updated visit documentation.
15. The coder codes the record from the EHR and drops the bill.

The revised scenario describes a **physician shadowing** process, in which the CDS's involvement in reviewing documentation before and after the visit offers a learning experience for the provider. After the CDS and provider work together, the clinical documentation and query process will become more efficient, and less re-review of the record by the CDS after a visit will be required.

Specialty-Specific Diagnosis Queries

Query templates should be designed to meet the needs of each specialty, and physician specialty leaders who are educated in the compliant query process should be included in the development of the templates so that each agrees with the basic template format and specific questions. Examples of specialty-specific diagnosis queries are provided in the figures 15.2 through 15.9.

Figure 15.2. Cardiology query example

Dear (Dr. Jones):

Arrhythmia was documented in the progress note of 11/8. *Example scenario:* 85-year-old female patient presents with rapid pulse, irregular heartbeat with flutter. The patient's caregiver reports recent confusion. The patient says she is light-headed and is short of breath. The progress note reveals a diagnosis of arrhythmia. The patient states that she has had these symptoms for three weeks.

Based on the clinical indicators and your professional judgment, please complete by selecting one of the options below.

- Paroxysmal atrial fibrillation
- Persistent atrial fibrillation
- Long-standing persistent atrial fibrillation
- Permanent atrial fibrillation
- Chronic atrial fibrillation
- Nonvalvular atrial fibrillation
- Unable to determine
- No further clarification

Source: AHIMA 2017.

Figure 15.3. Emergency medicine query example

Dear (Dr. Jones):

High blood alcohol level was identified in the ED note of 9/7. *Example scenario:* This 25-year-old man presents after an automobile accident with a blood alcohol level of 1.0. The patient's friend reports that he has had frequent emergency department visits related to alcohol use.

Based on the clinical indicators and your professional judgment, please complete by selecting one of the options below.

- Alcohol abuse (if so, please specify any associated mood disorder, intoxication, or withdrawal)
- Alcohol dependence (if so, please specify any associated mood disorder, intoxication, or withdrawal)
- Alcohol use (if so, please specify any associated mood disorder, intoxication, or withdrawal)
- Other explanation of clinical findings (please provide further clarification if selected)
- Unable to determine
- No further clarification needed

Source: AHIMA 2017.

Figure 15.4. Endocrinology, nutritional disease query example

Dear (Dr. Jones):

(*Example scenario:* This 89-year-old woman presents with a history of a recent 25 lb. weight loss and loss of appetite over the past month. The patient was recently placed in assisted living, and caretakers report that she is frequently missing meals. Her BMI [body mass index] is reported at 18; her albumin is 2.2 grams per deciliter [g/dL].)

Based on the clinical indicators and your professional judgment, choose an item. Please complete by selecting one of the options below.

- Mild protein-calorie malnutrition
- Moderate protein-calorie malnutrition
- Severe protein-calorie malnutrition
- Kwashiorkor
- Marasmus kwashiorkor
- Findings of no clinical significance
- Other explanation of clinical findings (please provide further clarification if selected)
- Unable to determine
- No further clarification needed

Source: AHIMA 2017.

Figure 15.5. Infectious disease query example

Dear (Dr. Jones):

Altered mental status and urosepsis were noted in the progress note of 6/9. (*Example scenario:* This 65-year-old man presents with a temperature of 102°F; WBC [white blood cell count] performed today: 14,000; pulse rate of 95; respiratory rate of 22. The patient's caregiver reports that the patient was confused. The provider notes altered mental status and urosepsis.)

Based on the clinical indicators and your professional judgment, please complete by selecting one of the options below.

- Urinary tract infection only
- Sepsis secondary to urinary sources
- Other explanation of clinical findings (please provide further clarification if selected)
- Other explanation of clinical findings (please provide further clarification if selected)
- Unable to determine
- No further clarification needed

Source: AHIMA 2017.

Figure 15.6. Internal medicine query example

Dear (Dr. Jones):

Hypotension, light-headedness and abnormal hemoglobin were noted in the progress note of 4/2. (*Example scenario:* This 47-year-old woman presents with a history of gastric ulcer currently being treated with Nexium. The patient's hemoglobin level is 9.0 g/dL. The patient also complained of light-headedness, palpitations, and headache. The patient is hypotensive with a BP [blood pressure] of 87/58 mmHg.)

Based on the clinical indicators and your professional judgment, please complete by selecting one of the options below.

- Acute blood loss anemia
- Chronic blood loss anemia
- Anemia of chronic disease (if so, please specify the chronic disease)
- Anemia due to antineoplastic chemotherapy
- Anemia due to end-stage renal disease
- Drug-induced aplastic anemia
- Other type of anemia (please provide further clarification if selected)
- Findings of no clinical significance
- Other explanation of clinical findings (please provide further clarification if selected)
- Unable to determine
- No further clarification needed

Source: AHIMA 2017.

Figure 15.7. Oncology query example

Dear (Dr. Jones):

A history of adenocarcinoma with recent weight loss was documented in the progress note of 4/19. (*Example scenario:* This 75-year-old female patient presents with a history of adenocarcinoma of the small intestine 1 year ago. The tumor was surgically removed when diagnosed a year ago. The patient has recently experienced unexplained weight loss of 20 lbs and complains of weakness, fatigue, and tarry stools.)

Based on the clinical indicators and your professional judgment, please complete by selecting one of the options below.

- The malignancy has been cured (it is only described as a history note).
- The malignancy is in remission.
- The malignancy is a current diagnosis (patient is still receiving treatment or tumor is still present).
- Other explanation of clinical findings (please provide further clarification if selected)
- Unable to determine
- No further clarification needed

Source: AHIMA 2017.

Figure 15.8. Orthopedics and pain management query example

Dear (Dr. Jones):

Repeated requests for refills of narcotic pain medicine were documented in the progress note of 12/14. (*Example scenario:* This 35-year-old man was seen for a follow-up visit after a lower lumbar injury during an automobile accident several months ago. The patient continues to have back pain and has requested increasing dosages of narcotic pain medicine over the past few visits. The patient is confused and less alert than in the past and also complains of fatigue. Physician exam reveals constricted pupils.)

Based on the clinical indicators and your professional judgment, please complete by selecting one of the options below.

- Narcotic abuse (if so, please specify any associated mood disorder, intoxication, or withdrawal)
- Narcotic dependence (if so, please specify any associated mood disorder, intoxication, or withdrawal)
- Narcotic use (if so, please specify any associated mood disorder, intoxication, or withdrawal)
- Other explanation of clinical findings
- Unable to determine
- No further clarification needed

Source: AHIMA 2017.

Figure 15.9. Neurology query example

Dear (Dr. Jones):

Difficulties with concentration and memory were reported in progress note of 3/20. (*Example scenario:* This 90-year-old male patient presents with difficulty concentrating, memory loss, and confusion. The caretaker reports a short attention span, lack of motivation, and depression. The progress note specifies a diagnosis of memory loss. The patient is being treated with an anxiolytic [midazolam], and the caretaker reports recent behavioral issues.)

Based on the clinical indicators and your professional judgment, please complete by selecting one of the options below.

- Pre-senile dementia
- Senile dementia
- Vascular dementia
- Alzheimer dementia
- Lewy body dementia
- Other type of dementia (please specify)
- Other explanation of clinical findings (please provide further clarification if selected)
- Unable to determine
- No further clarification needed

Source: AHIMA 2017.

Chapter 15 Review Exercises

1. The query process with outpatient CDI is similar to the inpatient CDI query process in which of the following ways?
   a. Both result in high-quality clinical documentation.
   b. Both must be initiated following the patient encounter.
   c. Both require the assistance of non-physician clinicians.
   d. Both are used frequently in physician practice documentation workflows.

2. In the outpatient setting, queries may be submitted for multiple purposes, including to_____.
   a. Compare the charge capture document to the clinical record
   b. Seek clarification on signs, symptoms, and clinical indicators
   c. Train the physician advisor in provider communication skills
   d. Educate nonprovider clinicians in quality metrics submission

3. At present, the manager of a CDI program tracks two query metrics: case review volume and query rate. However, she is interested in gaining a bigger-picture view about the efficiency and effectiveness of CDS activities, such as clinical documentation queries. Considering this goal, which of the following data points would provide the *greatest* benefit if added to the metrics she already tracks?
   a. Number of provider responses
   b. Number of cases reviewed by the CDSs
   c. Number of CDS hours spent in provider education sessions
   d. Number of CDS hours spent developing CDI-related training materials

4. Each entry in the outpatient record should include all conditions that coexist at the time of the encounter or_____.
   a. That affect the treatment received
   b. Were assigned an HCC code at a previous visit
   c. Were included as part of the hospital discharge summary
   d. Are listed in the hospital medication administration record

5. Which of the following scenarios would be *most likely* to result in a problematic query?
   a. The CDS submitted a handwritten query.
   b. The CDS generated the query prior to the patient encounter.
   c. The CDS removed an impertinent part of the query from prior to submission.
   d. The CDS combined elements from multiple query templates to create a custom template.

6. Query metrics are important to evaluate the efficiency and effectiveness of clinical documentation queries. The ratio calculated to determine provider accord rate and the recommended addition to the clinical documentation is the
   a. Query rate
   b. Response rate
   c. Agreement rate
   d. Educational rate

7. Each entry in the outpatient record should support the intensity of patient evaluation and treatment and describe the thought process and complexity of _____.
   a. Clinical indicators
   b. Medical decision making
   c. Past family and social history
   d. Pre-visit query communications

8. Query templates may be used for query development as part of the outpatient CDI process. Which of the following is *not* among the benefits of using query templates?
   a. Leading the provider to the correct diagnosis
   b. Promoting high-quality clinical documentation
   c. Guiding the CDS in developing compliant queries
   d. Accommodating the documentation needs of physicians in specialty areas

9. Which of the following would represent a reason for query submission as part of the outpatient CDI process?
   a. Present on admission (POA) indicator status
   b. Multiple clinical indicators supporting the same condition or procedure
   c. Uncertainty whether there is a cause-and-effect relationship between two conditions or organisms
   d. An underlying cause when admitted with symptoms and without a definitive diagnosis

10. A CDI manager is reviewing metrics for provider query participation and observes the following results:
    - Response rate = 95%
    - Agreement rate = 49%

    Which of the following would be the *most* logical conclusion based on the metrics provided?
    a. The provider lacks understanding of coding guidelines.
    b. Fluctuating case volumes have skewed the data for the period.
    c. The CDS has been unable to gain the cooperation of the provider.
    d. The CDI program has reached maturity and query rates have declined.

References

American Health Information Management Association (AHIMA). 2017. AHIMA query toolkit. http://bok.ahima.org/PdfView?oid=302140.

American Health Information Management Association (AHIMA). 2016. Practice brief: Guidelines for achieving a compliant query practice (2016 update). http://library.ahima.org/doc?oid=301357#.Wut8nYgvzcs.

American Health Information Management Association (AHIMA). 2011. Fundamentals of the legal health record and designated record set. *Journal of AHIMA* 82(2): expanded online version. http://library.ahima.org/doc?oid=104008#.WrKG-y7wbIU.

Combs, T. 2016. Measuring CDI productivity. Documentation Detective blog. *Journal of AHIMA* website. http://journal.ahima.org/2016/03/23/measuring-cdi-productivity./

Hess, P. 2015. *Clinical Documentation Improvement: Principles and Practice*. Chicago, IL: AHIMA.

Expanding the Outpatient CDI Program 16

Learning Objectives

- Explain the importance of stakeholder buy-in when expanding the outpatient CDI program into new settings.

- Describe the expansion of outpatient clinical documentation improvement (CDI) into the emergency and observation services departments.

Key Terms

Admission to observation
Hospital Readmissions Reduction Program (HRRP)
InterQual or Milliman Admission Criteria

Observation services
Two-midnight rule

The seven criteria for high-quality clinical documentation (legibility, reliability, precision, completeness, consistency, clarity, and timeliness) apply to clinical documentation in all settings (refer to chapter 1). After an outpatient clinical documentation improvement (CDI) program is rolled out to the outpatient clinic and physician practice settings, the program can expand to the emergency department (ED) and observation services. Such expansion to other outpatient settings is essential for an overarching CDI program covering the continuum of care.

Areas for CDI expansion should be selected based on the service-line offerings, volume, revenue impact, and known clinical documentation and claims submission issues. Based on these criteria, most healthcare entities will find it reasonable to include the ED and observation settings as next steps. Short-stay admissions denied by the payer for medical necessity should be included in the CDI program for the ED and observation services. These denials can occur due to a missing patient status order or missing two-midnight stay criteria. Some patients who were admitted for short stays perhaps should have been treated in an outpatient setting. After case review and root cause analysis of the denials, the outpatient clinical documentation specialist (CDS) can provide training to physicians on these guidelines to decrease denials for these areas.

As with other outpatient service areas, the *International Classification of Diseases, Tenth Revision, Clinical Modification* (ICD-10-CM) is used to code diagnoses, and the Current Procedural Terminology (CPT) and Healthcare Common Procedure Coding System (HCPCS) are used to code procedures. To ensure high-quality clinical documentation supporting the codes, the outpatient CDS must be familiar with the guidelines for these classifications systems. Refer to chapter 3 for more information on guidelines for ICD-10-CM and CPT/HCPCS.

Organizational and Stakeholder Adoption

Each new setting incorporated into the outpatient CDI program offers distinctive documentation challenges. Stakeholders in a particular setting are likely aware of these challenges and may have ideas about solutions that could mitigate risk in these areas. Prior to expanding into a new area, the CDI program manager should arrange a meeting between the CDI steering committee and the stakeholders in the new setting to discuss the program and seek buy-in from the stakeholders. It is generally more efficient to use existing steering committee meetings for this purpose, rather than creating a new set of CDI program-related meetings. For example, in the case of the ED, the medical staff leader of the ED and the ED administrative manager should be invited to meet with the steering committee to discuss the expanded program. Before the meeting, the CDI program manager can interview some of the stakeholders to determine some high-volume clinical documentation issues and perhaps identify a clinical example for presentation at the meeting. At the meeting, the brief presentation by the CDI steering committee chair or CDI manager should address the following:

- Known clinical documentation and claims submission challenges in the ED
- A clinical case example of the known CDI challenges
- The new process for incorporating a CDS into the ED clinical documentation workflow
- CDS coverage for the ED and observation areas

- Provider training for the new program
- Creation of an ED CDI taskforce to jump-start implementation of the CDI program and develop a detailed workplan, policies and procedures, and areas of focus

At the end of the CDI steering committee meeting, the chair should reflect upon the importance of the CDI program expansion to the healthcare organization and share some of the success stories already realized through the initial CDI program. These successes should focus on the following:

- Improved clinical documentation for patient care and provider collaboration
- Improved quality scores and publicly available quality data
- Accurate severity scores showing the level of care provided at the facility
- Accurate revenue and fewer denials because clinical documentation is complete, and patient status orders and claims submission are accurate

Whenever possible, the chair of the CDI steering committee should present metrics and dashboards reflecting success in these areas during the meeting with stakeholders. It is important that the chair gives this presentation to encourage buy-in and confirm the importance of the outpatient CDI program to meet the healthcare organization's mission, vision, goals, and objectives. CDI programs with high-level visibility are more sustainable. Refer to chapters 5 and 8 for more information on the steps and tasks involved in the implementation of the CDI program, and chapter 6 for more information on metrics.

Emergency Department

After the implementation of CDI to outpatient clinics and professional practices is complete, high-risk issues related to clinical documentation in the ED may become a CDI program priority. In this case, the ED may be among the first departments to be included in outpatient CDI. Clinical documentation gaps in the ED can result in medical necessity denials, inaccurate coding of outpatient claims, and problems with inpatient diagnosis-related group (DRG) assignment. Because the ED is often the first location where the patient is seen before he or she is transferred to other sites and levels of service, clinical documentation in the ED must "fully support the evaluation and management [E/M] level and the outcome of the visit. Emergency room providers must fully document the reason for discharging or admitting the patient. The ED note is an important part of the patient story" (Combs 2016).

The CDI process in the ED should include evaluation of clinical documentation to support the following critical areas and any procedure(s) or service(s) provided:

- Admission documentation
- Critical care documentation
- Charge capture
- Observation status, especially if the observation unit is housed in the ED (for example, a chest pain observation unit)
- E/M level

Admission Documentation

When a patient is admitted for observation or acute care through the ED, it is critical to accurately capture the clinical picture and treatment during the entire ED stay. This information is needed to assign the principal diagnosis for the ED visit and provide evidence of the medical necessity for admission. Payers may deny claims if there are gaps or inconsistencies between the emergency physician's documentation and that of the attending physician who takes over care on admission. One issue may be documentation related to patient acuity. The emergency physician documents the patient's acuity on arrival at the ED, and the attending physician documents the patient's acuity on admission. If the physicians' assessments of acuity differ and there is inadequate documentation of treatment given in the ED to explain the change in acuity, that documentation gap could lead to a denial.

Case Example

> The patient arrives at the ED with clinical indicators for sepsis, and the emergency physician documents a suspected diagnosis of sepsis. The patient is given intravenous (IV) antibiotics and remains in the ED for 48 hours prior to admission. When the patient is admitted and blood is drawn for diagnostic laboratory tests, the attending physician's documentation indicates a diagnosis of pneumonia. If the documentation does not include the clinical indicators observed by the emergency physician when the patient first arrived at the ED or capture the ED interventions, the clinical record will be incomplete and inconsistent and may not support the medical necessity of admission.

At the time of admission by the attending physician, the utilization review (UR) nurse uses **InterQual or Milliman admission criteria** to validate clinical indicators for admission for commercial payers. InterQual and Milliman are clinical criteria used to determine medical necessity for various sites of service, such as inpatient admission, observation services, the intensive care unit (ICU), step-down units, and discharge. Government payers, such as Medicare, use Centers for Medicare and Medicaid Services (CMS) guidance to determine medical necessity (for example, the two-midnight rule, which is explained later in this chapter). However, the UR and clinical teams in the ED are often busy at the time of the patient admission and may not have the time or resources to adequately assess and document the patient's admission rationale. Furthermore, the UR team may not be available during off-hours or weekends to review the admission criteria. In any of these cases, an admission denial can occur.

The outpatient CDS should be included in discussions between the ED and the denials management department regarding the root causes of admission denials. The outpatient CDS can be an extra set of eyes to review the documentation. A retrospective review of cases for a specific diagnosis denials trend may reveal patterns in clinical documentation gaps. The trend could be the result of incomplete documentation of clinical criteria or incomplete documentation of the emergency provider's medical decision making process at the time of the admission.

Once patterns and root causes are identified, the outpatient CDS can present education for the UR nurses and ED providers on complete and specific admission documentation. The outpatient CDS can also educate the attending physician staff on inconsistencies noted in the documentation from the ED physician as compared with that of the attending. A peer-to-peer conversation between providers may be needed to determine why a patient was admitted from the ED and ensure that this decision is adequately reflected in the ED and transfer documentation.

The Affordable Care Act established the **Hospital Readmissions Reduction Program (HRRP)**, which requires CMS to reduce payments to Inpatient Prospective Payment System (IPPS) hospitals with excessive readmissions. Readmission is defined as "an admission to a subsection (d) hospital within 30 days of a discharge from the same or another subsection (d) hospital." Subsection (d) hospitals are short-term, inpatient acute-care hospitals. Thus, the HRRP program "provides a strong financial incentive for hospitals that improve communication and care coordination efforts, and better engage patients and care givers during post-discharge planning" (QualityNet 2017).

For HRRP, CMS has targeted the readmission of patients with certain conditions. The six measures of focus beginning in fiscal year 2018 are as follows (CMS 2017a):

- Acute myocardial infarction
- Heart failure
- Pneumonia
- Chronic obstructive pulmonary disease
- Coronary artery bypass graft
- Total hip arthroplasty and total knee arthroplasty

For each applicable condition, CMS has a methodology to compare the hospital's readmission rate to the national average and calculate any readmission payment adjustment if the hospital's rate is deemed excessive. The calculations account for differences in case mixes among hospitals by adjusting for variables, such as age, comorbid diseases, and indicators of patient frailty, that are clinically relevant and have relationships with the outcome. Clinical documentation from outpatient records from the past 12 months may be used to determine which variables apply to specific patients.

To help the hospital avoid negative payment adjustments for excessive readmissions, the outpatient CDS can clarify less-specific diagnostic information in outpatient clinical documentation related to readmission measures. Improved documentation and more accurate coding of clinical records from the ED and observation services may decrease the number of patients categorized as having conditions targeted by the HRRP program. More information on HRRP as well as the data correction process, scoring, and payment adjustment methodology may be found on the CMS website (CMS 2017a).

Critical Care Documentation

To ensure accurate billing of services to payers, clinical documentation in the ED must support the E/M CPT codes assigned to patients' claims. Among the frequently assigned codes in the ED are the critical care CPT codes. To assess the clinical documentation for critical care, the outpatient CDS should verify compliance with the CPT guidelines for use of critical care codes. The critical care CPT guidelines are found in the Critical Care Services section of the Evaluation and Management Code chapter of the most recent version of the CPT manual published by the American Medical Association (AMA 2018). These guidelines are used for professional fee coding and billing. The CPT manual specifies that specific procedures are included in the critical care codes 99291 (initial 30–74 minutes) and 99292 (each additional 30 minutes) and may not be reported separately. These included procedures are as follows:

- Interpretation of cardiac output measurements (93561, 93562)
- Chest x-rays (71010, 71015, 71020)
- Pulse oximetry (94760, 94761, 94762)
- Blood gases
- Information date stored in computers, such as electrocardiograms, blood pressure, and hematologic data (99090)
- Gastric intubation (43752, 42753)
- Temporary transcutaneous pacing (92953)
- Ventilatory management (94002–94004, 94660, 94662)
- Vascular access procedures (36000, 36410, 36415, 36591, 36600)

The outpatient CDS should use these CPT manual guidelines to assist in provider education and to audit the accuracy of coding and claims submission in the professional practice setting. Additionally, the CDS should review CMS guidance for hospitals in Chapter 4, Section 160.1, of the Medicare Claims Processing Manual, which specifies that hospitals are required to provide at least 30 minutes of critical care services to support CPT code 99291. Hospitals also must report all ancillary services separately from the critical care codes (CMS 2017b), even though CMS bundles these services into the critical care code in the ambulatory payment classification (APC) of the Outpatient Prospective Payment System (OPPS). In other words, even though the individual service items are coded and submitted on the Medicare claim, the payment for them is packaged as part of reimbursement for the critical care code.

Hospitals are required to report face-to-face critical care time provided by physicians or hospital staff. When multiple staff members or physicians provide services simultaneously, their time is only counted once (CMS 2008a). For example, if a physician and nurse work together to treat a critically ill patient for 30 minutes, only one 99291 code is submitted for payment because the same period cannot be billed twice by two physicians and/or staff. Keeping the reporting requirements in mind, the outpatient CDS can review a sample of ED critical care cases to determine whether the clinical record accurately reflects the time spent by physicians and hospital staff providing critical care services.

Charge Capture

The E/M code for ED level of service is based on the resources consumed in the ED when they are not otherwise separately payable (CMS 2008b). This means that where services are considered separately payable, they may be reported on the claim and will not be bundled in the ED E/M level payment. CMS further clarifies the following in the 2008 OPPS final rule: "In the absence of national visit guidelines, hospitals have the flexibility to determine whether or not to include separately payable services as a proxy to measure hospital resource use that is not associated with those separately payable services" (CMS 2008b). In other words, because there are no CMS guidelines for facility E/M codes for

ED services, hospitals are free to create their own criteria for what resources to include in the E/M code assignment. These criteria may include services that have a separately payable CPT code that can reflect the intensity of the treatments performed. Clinical documentation should support separately payable services as they relate to the ED level of service assignment (ACEP 2011).

When procedures are reported with an E/M level code, modifier -25 must be appended to allow for payment of the code. The Office of Inspector General of the US Department of Health and Human Services in conjunction with the US Department of Justice has historically monitored the use of modifier -25 (Lojewski 2008). Modifier -25 may be used when the service to be separately coded meets the definition of a significant, separately identifiable E/M service according to the CPT manual. CMS Transmittals A-00-40 and A-01-80 further clarify this guidance (CMS 2000; CMS 2002). CDS staff should be familiar with the outpatient CPT/HCPCs modifiers and the documentation required to support them.

To validate compliance with these charge capture guidelines, the outpatient CDS should review a sample of ED clinical records and the corresponding UB-04 (hard-copy facility claims) or CMS1500 (professional claims) forms to confirm that each separately billable procedure is reported. Some of the more frequent coding problems are listed in table 16.1.

Table 16.1. Common problems in emergency department coding

Topic	Example
Infusion and injection	Multiple infusions and injections are often provided during one ED encounter. It is not unusual to find that some infusions and injections provided to the patient are not coded on the claim with a corresponding CPT code.
Splint and cast application	When patients are treated for sprains or other diagnoses requiring a splint or cast application, codes for these services may be incorrectly omitted from the claim.
Fracture and dislocation repair	Fractures and dislocations are coded using ICD-10-CM codes to reflect the diagnosis; however, in some cases, the CPT code for the repair is not reported on the claim.
Accurate CPT code for laceration repair	Clinical documentation specifying the length and depth of laceration repair is often inadequate for accurate CPT code assignment.
Respiratory therapy	Respiratory therapy services such as nebulizer and spirometry mentioned in the nursing notes or respiratory therapy flowsheet may be incorrectly omitted from the claim.
E/M code level	E/M code levels that do not meet the criteria established for the reported level are often incorrectly coded on the claim.

E/M Levels

The following are E/M codes for ED services (AMA 2018):

- 99281 Emergency department visit for the evaluation and management of a patient which requires a problem-focused history; problem-focused exam and straightforward medical decision making
- 99282 Emergency department visit for the evaluation and management of a patient which requires an expanded problem-focused history; expanded problem-focused exam and medical decision making of low complexity

- 99283 Emergency department visit for the evaluation and management of a patient which requires an expanded problem-focused history; expanded problem-focused exam and medical decision making of moderate complexity
- 99284 Emergency department visit for the evaluation and management of a patient which requires a detailed history; detailed exam and medical decision making of moderate complexity
- 99285 Emergency department visit for the evaluation and management of a patient which requires a comprehensive history; comprehensive exam and medical decision making of high complexity

While these E/M codes are used for ED services, there are no national standard criteria for assigning them to ED visits. Therefore, hospitals are permitted to establish their own guidelines.

Since the implementation of the Outpatient Prospective Payment System (OPPS), the Centers for Medicare and Medicaid Services (CMS) has required hospitals to report facility resources for emergency department (ED) visits using CPT evaluation and management (E/M) codes. However, CMS recognized that CPT E/M codes do not adequately describe the intensity and range of ED services by hospitals because the CPT E/M codes reflect physician activities. Therefore, CMS instructed hospitals to develop their own internal guidelines for reporting E/M visits (Lojewski 2008).

The assignment of E/M levels to services provided in the ED is based on a set of criteria that is defined by the healthcare organization that manages the ED. The following basic models are used to develop ED E/M levels:

- *Staff interventions/point system:* Guidelines from the American Hospital Association and American Health Information Management Association (Lojewski 2008) and the American College of Emergency Physicians (ACEP) guidelines (ACEP 2011) are based on complexity and time of the interventions. As the care interventions by either providers or staff become more complex, a higher level is reported. For example, an organization can establish criteria to assign points to services provided that are not separately billable, such as taking vital signs, obtaining a clean catch urine sample, or social worker intervention for a behavioral health patient. Then, the points for a patient encounter are added together, and the E/M level is assigned based on its correspondence with a point range preassigned in the organization's criteria.
- *Time spent with the patient:* The ED E/M level increases as the time increases.
- *Patient severity:* As the severity of the patient and medical decision making complexity increases, the ED E/M level increases. The standard CPT ED E/M-level descriptions listed at the start of this section are an example of this category because the E/M code level is based on the complexity of the case and the severity of the patient.

An important point to remember when hospital ED managers develop ED-level criteria is that the guidelines should reflect the resources used, and the code assignment should relate to the intensity of hospital resources. The E/M level reported by the hospital will not necessarily equate to the level reported by the physician for physician services provided for the same encounter (Lojewski 2008).

CMS provides guidance for internal hospital criteria development (Lojewski 2008; Federal Register 2006). The criteria should achieve the following:

- Follow the intent of the CPT code descriptor—the guidelines should be designed to reasonably relate the intensity of hospital resources to the different levels of effort represented by the [standard descriptions of codes 99281–99285]
- Be based on hospital facility resources, not physician resources
- Be clear to facilitate accurate payments and be usable for compliance purposes and audits
- Meet HIPAA [Health Insurance Portability and Accountability Act] requirements
- Require only documentation that is clinically necessary for patient care
- Not facilitate upcoding
- Be written or recorded, be well documented, and provide the basis for selection of a specific code
- Be applied consistently across patients in the clinic or emergency department to which they apply
- Not change with great frequency
- Be readily available for a fiscal intermediary (or, if applicable, MAC [Medicare Administrative Contractor]) review
- Result in coding decisions that could be verified by other hospital staff, as well as outside resources

To support the outpatient CDI effort in the ED, the CDS should conduct a review of 25 to 30 records per provider and determine whether the clinical documentation and code assignment correspond to the organization's guidelines for E/M code assignment. This sample size is a subjective sample often used in healthcare coding audits to determine the need for further analysis and review.

E/M Level Benchmarking

In addition to auditing the accuracy of E/M code assignment in the ED, the outpatient CDS can analyze how the E/M-level data distribution for the ED compares with the national distribution found in the Part B National Summary Data File, which lists the volume for each CPT code (CMS 2015). The file is updated annually, but there is a delay in availability of the data. In figure 16.1, the national ED E/M code distribution is a bell-shaped curve. Through this analysis, the outpatient CDS can determine, for example, whether the facility's code volume for E/M level 5 (99285) code volume is higher or lower than the national distribution. If it is and there is no evident reason to explain the deviation, the CDS can then perform a root cause analysis. Additional case audits may determine why the distribution varies from the national average.

Chapter 16 Expanding the Outpatient CDI Program

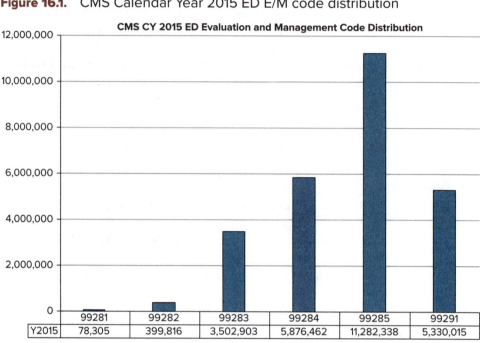

Figure 16.1. CMS Calendar Year 2015 ED E/M code distribution

	99281	99282	99283	99284	99285	99291
Y2015	78,305	399,816	3,502,903	5,876,462	11,282,338	5,330,015

Source: CMS 2015.

ACEP conducted a study comparing the Emergency Severity Index (ESI) with the CMS claims file ED E/M code frequency data (Wiler et al. 2011). ESI is a five-level, criteria-based triage tool that classifies patients from low to high priority (urgency) and assists providers in the identification of patients needing urgent treatment (Gilboy et al. 2011). The study objectives were to (1) compare ESI levels with ED E/M code levels to determine the possible correlation of these code sets; (2) identify factors that may alter the correlation; and (3) predict E/M code-related charges (Wiler et al. 2011). The study found that "the Emergency Severity Index triage scores and Evaluation and Management codes are moderately correlated and can be used to moderately predict expected ED Evaluation and Management codes" (Wiler et al. 2011). Figure 16.2 plots the ESI triage acuity assignment for three categories of hospitals included in the research study:

- Site A: Suburban university-affiliated
- Site B: Suburban community
- Site C: Urban university

Figure 16.2 reflects a distribution skewed toward the higher levels of ED E/M codes. Figure 16.3 shows ESI distributions for the research study sites. The graph includes the ESI Triage categories 1 through 5 and the corresponding volume for each category and site. Overall, the graph points out that ESI Triage level 3 is the highest volume code used in the study. Although the research study finds a moderate correlation between the ESI levels and the ED E/M code levels, the type of facility categorization affects the distribution of the data among levels. The ESI-level distribution is more closely aligned with a bell-shaped curve than the E/M-level distribution, which is skewed slightly toward the higher ED E/M levels.

The CDI manager and team should consider studying the correlation between ESI and ED E/M code data for the healthcare organization. If facility-specific data

Figure 16.2. ACEP Study CPT E/M Codes

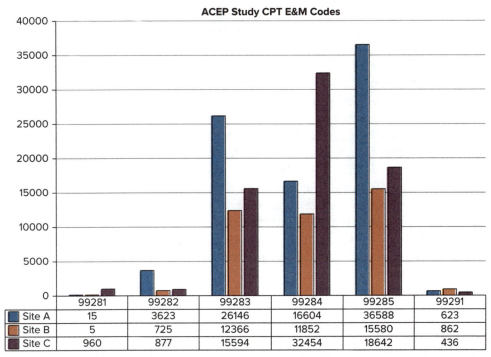

Source: Wiler et al. 2011.

Figure 16.3. ACEP study ESI Triage acuity assignment

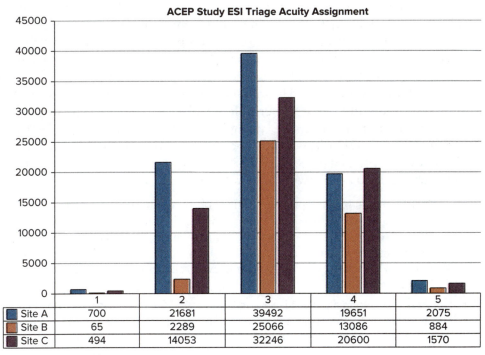

Source: Wiler et al. 2011.

distribution is skewed to a higher- or lower-level distribution when compared with a bell curve, the CDI team should evaluate the root cause of this skew and determine whether the current ED E/M data are accurate. This correlation can be conducted using facility ESI and E/M volumes. If the findings of the CDI team suggest that the coders and/or physicians are assigning the E/M levels incorrectly, education should be provided to address this issue. If E/M levels are assigned automatically by electronic health record software, the criteria for assignment and the software's crosswalk between clinical interventions and the ED E/M codes should be assessed and any errors corrected. For example, if the number of points assigned to vital signs in the ED is too high, the E/M code could be higher than is warranted.

CMS monitors facility E/M volumes for distributions that deviate from the national average distribution. Therefore, it is important to monitor the facility distribution to determine where it may deviate from the bell curve and national averages. A clinical record sample review will provide insight for the outpatient CDS about which clinical interventions may be skewing the E/M data. The assigned weight for each ED E/M tool criterion may need to be assessed and modified. The outpatient CDS can analyze facility-specific ESI and ED E/M level data to prepare steering committee and CDI taskforce meeting presentations on the accuracy of E/M codes within the health system's ED(s).

Observation Services

Observation services can be one of the areas to include in the expanded outpatient CDI program. Improved clinical documentation for patients in observation services can reduce denials, decrease unnecessary admissions and readmissions, and decrease revenue losses related to clinical documentation gaps. Observation services can be defined as a "set of specific, clinically appropriate services, which include ongoing short-term treatment, assessment, and reassessment" (CMS 2016a Section 20.6). When patients are treated in the ED and require an extended period of treatment to determine the final disposition to home or admission, observation services are often ordered by the ED physician (CMS 2016a Section 20.6). The initial observation care may be billed by the facility and by the physician responsible for observation care. The physician should report observation services using CPT codes from the ranges 99218 to 99220 and 99224 to 99226. The facility should report observation services using HCPCS Level II codes G0378 and G0379. For facility billing purposes, these G codes are reported as follows (Hapner 2010):

- G0378 is assigned by a hospital per hour of observation services when a patient presents to the facility through the emergency department, ancillary departments, and/or ambulatory surgery and something occurred that necessitated the patient being placed in observation status. This code is reported per hour up to 48 hours for Medicare patients. Note, however, that the time limit may vary for other commercial payers.
- G0379 is used when a patient is sent to the hospital from a community physician and bypasses the emergency department. This is reported once per encounter and then G0378 is assigned in addition for each hour the patient is in observation status.

Clinical records for observation services include the following elements (CMS 2016a Section 20.6):

- Time and dates in observation status
- Documentation that the attending and billing physician was present and performed the services
- A written order referring the patient to observation signed in a timely manner
- Documentation in the progress discharge notes by the attending and billing physician

In rare cases, the observation service will span more than 48 hours; however, in most cases, duration of service is less than 24 hours (CGS Administrators 2017).

The outpatient CDS should review a sample of observation clinical records and compare them to the UB-04 or CMS 1500 claim form to determine whether the appropriate codes were reported based on the clinical documentation. The following sections discuss key components of the clinical documentation that are essential for accurate and compliant observation coding.

Observation Services Dates and Times

The clinical record should differentiate the date and time that the patient arrived in the observation bed from the date and time that the patient arrived in the ED or outpatient setting. The date and time of placement in the observation setting should not be prior to the date and time of the physician order for that placement. The nursing notes, physician order, physician progress notes, and other portions of the record should be consistent and reflect the timing of the physician order and placement of the patient in the observation bed. Observation time begins when the nurse initiates treatment after the patient status is changed to observation.

The same levels of consistency and detail are required for the observation discharge time. When calculating the total hours in observation for the final claim submission, the physician order must be placed prior to the patient's discharge from observation. The patient's clinical record should reflect when observation services are discontinued. This information may be recorded by a nurse's note documenting the last services provided or by the medication record showing the last date and time of medication administration. Times should be rounded to the nearest hour. The time in which patients are simply waiting for transportation cannot be counted as observation services time. For detailed instruction on observation services billing and claims submission, refer to the following Medicare publications:

- Medicare Benefit Policy Manual, chapter 1, section 10 (CMS 2017c)
- Medicare Claims Processing Manual, chapter 30, section 20 (CMS 2017d)
- Medicare Claims Processing Manual, chapter 4, section 290 (CMS 2017e)

Case Example

Observation services were provided between 8:00 a.m. and 6:00 p.m., according to the nursing notes, and the patient was discharged home at 11:15 p.m. after observation care was completed. The hours of observation reported on the UB-04 claim form would be 105 units representing 510 hours of observation. It should be noted that "Medicare has an 8-hour minimum for physicians reporting the observation same-day-discharge codes 99234-99236" (ACEP 2017).

Regarding routine monitoring, observation services should not be billed concurrently with diagnostic or therapeutic services for which active monitoring is a part of the procedure (for example, colonoscopy or chemotherapy) (CMS 2017e Section 290; CMS 2016a Section 20.6). Hospitals may use the beginning and ending times for the monitoring services and add the total length of time for observation services together to determine the total number of observation hourly units to report on the claim using HCPCS code G0378 (Hospital observation service, per hour) (CMS 2017e Section 290; CMS 2016a Section 20.6). A hospital may also deduct the average length of time of the interrupting procedure from the total duration of time that the patient receives observation services.

CMS provides specific guidance related to composite APCs. Composite APCs allow facilities to bill as a single payment a comprehensive diagnostic or treatment service that would otherwise be billed with multiple HCPCS codes (CMS 2017e Section 290; CMS 2016a Section 20.6). The 2018 OPPS Final Rule identifies the specific composite APC that is assigned when criteria are met for services billed on the same date of service. The list may be found in appendix 16A of this text (CMS 2018)

The outpatient CDS should review observation services clinical records and corresponding claims to determine whether observation services falling under composite APC guidelines are documented and coded correctly.

Provider Orders and Documentation in Observation Services

The payment for an initial observation care code should be billed by the physician who orders the service. Other consulting physicians should bill for outpatient services using the corresponding CPT code for the service provided (CMS 2017e).

CMS provides specific guidance related to physician orders for observation services: "Observation services are covered only when provided by the order of a physician or another individual authorized by State licensure law and hospital staff bylaws to admit patients to the hospital or to order outpatient services" (CMS 2017e Section 290; CMS 2016a Section 20.6). Observation time begins at the clock time documented in the clinical order and must correspond to the time of the physician order (CMS 2017e Section 290; CMS 2016a Section 20.6).

CMS specifically states that "general standing orders for observation services following all outpatient surgery are not recognized" (CMS 2017e Section 290; CMS 2016a Section 20.6). In addition, "hospitals should not report as observation care, services that are part of another Part B service, such as postoperative monitoring during a standard recovery period (e.g., 4-6 hours), which should be billed as recovery room services" (CMS 2017e Section 290; CMS 2016a Section 20.6). When a patient undergoes diagnostic testing as a hospital outpatient, "routine preparation services furnished prior to the testing and recovery afterwards are included in the payments for those diagnostic services" (CMS 2017e Section 290; CMS 2016a Section 20.6).

Medicare requires a valid admission order for acute care inpatient admission. The term *inpatient* should be used in the admission order to clarify the intent for payment under Medicare Part A. When an observation admission is appropriate instead of an acute care inpatient admission, the order should clearly state **admission to observation**. The exact wording of the order should follow the medical staff rules and regulations at the individual facility.

According to CMS's **two-midnight rule**, the clinical documentation for an inpatient admission should reflect that the attending provider expects the patient to require at least two midnights in the hospital for medically necessary hospital care or the physician has determined that the admission is appropriate based on clinical judgment regardless of whether the two midnights are expected. This rule was put in place to decrease the number of unnecessary observation services and to incentivize efficient healthcare delivery. Under CMS's two-midnight rule, the physician is not required to specify precisely how long the patient will stay, but the clinical documentation reflecting medically necessary observation care for two midnights must be available in the clinical record to validate compliance with this rule. There are three exceptions to this rule (CMS 2017c Section 10; CMS 2017f Section 6.5):

- Procedures on the CMS list of "inpatient only" procedures
- CMS-identified procedures that qualify for a national exception to the two-midnight rule
- Case-by-case exceptions to the two-midnight rule because clinical documentation demonstrates the admitting physician or practitioner's judgment that the patient requires inpatient care

Figure 16.4 provides the CMS guidelines for the two-midnight rule workflow.

The CDS can assist to ensure a valid inpatient or observation patient order using these guidelines:

- Validate the admission order and determine whether the wording reflects admission to inpatient or admission to observation. Keep in mind that nonprovider practitioners may place the admission status order.
- When inpatient admission to acute care is planned, make sure that the documentation related to the two-midnight rule is clear and complete.
- Notify the UR staff if a decision is made before the patient is discharged to change the patient status back to outpatient.
- When the UR committee makes a determination related to the site of service, verify that the physician documentation is consistent with the committee determination and that the order reflects the level of care change.

    Example: The provider's progress note states, "Change order for patient status from inpatient to outpatient."

- Notify the stakeholder departments, such health information management and the business office, to ensure that the patient's account site of service is correct when changed from inpatient to outpatient or outpatient to inpatient.
- If the patient site of service is changed from inpatient to outpatient and the requirements for condition code 44 are not met, contact the UR committee to ensure that the case is reviewed and procedural guidelines for condition code 44 are met.
- Educate providers to document an outpatient or observation order when they are uncertain of the patient's progression to recovery. It is easier to change a patient status from outpatient to inpatient than inpatient to outpatient.

Figure 16.4. CMS's two-midnight rule for inpatient admission claims

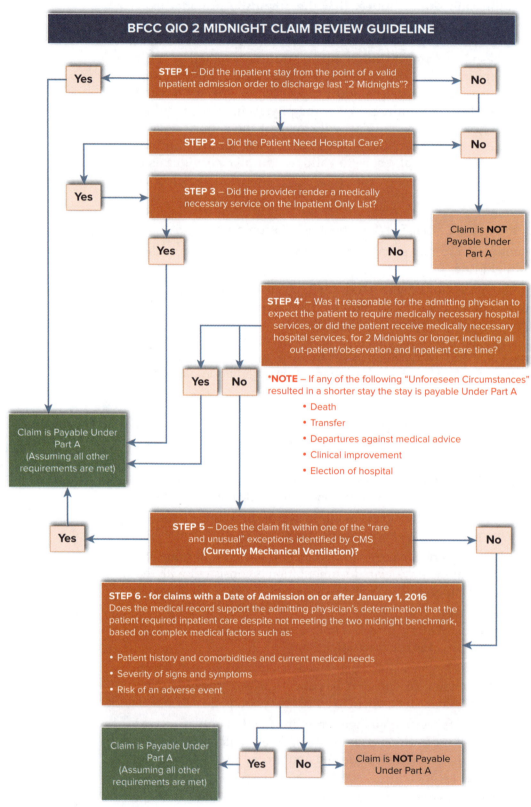

Source: CMS 2016b.

Other Observation Services Documentation

The coding of observation services accounts can be time-consuming and often difficult because of clinical documentation gaps. The outpatient CDI can help ensure that all required documentation is complete and specific prior to the coding and final bill process.

Areas of focus for observation case documentation include the following:

- *Injections and infusions:* For each injection and infusion, the start time, stop time, administration details, medication name, and dosage should be included in the clinical record.
- *Procedures:* Documentation for each procedure performed should be specific as to the site of service (bedside versus another clinical area), body site, depth, procedure description, provider, date, and time. Documentation of wound debridement and laceration repairs requires specificity for length and depth of debridement or repair. Lesion removal documentation requires number of lesions, size, and type of lesion. Also, when counting observation hours, time is extracted when the patient undergoes a procedure.
- *Diagnosis specificity:* The diagnosis documentation should include information adequate to meet the ICD-10-CM specificity requirements. The reason for admission or encounter should be clearly stated, and secondary diagnoses should be clearly documented. A differentiation should be made regarding history of conditions, chronic conditions, and current acute conditions.

Chapter 16 Review Exercises

1. Which of the following should be included in a brief presentation by the CDI steering committee chair or CDI manager at the start of the expansion project?
   a. A detailed review of the project budget
   b. A presentation of a clinical case example of the area of focus
   c. An analysis of E/M code accuracy in the health system's ED
   d. A discussion on complete and specific admission documentation

2. At the end of the CDI steering committee meeting to discuss expansion, the chair should reflect upon the importance of the CDI program expansion and share some of the success stories already realized through the initial CDI program. Which of the following would *least* likely be among the CDI program successes discussed?
   a. Increased revenue
   b. Improved quality scores
   c. More accurate severity scores
   d. Improved clinical documentation

3. Which of the following *best* describes a similarity between InterQual or Milliman admission criteria and the two-midnight rule?
   a. Both are used to determine medical necessity.
   b. Both are used to predict expected ED E/M codes.

c. Both are used for professional fee coding and billing.
d. Both are used to clarify the intent for payment under Medicare Part A.

4. HRRP aims to reduce excessive readmissions primarily by which of the following means?
   a. Legal penalties
   b. Financial incentives
   c. On-site provider education
   d. Nationwide standards for E/M code assignment in the ED

5. If the patient site of service is changed from inpatient to outpatient and the requirements for condition code 44 are not met, who should be contacted to ensure that the case is reviewed and procedural guidelines for condition code 44 are met?
   a. CDI taskforce
   b. Care manager
   c. Physician advisor
   d. Utilization review committee

6. A healthcare facility has observed a steady rise in medical necessity denials for admissions and problems related to inpatient DRG assignment. Leadership at the facility has decided to address these issues through an expansion of the facility's existing CDI program. In which of the following settings would CDI program expansion be most likely to correct the issues identified?
   a. ED
   b. Outpatient clinic
   c. Observation services
   d. Professional practice

7. Which of the following describes the primary benefit of the two-midnight rule?
   a. It simplifies the process for changing patient status.
   b. It decreases the number of unnecessary observation services.
   c. It eliminates the need for the UR staff to review admission criteria.
   d. It allows physicians to be more precise in documenting how long a patient will stay.

8. Which of the following is *least* likely to be a factor in choosing a new setting for CDI program expansion?
   a. Potential revenue impact
   b. Current service line offerings
   c. Known claims submission issues
   d. Analysis of competing facilities' CDI programs

9. In the context of the two-midnight rule, which of the following would be *most* likely to result in denial of an inpatient admissions claim under Medicare Part A?
   a. The patient did not need hospital care.
   b. The inpatient stay from admission to discharge did not last two midnights.
   c. The claim did not constitute a rare and unusual exception as defined by CMS.

d. It was not reasonable for the admitting physician to expect the patient to require medically necessary hospital services.

10. Discussions about the root causes of admission denials should include all but whom among the following?
    a. UR nurses
    b. Outpatient CDS
    c. ED representatives
    d. Denials management department representatives

References

American College of Emergency Physicians (ACEP). 2017. Observation care payments to hospitals FAQ. https://www.acep.org/Clinical---Practice-Management/Observation-Care-Payments-to-Hospitals-FAQ/#sm.00017kosewz9nejey622868gd36xs.

American College of Emergency Physicians (ACEP). 2011. ED facility level coding guidelines. https://www.acep.org/Content.aspx?id=30428#sm.001a29ciu1d3we1k11gbkg15jzi29.

American Medical Association (AMA). 2018. *CPT 2018 Professional*. Chicago: AMA.

CGS Administrators, LLC. 2017. Fact sheet: observation services CPT codes: 99218–99220, 99224–99226. https://www.cgsmedicare.com/partb/mr/pdf/observation_serv_factsheet.pdf.

Centers for Medicare and Medicaid Services (CMS). 2018. Hospital Outpatient Prospective Payment—notice of final rulemaking (NFRM) with comment period. https://www.cms.gov/Medicare/Medicare-Fee-for-Service-Payment/HospitalOutpatientPPS/Hospital-Outpatient-Regulations-and-Notices-Items/CMS-1678-FC.html.

Centers for Medicare and Medicaid Services (CMS). 2017a. Readmission Reduction Program (HRRP). https://www.cms.gov/medicare/medicare-fee-for-service-payment/acuteinpatientpps/readmissions-reduction-program.html.

Centers for Medicare and Medicaid Services (CMS). 2017b. Medicare Claims Processing Manual. Chapter 4: Part B hospital (including inpatient Hospital Part B and OPPS). Section 160: Clinic and emergency visits. https://www.cms.gov/Regulations-and-Guidance/Guidance/Manuals/Downloads/clm104c04.pdf.

Centers for Medicare and Medicaid Services (CMS). 2017c. Medicare Benefits Policy Manual. Chapter 1: Inpatient hospital services covered under Part A. Section 10: Covered inpatient hospital services covered under Part A. https://www.cms.gov/Regulations-and-Guidance/Guidance/Manuals/Downloads/bp102c01.pdf.

Centers for Medicare and Medicaid Services (CMS). 2017d. Medicare Claims Processing Manual. Chapter 30: Financial liability protections. Section 20: Limitation on liability (LOL) under §1879 where Medicare claims are disallowed. https://www.cms.gov/Regulations-and-Guidance/Guidance/Manuals/Downloads/clm104c30.pdf.

Centers for Medicare and Medicaid Services (CMS). 2017e. Medicare Claims Processing Manual. Chapter 4: Part B hospital (including inpatient Hospital Part B and OPPS). Section 290: Outpatient observation services. https://www.cms.gov/Regulations-and-Guidance/Guidance/Manuals/downloads/clm104c04.pdf.

Centers for Medicare and Medicaid Services (CMS). 2017f. Medicare Program Integrity Manual. Chapter 6. Medicare contractor medical review guidelines for specific services. Section 6.5: Medical review of inpatient hospital claims for Part A payment. https://www.cms.gov/Regulations-and-Guidance/Guidance/Manuals/Downloads/pim83c06.pdf.

Centers for Medicare and Medicaid Services (CMS). 2016a. Medicare Benefit Policy Manual. Chapter 6: Hospital services covered under Part B. Section 20.6 Outpatient observation services. https://www.cms.gov/Regulations-and-Guidance/Guidance/Manuals/Downloads/bp102c06.pdf.

Centers for Medicare and Medicaid Services (CMS). 2016b. BFCC QUI 2MN policy decision guideline. http://www.cms.gov/Research-Statistics-Data-and-Systems/Monitoring-Programs/Medicare-FFS-Compliance-Programs/Medical-Review/Downloads/-Policy-Decision-Guideline-Temporary-Suspension-of-Two-Midnight-Reviews.pptx.

Centers for Medicare and Medicaid Services (CMS). 2015. Part B National Summary Data File (Previously known as BESS). https://www.cms.gov/Research-Statistics-Data-and-Systems/Downloadable-Public-Use-Files/Part-B-National-Summary-Data-File/Overview.html.

Centers for Medicare and Medicaid Services (CMS). 2011. Critical care services. https://www.cms.gov/Regulations-and-Guidance/Guidance/Manuals/Downloads/clm104c04.pdf

Centers for Medicare and Medicaid Services (CMS). 2008a. OPPS visit codes: Frequently asked questions. https://www.cms.gov/medicare/medicare-fee-for-service-payment/hospitaloutpatientpps/downloads/opps_qanda.pdf.

Centers for Medicare and Medicaid Services (CMS). 2008b. Final changes to the Hospital Outpatient Prospective Payment System and CY 2008 payment rates. https://www.cms.gov/Medicare/Medicare-Fee-for-Service-Payment/HospitalOutpatientPPS/Hospital-Outpatient-Regulations-and-Notices-Items/CMS1204971.html.

Centers for Medicare and Medicaid Services. 2006. Medicare: Hospital Outpatient Prospective Payment System and CY 2007 payment rates; proposed rule. *Federal Register* 71(163):49505–49977.

Centers for Medicare and Medicaid Services (CMS). 2002. Medicare program; Changes to the Hospital Outpatient Prospective Payment System and calendar year 2003 payment rates; and changes to payment suspension for unfiled cost reports. *Federal Register* 67(154):52133–52240.

Centers for Medicare and Medicaid Services (CMS). 2000. Further information on the use of modifier -25 in reporting hospital outpatient services. Transmittal A-00-40. https://www.cms.gov/Regulations-and-Guidance/Guidance/Transmittals/downloads/A0040.pdf.

Combs, T. 2016. CDI is expanding as need for quality documentation grows. *Journal of AHIMA* blog. http://journal.ahima.org/2016/06/23/cdi-is-expanding-as-need-for-quality-documentation-grows.

Gilboy, N., T. Tanabe, D. Travers, and A.M. Rosenau. 2011. Emergency Severity Index (ESI): A triage tool for emergency department care, version 4. Implementation handbook 2012 edition. AHRQ publication No.12-0014. https://www.ahrq.gov/sites/default/files/wysiwyg/professionals/systems/hospital/esi/esihandbk.pdf.

Hapner, P. 2010. Observation services. 2010. AHIMA Convention Proceedings, September 2010. http://library.ahima.org/doc?oid=105977#.WmVeAqjtzIU.

Lojewski, T. 2008. Principles for emergency department coding guidelines. *Journal of AHIMA* 79(9):76–78.

QualityNet. 2017. Hospital Readmissions Reduction Program Overview. https://www.qualitynet.org/dcs/ContentServer?c=Page&pagename=QnetPublic%2FPage%2FQnetTier2&cid=1228772412458.

Wiler, J., R. Poirier, H. Farley, W. Zirkin, and R.T. Griffey. 2011. Emergency Severity Index Triage system correlation with emergency department evaluation and management billing codes and total professional charges. *Academic Emergency Medicine* 18(11):1161–1166. doi: 10.1111/j.1553-2712.2011.01203.x.

Glossary

837i Form for submitting claims in electronic format in an outpatient setting facility.

837p Industry standard form used for electronic billing to payers in the physician practice setting.

Admission for observation An order by a physician to place a patient in admission status to monitor a patient's condition over a period, during which the patient is considered an outpatient, to determine whether he or she meets the criteria for admission to a hospital as an inpatient or be discharged.

Advanced Alternative Payment Models (Advanced APMs) A subset of APMs that allow practices to take the risk (receive less payment) or receive bonus payments related to patient outcome.

Advancing Care Information (ACI) One of the four performance categories under the Merit-based Incentive Payment System (MIPS), which was created as part of the Medicare Access and CHIP Reauthorization Act (MACRA) and the Quality Payment Program (QPP). Previously referred to as *meaningful use*, ACI replaces the Medicare electronic health record (EHR) incentive program.

Agency for Healthcare Research and Quality (AHRQ) An organization that aims to find evidence to improve the safety, quality, accessibility, equitability, and affordability of healthcare and promote the use of such evidence.

AHIMA Registered HIM Apprenticeship Program A health information management (HIM) program, sponsored by the American Health Information Management Association (AHIMA) and certified by the US Department of Labor, that includes a paid position that students can use to transition into an HIM career; roles that are available in the program include hospital coder, CDI specialist, business analyst, and data analyst (AHIMA 2016a).

Alert A message in the EHR regarding a specific condition, ongoing treatment, or management that appears when a provider accesses a specific patient's account.

Alternative Payment Model (APM) A payment approach, developed in partnership with the clinician community, that provides added incentives to clinicians to provide high-quality and cost-efficient care (CMS 2017a).

Ambulatory payment classification (APC) The Outpatient Prospective Payment System applicable to hospitals.

Ambulatory payment classification (APC) weight A number assigned to each APC that, when multiplied by an annually designated conversion factor, identifies the payment by the Centers for Medicare and Medicaid Services (CMS) for the specified APC.

Audit and feedback   Educational intervention that summarizes clinical performance in patient care over a specified period based on medical records, computerized databases, patient surveys, or observation (Mostofian et al. 2015).

Big data   The concept of large volumes of complex and diverse data or data sets that are so large or complex that traditional data-processing applications are inadequate.

Bloom's taxonomy   Categorization of levels of learning from low (knowledge, comprehension, and application) to high (analysis, evaluation, and creation).

Case review   The process of reviewing a patient's clinical record and assessing the completeness and specificity of the clinical documentation.

CDI steering committee   A governance committee for the clinical documentation improvement (CDI) program. It is made up of the facility or health system executive-level leaders and selected department directors whose purpose is to provide visibility for the program and resources needed to implement and maintain the program functions.

CDI taskforce   Working committee representing the teams that are actively involved in the CDI program; its members are responsible for day-to-day management of the clinic or practice operations and corresponding support departments affected by CDI.

CDM number   A unique identifier code designated to identify the department of the hospital or healthcare facility within the charge description master (CDM), also known as the *chargemaster*. This number is important when determining volume for a specific Current Procedural Terminology (CPT) code on the chargemaster.

Certified clinical documentation specialist (CCDS)   A credential awarded by the Association of Clinical Documentation Improvement Specialists (ACDIS) that elevates an individual's professional standing as a specialist in clinical documentation.

Certified coding associate (CCA)   An AHIMA credential awarded to entry-level coding professionals who have demonstrated skill in classifying healthcare data by passing a certification exam.

Certified coding specialist (CCS)   An AHIMA credential awarded to individuals who have demonstrated skill in classifying healthcare data from patient records, generally in the hospital setting, by passing a certification exam.

Certified coding specialist–physician-based (CCS-P)   An AHIMA credential awarded to individuals who have demonstrated coding expertise in physician-based settings, such as group practices, by passing a certification examination.

Certified medical assistant (CMA)   A credential for an individual with training in medical assistance through a postsecondary program accredited by the US Department of Education or the Council for Higher Education who has passed the Certifying Board of the American Association of Medical Assistants exam (AAMA 2017).

Certified outpatient coder (COC)   A credential that certifies a coder's knowledge of specialized payments regarding ambulatory surgery centers or hospital outpatient billing, proficiency in accuracy of medical codes for diagnoses, procedures, and services performed in outpatient settings. It was formerly called *certified professional coder–hospital outpatient*, and the training program is sponsored by the American Academy of Professional Coders (AAPC).

Certified professional coder (CPC)   A credential sponsored by the AAPC that certifies that the coder has proven mastery of all code sets (CPT, ICD-10-CM, and HCPCS Level II), evaluation and management principles, surgical coding, and adherence to documentation and coding guidelines.

Chargemaster A comprehensive listing of the prices of items that are billed by a facility to a patient or on the UB-04 claim to the patient's health insurance company. Also known as *charge description master* (CDM).

Chief compliance officer A designated individual who monitors the compliance process at a healthcare facility.

Chief financial officer (CFO) The highest-ranking executive of finance for the health system or facility.

Chief information officer (CIO) The highest-ranking executive of information technology services within the health system or facility.

Chief medical officer (CMO) The highest-ranking executive of the medical staff.

Children's Health Insurance Program (CHIP) An insurance program funded through the states as well as the federal government that provides low-cost health coverage to eligible uninsured children (up to age 19 years) and pregnant women; eligibility is determined by the states and is based on financial need.

Claim Adjustment Reason Code (CAs or CARCs) Codes used to provide additional explanation for an adjustment, implying that the payer must communicate why a claim or service line was paid differently than it was billed.

Claims edits Flags or error messages identified by a claims scrubber.

Claims scrubber Medical billing software that edits and validates claims for clean claims submission.

Clarity A criterion for high-quality clinical records; it means the record is understandable and distinct, without any illegible or unclear clinical documentation.

Clinical documentation Any manual or electronic notation (or recording) made by a physician or other healthcare clinician related to a patient's medical condition or treatment.

Clinical documentation improvement practitioner (CDIP) A credential awarded by AHIMA to individuals who have achieved specialized skills in CDI.

Clinical nurse specialist (CNS) A healthcare professional with a bachelor's degree in nursing, as well as a master's or doctorate degree from a CNS program.

CMS 1450 Another term for Uniform Bill-04 (UB-04), a hard-copy claim form suitable for use in billing multiple third-party payers in both inpatient and outpatient settings.

CMS 1500 The standard paper claim form used to bill Medicare fee-for-service claims, and the counterpart of the 837p used for electronic billing. The form includes demographic and patient payer-specific information as well as the ICD-10-CM and CPT/HCPCS codes corresponding to the patient's diagnosis and treatment.

Completeness A criterion for high-quality clinical records; it means the record has the required content to provide a complete clinical picture of the patient encounter.

Compliant query A query that meets the AHIMA industry-standard guidelines outlined the AHIMA Query Toolkit.

Comprehensive APC (C-APC) An APC (ambulatory payment classification) that has a primary service with a high cost, whereby that cost is a large portion of the cost of the patient encounter; it is similar to a diagnosis-related group (DRG) in that there is an all-inclusive rate for a group of related services.

Computer-assisted coding (CAC) The process of extracting and translating dictated and subsequently transcribed free-text data (or dictated and then computer-generated discrete data) into diagnostic and procedural codes of varying classifications for billing and coding purposes.

Computerized decision support system data Metrics, trends, and other data used by computerized decision support systems to improve clinical decision making.

Conditions for Coverage (CfCs) The minimum health and safety standards issued by CMS with which providers and suppliers of health services must comply to qualify for Medicare certification and reimbursement.

Conditions of Participation (CoPs) The CMS requirements that hospitals and critical access hospitals must meet to participate in Medicare and Medicaid programs.

Consistency A criterion for high-quality clinical documentation; it means that the documentation does not include contradictory statements from providers.

Continuing medical education (CME) Educational activities for physicians, typically in the areas of medical science and public health, conducted for the purpose of increasing professional practice knowledge and skills (ACCME 2017).

Critical thinking Thinking that involves validating information, identifying exceptions, analyzing trends, considering what is not there, thinking "outside the box," and being creative, while being open to new information and alternative explanations as well as unbiased consideration of what one presumes to be true about a given situation or problem before drawing a conclusion (Hess 2015).

Current Procedural Terminology (CPT) A comprehensive, descriptive list of terms and associated numeric and alphanumeric codes used for reporting diagnostic and therapeutic procedures and other medical services performed by physicians in the outpatient setting; published and updated annually by the American Medical Association (AMA 2018).

Deidentification Removal of information or data from a patient's record that can be used to identify a patient in order to protect the privacy of the patient's identity.

Denials trend analysis The process of analyzing denials frequency data by category and determining trends for high-volume denials.

Designated record set A set of clinical record information that includes medical diagnostic and treatment information, as well as billing information related to enrollment, payment, and claims adjudication for the insurance payer.

Diagnosis-related groups (DRGs) A statistical system that CMS uses to classify inpatient care services for reimbursement; under the Prospective Payment System, hospitals are paid a set fee for treating patients in a single DRG category, regardless of the actual cost of care for the individual.

Electronic health record (EHR) A record of an individual's health-related information stored electronically that can be shared across different healthcare settings.

Encounter summary A summary of a patient's clinical information related to the diagnosis, treatment, prognosis, and instructions for follow-up care.

Evidence-based clinical practice guidelines Explicit statements that have been systematically developed from scientific evidence and clinical expertise to answer clinical questions and guide clinical decision making.

Evidence-based medicine (EBM) The practice of medicine informed by the best scientific data available; it pursues optimal outcomes by relying on three key types of knowledge: research-based evidence, clinical expertise, and the patient's values and preferences.

Executive sponsor   The leader of a multidisciplinary healthcare team who is responsible for the guidance and success of a project.

Fee-for-service payment methodology   A payment model in which providers are reimbursed based on the volume of services they perform for patients.

Foundational interoperability   Provision of data exchange from one information technology (IT) system to be received by another; this type of interoperability does not require the ability for the receiving IT system to interpret the data (HIMSS 2013).

Geographic practice cost index (GPCI)   An index developed by the CMS to adjust relative value units (RVUs), which are national averages, to reflect local costs when calculating accurate Medicare payment for a service done in the physician practice setting that is assigned a CPT code. It was developed by CMS to measure the differences in resource costs among fee-schedule areas, compared with the national average in the three components of the RVU.

Glasgow Coma Scale   A scale that uses a point system to assess a patient's responses from three categories: eye opening response, verbal response, and motor response; it may be part of a neurological assessment to provide an objective review of a patient's level of consciousness.

Goals   Statements that explain what a program will accomplish; it is a destination rather than a measurement of the program's achievements.

Governance structure   Overall framework for the leadership and oversight of a program, such as an outpatient CDI program.

HCC suspecting   The process of using a natural language processing (NLP) engine to scan clinical documentation for potential chronic illnesses that are categorized in Hierarchical Condition Categories (HCCs).

Health Information Technology for Economic and Clinical Health (HITECH) Act   A law created to promote the adoption and meaningful use of health IT in the United States; it authorizes the Office of the National Coordinator for Health Information Technology (ONC) to coordinate nationwide efforts to implement and use the most advanced health IT and the electronic exchange of health information.

Health Insurance Portability and Accountability Act (HIPAA)   The law that enforces and mandates the adoption of the federal privacy protections for individual patient information, including national standards for electronic healthcare transactions and security (HHS 2017).

Health IT Standards Committee (HITSC)   A committee that makes changes recommended to the National Coordinator for Health to comply with the standards, implementation, and criteria certification related to electronic healthcare data exchange.

Health Level Seven International (HL7)   A set of standards for the exchange, integration sharing, and retrieval of electronic health information.

Healthcare Common Procedure Coding System (HCPCS)   A billing system published and used by the CMS that reports outpatient and physician services.

Healthgrades   An organization that provides online information on hospitals, physicians, and healthcare providers to help consumers search for and select providers based on the providers' experience and their ratings for patient satisfaction and quality of care.

Hierarchical Condition Category (HCC) A payment model used for Medicare Advantage plans that identifies patients with serious or chronic illnesses and assigns a risk factor score to each patient based upon a combination of the individual's health conditions and demographic details.

Hierarchical Condition Category codes (HCCs) Codes used by Medicare Advantage plans to predict healthcare costs based on chronic illness and demographics (CMS 2016a).

High-level technology assessment Conducted by the project manager in conjunction with the IT department, this assessment includes a review of current software tools to support denials management; software to perform HCC suspecting (HCC capture); and tools to support outpatient coding and coding compliance (such as encoders).

Hospital Outpatient Quality Reporting (OQR) Program A program established by the Tax Relief Act of 2006 that requires hospitals to submit data related to the quality of services provided in the outpatient setting.

Hospital Readmissions Reduction Program (HRRP) Rule established by the Affordable Care Act that requires the CMS to reduce payments to Inpatient Prospective Payment System (IPPS) hospitals with excessive readmissions.

Hybrid health record (HHR) Documentation of an individual's health information that is a combination of both handwritten (paper) and electronic formats.

Interdisciplinary team Team of subject matter experts and leaders who represent the many specialties, locations, and types of healthcare delivery settings involved in clinical documentation.

International Classification of Diseases, Tenth Revision, Clinical Modification **(ICD-10-CM)** A system used by physicians, other healthcare providers, payers, and others to code and classify diagnoses, signs, and symptoms in an inpatient or outpatient setting.

International Classification of Diseases, Tenth Revision, Procedure Coding System **(ICD-10-PCS)** A system used to classify or code procedures and treatments provided to a patient in an inpatient setting; used to track various health interventions by healthcare professionals.

Interoperability The ability of systems to exchange information and interpret data from other systems.

InterQual or Milliman admission criteria Clinical guidelines used to determine medical necessity for various healthcare services, such as inpatient admission, observation services, the intensive care unit, step-down units, and discharge.

The Joint Commission A not-for-profit organization that uses sets of standards to evaluate the quality of service delivery from healthcare entities such as hospitals, home care agencies, nursing care centers, behavioral healthcare centers, ambulatory care centers, and laboratory service providers.

Key performance indicator (KPI) A quantifiable measure used over time to determine whether some structure, process, or outcome in the provision of care to a patient supports high-quality performance measured against best-practice criteria.

Leapfrog Group A nonprofit organization that aims to promote healthcare quality and safety by collecting and reporting data about hospital performance.

Legal health record An official clinical record of healthcare services delivered by a provider.

Legibility A criterion for high-quality clinical documentation; it evaluates whether entries in the clinical record are readable.

Medically unlikely edit (MUE) The maximum units of service that a provider would report under most circumstances for a single Medicare Part B beneficiary on a single date of service; the CMS developed the MUE to reduce the paid-claims error rate for Medicare Part B claims.

Medicare Administrative Contractors (MACs) A private healthcare insurance company that has jurisdiction for Medicare Part A and Part B claims as well as for durable medical equipment (DME) and Fee-for-Service (FFS) claims for Medicare beneficiaries in a specific geographic region.

Medicare Advantage A program that provides Medicare recipients with more choices among health plans. This plan is also called Part C Medicare and is provided by private insurance companies to cover Medicare benefits (CMS 2017b).

Medicare Provider and Analysis Review (MedPAR) A database that contains information for 100 percent of Medicare beneficiaries using hospital inpatient services (CMS 2017c).

Medication Administration Record (MAR) A medical record that documents all medications taken during a patient's encounter.

Mission statement A written statement that sets forth the core purpose and philosophies of an organization or group; it defines the organization or group's general purpose for existing (AHIMA 2017).

Monitor, evaluate, address/assess, or treat (MEAT) An industry-accepted standard for clinical documentation to support HCC assignment.

National Uniform Billing Committee (NUBC) A national group responsible for identifying data elements and designing the UB-92; it publishes the Official UB-04 Data Specifications Manual and is the official source for UB-04 billing information.

National Uniform Claim Committee (NUCC) A national group that has developed a standard data set to be used in the transmission of noninstitutional provider claims to and from third-party payers. NUCC is responsible for approval of changes made to the 837p and CMS 1500 forms.

Needs assessment A type of evaluation, similar to cost–benefit analysis, in which the evaluator reviews the benefits of a project against the cost of the project, and assesses the political, operational, and resource issues related to the proposed project.

Nonphysician Provider (NPP) A midlevel provider who works under the supervision of an attending physician in both the inpatient and ambulatory settings.

Objectives Specific, measurable, achievable steps to meet a goal within a given time frame.

Observation services A set of specific, clinically appropriate services, which include ongoing short-term treatment, assessment, and reassessment (CMS 2016); hospital outpatient services offered to help a physician decide whether the patient needs to be admitted or discharged.

Office of Inspector General (OIG) An independent office in the US Department of Health and Human Services "tasked with detecting and preventing fraud, waste, and abuse; identifying opportunities to improve program economy, efficiency and effectiveness; and holding accountable those who do not meet program requirements or who violate federal healthcare laws" (OIG 2017).

Office of the National Coordinator for Health Information Technology (ONC) The principal federal entity charged with coordination of nationwide efforts to implement and use the most advanced health IT and the electronic exchange of health information.

OIG Work Plan Office of Inspector General plan, updated monthly, that outlines the focus for OIG reviews and investigations (including cases of fraud and abuse) in various healthcare settings.

Ongoing program monitoring The process of analyzing CDI program effectiveness by a program leader or sponsor, through the use of metrics related to HCC capture, coding gaps, and denials management; it includes discussions with key stakeholders about team progress and focus areas for future CDI.

Outpatient Prospective Payment System (OPPS) A payment system for hospital outpatient services billed to Medicare.

Outsourcing Assignment of core services or operations of the organization to a provider that focuses in that area of service or operation (Roberts et al. 2013).

Overdocumentation The practice of inserting false or irrelevant documentation to create the appearance of support for billing higher-level services.

Passive dissemination The act of distributing information, such as learning materials and data, without engaging in interactive discussion related to the distributed content.

Physician collaboration The process used to communicate with physicians in a healthcare facility. This process could be through e-mail, one-on-one meetings, group education, or delivery of educational materials such as newsletters and intranet blogs.

Physician orders Documentation of specific instructions for patient interventions such as medications, diagnostics tests, therapies, or other treatments.

Physician shadowing A process in which the CDS reviews a provider's clinical documentation before and after a patient's visit, thus offering a learning experience for the provider through the query process.

Population health The capture and reporting of healthcare data that are used for public health purposes. Population health initiatives allow healthcare providers to report infectious diseases, immunizations, cancer, and other reportable conditions to public health officials.

Practice plan administrator A subject matter expert in the operations of an owned medical practice, who works collaboratively with the physician specialty leaders and has a working relationship with most of the physicians in the network.

Preceptorship Program in which an experienced CDS (the preceptor) mentors and trains an inexperienced CDS in the guiding principles of CDI and the case review process. The trainee may be an employee of a contracting company until the completion of training, or the trainee may be an employee of the healthcare entity.

Precision A criterion for high-quality clinical records; it means that the record is accurate and well defined so that the details support the clinical picture from a diagnostic, as well as a treatment, perspective.

Progress notes Notes of clinical observations documented by physicians and other clinicians that are related to the patient diagnosis and subsequent treatments.

Project kickoff meeting A presentation by project leaders and a discussion by the key stakeholders of an outpatient CDI program; participants may include the executive leaders, medical staff leaders, HIM director, CDI project manager, and CDI program manager.

Project management   The process of defining project tasks, goals, and objectives; developing and tracking the project timeline; managing project resources; and planning and conducting activities that result in a successful project.

Project manager (PM)   Individual assigned to lead the project activities and keep the project on time and delivered as established in the project plan; he or she may be an existing employee of the health system or facility or may be a consultant hired to fill this role.

Project workplan (workplan)   A plan, formally reviewed and accepted by the stakeholders on the CDI steering committee and CDI taskforce, that provides a basis for all the tasks associated with the project and documents changes in tasks as they occur during the life of the project.

Prompt   EHR tool that automatically produces messages containing questions or additional information related to specific steps in the clinical documentation process, intended to help the provider ensure all relevant information is recorded.

Prospective Payment System (PPS)   A reimbursement methodology for Medicare payment that is based on a predetermined and fixed amount for services to treat a patient depending on the classification of that patient's diagnosis (such as the DRG or APC).

Protected health information (PHI)   "Information, including demographics, which relates to the individual's past, present, or future physical or mental health or condition, the provision of healthcare to the individual, or the past, present, or future payment for the provision of healthcare to the individual, that identifies the individual or for which there is a reasonable basis to believe can be used to identify the individual" (OCR 2015).

Query metrics   Parameters established by an outpatient CDI program, such as case review volume, response rate, agreement rate, and training sessions, for evaluating the efficiency and effectiveness of clinical documentation queries.

Query templates   Templates that can be used for query development, as long as they follow the policies and procedures of the healthcare entity and adhere to the AHIMA compliant query guidelines (AHIMA 2016b).

Rapid redesign   The process of evaluating and revising the workflow of a CDI program over a short period (one- to two-day discussion group); steps include visiting the pilot clinic(s) and evaluating the clinical documentation workflow.

Real-time computerized reminders   EHR prompts that become available to the user while using the EHR for clinical documentation.

Relative value units (RVUs)   Numbers assigned to a procedure that describe its difficulty and expense in relationship to other procedures by assigning weights to such factors as personnel, time, and level of skill; used for calculating reimbursement under physician fee schedules.

Reliability   A criterion for high-quality clinical documentation; it refers to clinical record content that is trustworthy, safe, and yielding the same result when repeated.

Research Data Assistance Center (ResDAC)   A CMS contractor that provides data to healthcare organizations and researchers (ResDAC 2017).

Research identifiable files (outpatient RIFs)   Files containing data elements such as diagnosis codes, HCPCS codes, dates of service, reimbursement amounts, outpatient provider numbers, revenue center codes, and beneficiary demographic information that are available for purchase from the ResDAC; patient-identifying information has been removed from these files.

Risk Adjustment Data Validation (RADV) An audit performed by CMS to verify that the clinical documentation is present to support each HCC submitted for payment on a claim.

Risk Adjustment Factor (RAF) score The sum of the HCC weights (tied to ICD-10-CM diagnosis codes) for a specific patient over a 12-month period; used to calculate reimbursement for patients enrolled in Medicare Advantage plans.

Risk-based payment methodologies Payment plans in which providers are reimbursed based on treatment outcomes, thereby increasing their financial incentive to use the most effective and cost-efficient services while decreasing their incentive to provide services that are less likely to improve outcomes.

Semantic interoperability The ability of two or more systems or elements to exchange information and use the information that has been exchanged (HIMSS 2013).

Semantic reasoning The use of software to make assertions or inferences based on a set of data within a data set, such as an EHR (Maarala et al. 2016).

Shared Nationwide Interoperability Roadmap Plan created by ONC that outlines the strategy and direction to be taken to improve an exchange of health information among systems across the nation.

Specific, measurable, attainable, relevant, time-bound (SMART) A mnemonic used to make objectives more powerful and measurable by defining them in terms that are specific, measurable, attainable, relevant, and time-bound.

Structural interoperability An intermediate level of interoperability that defines the structure or format of data exchange (that is, the message format standards) where there is a uniform movement of healthcare data from one system to another such that the clinical or operational purpose and meaning of the data are preserved and unaltered (HIMSS 2013).

Structured query language (SQL) A fourth-generation computer language that includes both DDL (data definition language) and DML (data manipulation language) components and is used to create and manipulate relational databases.

Tasks Messages in an EHR or other system to remind the provider about a required action related to a patient's condition.

Timeliness A criterion for high-quality clinical documentation; it refers to a clinical record that is available at the time it is needed for patient care delivery.

Treating providers Individuals licensed to practice medicine in a specific state and authorized by the medical staff bylaws. Types of treating providers include doctors of medicine, doctors of osteopathy, nurse practitioners, and physician assistants.

Two-midnight rule The CMS rule that specifies that the clinical documentation for an inpatient admission should reflect that the attending provider expects the patient to require at least two midnights in the hospital for medically necessary hospital care or the physician has determined that the admission is appropriate based on clinical judgment regardless of whether the two midnights are expected.

UB-04 Uniform Bill format A uniform institutional provider hard-copy claim form suitable for use in billing multiple third-party payers in both inpatient and outpatient settings.

Virtual private network (VPN) A technology that allows users to securely access a facility's or practice's clinical records through a facility intranet that must include security levels to satisfy HIPAA requirements. This technology allows providers to use laptops and other personal "smart" devices for clinical documentation.

Vision statement An organization's statement that clearly and concisely describes the purpose of a group, team, or program and why that purpose is important; this statement is directional and future-focused, reflecting the values of the stakeholders.

Vital signs flowsheet A chart that documents a patient's height, weight, temperature, pulse, respiration, oxygen level, blood pressure, and position, over time.

World Health Organization (WHO) The United Nations specialized agency created to ensure the attainment by all peoples of the highest possible levels of health; WHO is responsible for multiple international classifications, including the 10th revision of the *International Statistical Classification of Diseases and Related Health Problems* (ICD-10) and *International Classification of Functioning, Disability, and Health* (ICF).

References

Accreditation Council for Continuing Medical Education (ACCME). 2017. CME content: definition and examples. http://www.accme.org/requirements/accreditation-requirements-cme-providers/policies-and-definitions/cme-content-definition-and-examples.

American Association of Medical Assistants (AAMA). 2017. What is a CMA (AAMA)? http://www.aama-ntl.org/medical-assisting/what-is-a-cma#.WkFgyt_tzIU.

American Health Information Management Association (AHIMA). 2017. Clinical Documentation Improvement: Overview. http://www.ahima.org/topics/cdi.

American Health Information Management Association (AHIMA). 2016a (Oct. 7). $7 million award to create new career opportunities through apprenticeships (press release). Chicago, IL: AHIMA.

American Health Information Management Association (AHIMA). 2016b. Practice brief: Guidelines for achieving a compliant query practice (2016 update). http://library.ahima.org/doc?oid=301357#.Wut8nYgvzcs.

American Medical Association (AMA). 2018. *Current Procedural Terminology, Professional Edition 2018.* Chicago: AMA.

Centers for Medicare and Medicaid Services (CMS). 2017a. Quality Payment Program. https://qpp.cms.gov.

Centers for Medicare and Medicaid Services (CMS) Glossary. 2017b. https://www.cms.gov/apps/glossary/default.asp?Letter=ALL&Language=English.

Centers for Medicare and Medicaid Cervices (CMS). 2017c. MEDPAR. https://www.cms.gov/Research-Statistics-Data-and-Systems/Statistics-Trends-and-Reports/MedicareFeeforSvcPartsAB/MEDPAR.html.

Centers for Medicare and Medicaid Services (CMS). 2016a. March 31, 2016, HHS-operated risk adjustment methodology meeting discussion paper. https://www.cms.gov/CCIIO/Resources/Forms-Reports-and-Other-Resources/Downloads/RA-March-31-White-Paper-032416.pdf.

Centers for Medicare and Medicaid Services (CMS). 2016b. Medicare Benefit Policy Manual. Chapter 6: Hospital services covered under Part B: Section 20.6 outpatient observation services. https://www.cms.gov/Regulations-and-Guidance/Guidance/Manuals/Internet-Only-Manuals-IOMs-Items/CMS012673.html.

Healthcare Information and Management Systems Society (HIMSS). 2013. What is interoperability? http://www.himss.org/library/interoperability-standards/what-is-interoperability.

Hess, P.C. 2015. *Clinical Documentation Improvement: Principles and Practice.* Chicago: AHIMA Press.

Maarala, A., X. Su, and J. Riekki. 2016. Semantic reasoning for context-aware internet of things applications. *Internet of Things Journal.* https://arxiv.org/ftp/arxiv/papers/1604/1604.08340.pdf.

Mostofian, F., C. Ruban, N. Simunovic, and M. Bhandari. 2015. Changing physician behavior: What works. *American Journal of Managed Care* 21(1):75–84.

Office of Civil Rights (OCR), US Department of Health and Human Services. 2015. Guidance regarding methods for de-identification of protected health information in accordance with the Health Insurance Portability and Accountability Act (HIPAA) Privacy Rule. https://www.hhs.gov/hipaa/for-professionals/privacy/special-topics/de-identification/index.html#protected https://www.hipaa.com/hipaa-protected-health-information-what-does-phi-include.

Office of Inspector General (OIG), US Department of Health and Human Services. 2017. HHS OIG Work Plan 2017. https://oig.hhs.gov/reports-and-publications/archives/workplan/2017/HHS%20OIG%20Work%20Plan%202017_508.pdf.

Research Data Assistance Center (ResDAC). 2017. https://www.resdac.org.

Roberts, J.G., J.G. Henderson, L.A. Olive, and D. Obaka. 2013. A review of outsourcing of services in healthcare organizations. *Journal of Outsourcing and Organizational Information Management* 2013(2013):985197. doi: 10.5171/2013.985197.

US Department of Health and Human Services (HHS). 2017. HIPAA for Professionals. https://www.hhs.gov/hipaa/for-professionals/index.html.

World Health Organization (WHO). 2017. http://www.who.int/en/.

Index

Abuse prevention and detection, with outpatient clinical documentation, 10
Accessibility, 90
Accreditation standards, 24
Active learning, 277
    in CME, 290–292
Addendum B, of OPPS, 72–73
Administration information, 24
Admission denials, 350
Admission documentation, for emergency department, 350–351
Admission to observation, 360
Advanced Alternative Payment Models, 105–107
Advancing Care Information (ACI), 10, 103, 107–108
Advisors, physician, 249–251
Agency for Healthcare Research and Quality (AHRQ), 96, 99
Alerts, for electronic health record, 162
Allscripts, 51
Alphabetic Index, of ICD-10-CM, 56
Alternative Payment Model (APM), 105–107
Ambulatory clinic administrator, as CDI team member, 216
Ambulatory facility setting. *See also* emergency department
    CDI compliance in, 82
    coding in, 71–74
    evaluation and management coding in, 63–65
    hospital chargemaster, 74
    OIG guidance for hospitals, 83–84
Ambulatory payment categories
    methodologies for, 73
    Outpatient Prospective Payment System and, 72–73
Ambulatory Payment Classifications (APCs)
    CDI and accurate assignment of, 119
    CDI assessment program and errors in, 125, 127
    CDS training in, 268
    CMS regulations and, 72
    composite, 360
    in outpatient settings, 41–42
    SI codes and, 60–62
Ambulatory Payment Classifications (APCs) weights, 72
Ambulatory Revenue Manager, 179–181
Ambulatory surgery, outpatient record categories at, 36
American College of Emergency Physicians (ACEP)
    Emergency Severity Index compared with E/M code frequency data by, 356–358
    evaluation and management coding and, 75–76
American Health Information Management Association (AHIMA)
    ambulatory record documentation guidance from, 9–10
    Clinical Documentation Toolkit of, 267, 271
    compliant query, 336–337
    criteria for query submission by, 334–335
    interoperability and, 52–53
    online courses offered by, 267–268
    on purpose of CDI programs, 266–267
    query guidelines established by, 269–270
    Query Toolkit, 334, 336–337
    Standards of Ethical Coding, 92–93
American Health Information Management Association (AHIMA) Registered Health Information Management (HIM) Apprenticeship Program, 254–255
American Medical Association (AMA), Current Procedural Terminology and, 57
American Recovery and Reinvestment Act of 2009, problem lists and, 34
Analysis, as higher-order thinking, 277–278, 280, 282
Anesthesia record, 29–30, 36
Appeals, CDS expertise in, 262
Applicable Policies and Procedures, 90
Application, as lower-order thinking, 277–279
Apprenticeships, HIM, 254–255
Attendance, in CDI educational sessions, 296–297
Attending physicians, clinical documentation by, 37
Audit and feedback, physician CDI education using, 291–292
Audits
    of clinical documentation, 196
    HCC, 320
    OIG risk-adjustment data validation, 319–320
Automated claims reviews, for CDI assessment program, 124

Barriers to success, critical thinking for surmounting, 282–285
Big data, 166
Bilateral procedures, 142
Bloom's taxonomy, 277–282
Boot camps, CDI, 251
Brief encounters, medical necessity of, 43–44
Bundled payment revenue risks, 128–129
Bundling, 59

Cardiology query example, 341
Case review, 228
    as CDI workplan task, 231, 233
    CDS training in, 268–269
    medical coder education on, 321
Cash flow, CDI program staffing and, 249

Cash-flow issues, reimbursement and revenue generation and, 122–123
Centers for Disease Control and Prevention (CDC), 96, 99
Centers for Medicare and Medicaid Services (CMS)
  agencies of, 94, 96
  claims processing manuals of, 9
  clinical data for, 6
  clinical documentation impacts of, 97
  CMS 1500 form and, 51, 141
  compliance guidance from, 87
  electronic health records, 4
  E/M volume distribution monitoring by, 358
  Evaluation and Management Codes by Specialty file by, 147
  on evaluation and management coding, 63
  Healthcare Common Procedure Coding System and, 57
  Hospital Outpatient Quality Reporting Program, 99–101
  medical coder education on, 327–328
  medically unlikely edits program of, 142–143
  physician orders and, 33
  programs of, 96–97
  public health data from, 98–99
  quality measure scores by, 144
  regulatory requirements of, 7–8, 82
  relative value units revisions by, 65–66
  status indicator codes of, 60–62
  UB-04 form and, 51, 141
Cerner, 51
Certification standards, 24
Certified clinical documentation specialist (CCDS), as recommended CDS credential, 261–262
Certified coding associate (CCA), 43
  as recommended CDS credential, 261
Certified coding specialist (CCS), 43
  as recommended CDS credential, 261
Certified coding specialist–physician-based (CCS-P), 43
  as recommended CDS credential, 261
Certified Electronic Health Record Technology (CEHRT), 102–103
Certified medical assistants (CMAs), 294
Certified outpatient coder (COC), as recommended CDS credential, 261
Certified professional coder (CPC), as recommended CDS credential, 261
Certified risk adjustment coder (CRC), as recommended CDS credential, 262
Charge capture
  CDI assessment program and gaps in, 127, 129–131
  for emergency department, 352–353
  Revenue Integrity and, 181–182
Charge description, 138–139
Charge description master (CDM), 74
  for CDI assessment program, 123
  charge code for, 140–141
  charge description for, 138–140
  charge status for, 141
  for clinical documentation analysis, 138–141
  CPT or HCPCS codes for, 140
  department code for, 140
  medical coder education on, 326
  pilot program review of, 149
  revenue code for, 140
Charge description number (CDM), 140–141
Chargemaster, hospital. *See* charge description master
Charge status, 141

Chief compliance officer, 82–83
  DOJ memorandum and, 89–90
  in third-party medical billing companies, 85
Chief executive officer (CEO)
  in CDI program creation, 192–193
  as CDI team member, 212–214
Chief financial officer (CFO)
  accounts receivable days and, 124
  in CDI program creation, 192–193
  in CDI taskforce, 122
  as CDI team member, 212–214
Chief information officer (CIO), as CDI team member, 216
Chief medical officer (CMO), as CDI team member, 212–216
Children's Health Insurance Program (CHIP), 96
Chronic illness, CDS identification of, 71
Chronic obstructive pulmonary disease (COPD), EHR drop-down menu for, 162
Claim adjustment reason code (CA/CARC), 177
Claims, CDS expertise in, 262
Claims data
  for CDI assessment program, 123
  need for, 6
Claims denial. *See also* denials trend analysis
  admission documentation and, 350
  CDI and fewer, 119
  NCD and LCD based, 126–128
  reports of, 143
  tracking of, 176–178
Claims edit
  issues and CDI assessment program, 127–129
  medically unlikely edits, 142–143
  medical necessity edits, 142
  production of, 141
  trends for CDI assessment program, 124
  types of, 141–142
  workflow process for, 143
Claims editors, medical coder education on, 326
Claims in accounts receivable, CDI and fewer days in, 119–120
Claims scrubber, 124, 141–143
Clarity
  in clinical documentation, 17
  consultation reports and, 30
  operative and procedure reports and, 32
  of patient history and physical examination, 31
  of progress notes, 34
  query for, 334
Client responsible party, on CDI workplan, 226–227
Clinic administrative manager, as CDI team member, 217
Clinical coding specialist
  ICD-10-CM guidelines for, 56–57
  job description for, 54
Clinical data
  medical coder education on, 320
  need for, 6
  usage of, 5
Clinical documentation. *See also* clinical records; outpatient clinical documentation
  authors of, 37–40
  CDS training in, 268–269
  CMS impact on, 97
  coding and, 54–55
  definition of, 5
  electronic health records and potential risks with, 163–165
  evaluation and management coding and, 65
  implementing and overseeing activities to obtain, 196

interoperability of, 52–53
monitoring and auditing of, 196
query process and, 339–340
record type categorization in, 26–28
for relative value units, 66–67
risk adjustment data validation audit of, 70
sources of, 22–24
technology landscape for, 160–161
timing of review of, 120
types of, 24–26
uses of, 6–7
workflow redesign for, 148, 152–153
Clinical documentation analysis
charge code for, 140–141
charge description master for, 138–141
charge status for, 141
claims edits for, 141–143
coding audit reports for, 143
CPT or HCPCS code for, 138–140
data selection for, 138
denials trends and reports, 143
department code for, 140
focused clinical record review process, 151–153
HCC reports and audits for, 143–144
other HCPCS code utilization files, 145–147
outpatient research identifiable files for, 144–145
quality measure scores, 144
report on program data for, 153–154
revenue code for, 140
Clinical documentation assessment, as CDI workplan task, 234, 236
Clinical documentation improvement (CDI)
ambulatory compliance for, 82
benefits of, 119–120, 202
challenges of, 12–14
data report on, 153–154
documentation review timing and, 120
EHR interoperability and, 121
electronic health records and, 13, 161–163
evaluation and management coding and, 75
evidence-based medicine and, 11
feasibility of, 118–121
interoperability and, 52
Meaningful Use requirements for, 34
NLP applications for, 167
physician buy-in and, 121
physician executives and, 38
policies and procedures for, 90–91
potential barriers to, 120–121
query metrics for, 337–339
query process in, 334
rationale for improvements to, 4–7
recruiting professionals trained in, 249
risk adjustment data validation for, 70
ROI and, 118
staffing issues and, 120
technology and, 160
Clinical documentation improvement (CDI) assessment program
analysis of case review, 127–129
audit results for, 123
charge capture gaps, 127, 129–131
charge description master and physician practice fee schedules for, 123
claims data with codes for, 123
claims edit issues, 127–129
claims edit trends and reports, 124
CPT, HCPCS, and APC errors in, 125, 127, 130–131
data and area of focus for, 122–124
denials and, 124, 130–131
executive and key stakeholder buy-in for, 134
focused case review for, 124–127
HCC codes and, 125–127, 129
high-level work plan for, 131–134
medical necessity denials for, 126–128
ROI for, 129–131
steps in, 121
task force establishment for, 122
Clinical documentation improvement (CDI) compliance
analysis and remediation of underlying misconduct, 88–89
autonomy and resources, 89–90
CMS guidance on, 87
confidential reporting and investigation, 91–92
continuous improvement, periodic testing, and review, 92
DOJ compliance memorandum on, 87–92
Office of Inspector General guidance on, 83–87
OIG guidance for hospitals, 83–84
OIG guidance for individual and small group practices, 84–85
OIG guidance for third-party medical billing companies, 84–85
OIG Work Plan, 86–87
operational integration, 91
operationalization of, 93–94
policies and procedures for, 90
senior and middle management, 89
training and communications, 91
Clinical documentation improvement (CDI) education
on CDI in outpatient setting, 314–315
on CDI program components, 302–303
CME presentation content for, 297
on defining outpatient CDI, 299–300
educational session content for, 297
establishing group sessions for, 295
on HCC redesign process, 304
maximizing attendance for, 296–297
for medical coding professionals. *See* coder educational programs
on need for outpatient CDI, 302
for nonphysician providers, 292–295
for nonprovider clinicians, 294–296
on physician queries, 300–302
for physicians, 290–292, 295–296
on risk scores, 303–304
sample presentation for, 297–305
selecting instructors for, 296
on team-based approach to CDI, 298–299
on workflow redesign, 304–305
Clinical documentation improvement (CDI) expansion
admission documentation, 350–351
area selection for, 348
charge capture, 352–353
critical care documentation, 351–352
E/M codes for, 353–355
to emergency department, 349
E/M level benchmarking, 355–358
observation services, 358–359
observation services dates and times, 359–360
organizational and stakeholder adoption of, 348–349
other observation services documentation, 363
provider orders and documentation in observation services, 360–362

Clinical documentation improvement (CDI) interdisciplinary
    team
    characteristics of good teams, 219
    definition of, 210
    fostering collaboration among, 218–219
    identifying organizational leaders to be members of, 211–214
    need for, 210–211
    selection and roles of members of, 215–218
Clinical documentation improvement (CDI) leader, 215, 217
    CDI expansion and, 348–349
    DOJ memorandum on, 89
    Emergency Severity Index compared with E/M code
        frequency data and, 356–358
Clinical documentation improvement (CDI) pilot program, 118, 131
    data report on, 153–154
    data review for, 148
    findings and recommendations discussion for, 150
    focus area selection for, 148–149
    focused clinical record review process for, 151–153
    HCC capture monitoring for, 149
    HCPCS/CPT frequency report review, 149
    key stakeholder interviews for, 150
    root cause identification for, 150
    sample audit, 149–150
    site identification for, 147–148
    solution implementation for, 151
Clinical documentation improvement practitioner (CDIP), 43
    as recommended CDS credential, 261–262
Clinical documentation improvement (CDI) program
    CDS training in process and design of, 266–267
    goals and objectives of, 199–201
    governance structure of, 193–197
    implementation strategies for, 203–205
    key decision makers involved in, 192–193
    maintaining visibility of, 273–274
    mission statement of, 198–199
    need for interdisciplinary leadership team in, 210–211
    organizational communication about, 201–203
    origination of, 192
    project management for, 224–225
    ROI of, 192, 195, 211, 319
    staffing options for. *See* staffing
    success path of, 205
    sustainability of, 195, 273–274
    vision statement of, 197–199
Clinical documentation improvement (CDI) program director,
    selection of, 193
Clinical documentation improvement (CDI) steering committee
    CDI expansion and, 348–349
    as CDI workplan task, 231–232
    DOJ memorandum on, 89
    goals and objectives developed by, 199–201
    members of, 194, 212–216
    mission statement development by, 198–199
    phases in discussions of, 195
    program communication by, 201–203
    responsibilities of, 194–195
    vision statement development by, 197–199
Clinical documentation improvement (CDI) taskforce
    as CDI workplan task, 231–232
    DOJ memorandum on, 89
    establishment of, 122
    meeting frequency of, 196–197
    members of, 194, 212–214, 216–218
    responsibilities of, 196–197

Clinical documentation improvement (CDI) taskforce chair,
    215, 217
Clinical documentation improvement (CDI) team.
    See interdisciplinary CDI team
Clinical documentation improvement (CDI) workplan, 225–227
    clinical documentation assessment, 234, 236
    data analytics, 227–229
    high-level technology assessment, 234–235
    ongoing program monitoring, 239, 242
    on-site kickoff meeting and interviews, 228, 230
    outpatient and professional practice case review, 231, 233
    physician collaboration and education, 237, 239–240
    program governance and oversight, 231–232
    rapid redesign of clinical documentation workflow at pilot
        clinics, 234, 237–238
    rapid redesign of clinical documentation workflow in
        remaining clinics, 239, 241
Clinical documentation specialists (CDSs)
    admission documentation and, 350–351
    AHIMA Standards of Ethical Coding for, 92–93
    In ambulatory facility setting, 72
    anesthesia record and, 30
    areas of expertise for, 13–14
    charge capture and, 352–353
    charge description master and, 74, 139
    chronic illness identification by, 71
    clinical documentation improvement and, 13
    clinical editors and, 179
    CMS guidance for, 87
    code sets and, 51
    coding audit reports and, 143
    credentials for, 261–262
    critical care documentation, 351–352
    denials tracking by, 176–178
    diagnostic test results and, 30
    DocEdge Communicator and, 173–176
    emergency department record and, 28–29
    E/M level benchmarking, 355–358
    evaluation and management coding and, 63–65, 353–355
    Hierarchical Condition Categories review by, 69
    hiring and training of, 196
    ICD-10-CM guidelines for, 56–57
    in interdisciplinary CDI leadership teams, 210–211, 218
    job description for, 55, 263–264
    medication administration record and, 32
    observation services and, 359, 361
    OIG Work Plan and, 83, 86–87
    operative and procedure reports and, 32
    outpatient, 42–44
    outpatient coding and reimbursement systems, 40–41
    outsourcing and employed staff options for, 251–255
    pilot site data review by, 148
    preceptorships for, 254
    program data report by, 153–154
    progress notes and, 34–35
    query improvements and, 339–340
    query metrics and, 337–339
    query submission by, 334, 336
    readmissions and, 351
    recruitment of, 249
    reimbursement maximization by, 9
    relative value units and, 66–68
    sample case audit by, 149–150
    skills required of, 248–249, 261–262
    technology and, 160

vital signs flowsheet and, 35
workflow redesign and, 152–153
Clinical documentation specialist (CDS) training
   in CDI program process and design, 266–267
   CDS job description and, 263–264
   in communication, 285
   in critical thinking. *See* critical thinking
   in data review, 268
   in ICD-10-CM, CPT, HCPCS, APC, and HCC, 268
   in maintaining CDI program visibility, 273–274
   methodologies for, 260
   in metrics and trending, 270–273
   in outpatient clinical documentation case review, 268–269
   in physician advisor role, 270
   posttraining evaluation of, 274–275
   pretraining assessment for, 262–263
   in query process, 269–270
   self-evaluation for, 265–266
   skills required in outpatient settings and, 261–262
   topics, programs, and resources for, 266–267
Clinical Documentation Toolkit, AHIMA, 267, 271
Clinical documentation workflow, rapid redesign of, 234, 237–239, 241
Clinical editors, 124
   Ambulatory Revenue Manager, 179–181
   CDS expertise in, 262
   Revenue Integrity, 181–184
Clinical information, 24
Clinical nurse specialists (CNSs), 293
Clinical outcomes data, need for, 6
Clinical Practice Improvement Activities (CPIAs), 103
Clinical records
   anesthesia record, 29–30
   categorization of, 26–28
   consultation reports, 30
   diagnostic test results and, 30–31
   emergency department record, 28–29
   encounter summary, 31
   focused review process of, 151–153
   Glasgow coma scale, 29
   MEAT requirements for, 70
   medication administration record, 32
   need for, 6
   for observation services, 358–359
   operative and procedure reports, 32
   outpatient records by settings, 35–36
   patient history and physical examination, 31
   physician orders, 33
   problem list, 33–34
   progress notes, 34–35
   vital signs flowsheet, 35
Clinical staff, CDI education for. *See* clinical documentation improvement education
Clinic nurse manager, as CDI team member, 217
CMS 1450 form, 51
CMS 1500 form, 50–51, 141
Coder educational programs, 310
   on CDI focus areas, 321
   on CDI mastery for coders, 324
   on CDI program components, 315
   on claims editors, 326
   on clinical data requirements, 320
   on CMS quality programs for outpatient facilities, 327–328
   on common HCCs, 318

on conducting HCC audits, 320
on credentials for outpatient coders, 324
on data analytics, metrics, and trending, 328–329
on defining outpatient CDI, 314
on denials management, 326–327
educational session content for, 313
on growing demand for CDI to support risk adjustment, 318
on HCC and outpatient code assignment, 328
on HCC case review, 321
on HCC shadowing process, 316–317
on hospital chargemaster, 326
on need for outpatient CDI, 325
on OIG risk-adjustment data validation audit, 319–320
on outpatient coding and CDI resources, 324
on physician fee schedules, 325
on physician query process, 317–318
preparing for and running of, 312–313
on provider program adoption, 322
on risk scores, 319
on ROI of CDI program, 319
on team-based approach to CDI, 314
on technology for HCC capture, 323
on technology for outpatient CDI, 322
on workflow redesign, 323–324
Coding. *See also* clinical coding specialist
   AHIMA Standards of Ethical, 92–93
   in ambulatory facility setting, 71–74
   anesthesia record for, 30
   CDS expertise in, 261–262
   CDS training in, 268
   clinical documentation and, 54–55
   consultation reports for, 30
   CPT and HCPCS guidelines for, 57–62
   diagnosticians and, 38
   diagnostic test results for, 31
   in emergency department, 74–76, 353
   evaluation and management, 63–65
   experts in outpatient, 42–43
   guidelines for outpatient, 41–42
   ICD-10-CM guidelines for, 56–57
   National Correct Coding Initiative guidelines for, 59
   nonphysician practitioners and, 39
   nurses and, 39
   nutritionists and, 39–40
   outpatient, 40–41
   patient history and physical examination for, 31
   in physician practice, 63
   problem list and, 33
   process for, 50–52
Coding audit reports
   for CDI assessment program, 123
   for clinical documentation analysis, 143
Coding manager, as CDI team member, 218
Collaboration
   among interdisciplinary team members, 218–219
   physician, 237, 239–240
Colonoscopy coding example, 57–59
Communication
   about CDI program, 201–203
   CDS skills in, 262
   CDS training in, 285
Communication tools, in electronic health records, 165
Complementary and integrative medicine (CIM) practitioners, clinical documentation by, 40

Completeness
　in clinical documentation, 16–17
　nurses and, 39
　of patient history and physical examination, 31
　query for, 334
Compliance, 82. *See also* clinical documentation improvement compliance
　ambulatory CDI, 82
　coding, 92–93
Compliance program guidance, 82
Compliance role, 89
Compliance training, adding CDI education to, 292
Compliant query, 336–337
Component codes, 142
Composite APCs, for observation services, 360
Comprehension, as lower-order thinking, 277–279
Comprehensive APC (C-APC), 72
Comprehensive Care for Joint Replacement (CJR) Payment Model, 106–107
Comprehensive ESRD Care (CEC), 106
Comprehensive Primary Care Plus (CPC+), 106
Computer-assisted coding (CAC) software, 164
　applications of, 167–168
Computerized decision support system data, physician CDI education using, 292
Computerized reminders, physician CDI education using, 292
Concurrent case review, 151–153
Conditions for Coverage (CfCs), outpatient clinical documentation for, 7–8
Conditions of Participation (CoPs), outpatient clinical documentation for, 7–8
Conduct at the Top, 89
Congestive heart failure (CHF), EHR template for, 161–162
Consistency
　in clinical documentation, 17
　in observation services dates and times, 359
　in outpatient coding, 43
　query for, 334
Consultant responsible party, on CDI workplan, 226–227
Consultants, clinical documentation by, 37
Consultation reports, 30, 36
　responsibility for, 37
Continuing medical education (CME)
　CDI presentation content for, 297
　learning trends in, 290–292
Continuum of care
　clinical records for, 6
　guidelines for, 7–8
Contract-to-employed staff, CDI program staffing with, 253–254
Controls, for operational integration, 91
Conversion factor, in relative value units calculation, 65
Credentials
　for CDSs, 261–262
　for outpatient coders, 324
Critical care documentation, 351–352
Critical thinking
　defined, 275
　learning process and, 277–279
　need for, 276–277
　problem resolution with, 280–282
　problem resolution without, 279
　in surmounting barriers to success, 282–285
Current Procedural Terminology (CPT)
　for ambulatory facility setting, 72
　application of, 50

　categories of, 57
　CDI and accurate assignment of, 119
　CDI assessment program and errors in, 125, 127, 130–131
　CDS expertise in, 261
　CDS training in, 268
　for clinical documentation analysis, 138–140
　clinical documentation specialists and, 51
　code sections of, 57
　code sets of, 9
　coding guidelines for, 57–62
　colonoscopy example for, 57–59
　denials tracking by, 178
　in emergency department, 74–75, 351–352
　evaluation and management coding with, 63–65
　guidelines and specifications for, 51
　Healthcare Common Procedure Coding System and, 57–58
　medically unlikely edits and, 142–143
　in Medicare Physician Fee schedule, 65
　modifier validity, 141
　nail plate example for, 59–60
　for observation services, 358
　in outpatient settings, 42
　pilot program review of, 149
　quality of care and, 10
　relative value units and, 65
　research identifiable files and, 144–145
　top 200 Level I and II codes for, 146–147
Custom edits, 142
Customization, of existing CDI program, 203–204

Data analytics
　as CDI workplan task, 227–229
　medical coder education on, 328–329
Data mining, 167
Data review, CDS training in, 268
Decision makers, in CDI program creation, 192–193
Deidentification of records, 26
Deleted codes, claims edits and, 141
Dementia—Caregiver Education and Support, 144
Dementia—Cognitive Assessment, 144
Denials, CDS expertise in, 262
Denials database, 176–178
Denials management, medical coder education on, 326–327
DenialsNavigator, 176–178
Denials trend analysis
　CDI assessment program and, 124, 130–131
　for clinical documentation analysis, 143
Department code, 140
Department of Health and Human Services, US (HHS), healthcare regulation by, 94–95
Department of Justice, US (DOJ)
　analysis and remediation of underlying misconduct, 88–89
　autonomy and resources, 89–90
　compliance memorandum from, 87–88
　confidential reporting and investigation, 91–92
　continuous improvement, periodic testing, and review, 92
　operational integration, 91
　policies and procedures for, 90
　senior and middle management, 89
　training and communications, 91
Designated record sets
　clinical records in, 27–28
　contents of, 24–25
Designing Compliance Policies and Procedures, 90

Diagnosis-related group (DRG), in ambulatory facility setting, 72–73
Diagnosis-related revenue risks, 128–129
Diagnosis specificity, 363
Diagnostic Coding and Reporting Guidelines for Outpatient Services, of ICD-10-CM Official Guidelines for Coding and Reporting, 56–57
Diagnosticians, 38
Diagnostic test results, 30–31, 36
Dietitians. *See* nutritionists
Discharge summary, house staff responsibility for, 37
Discrete data, 165–166
Disease prevention and wellness, 96
Disposition, on CDI workplan, 226–227
Distinguished Hospital for Clinical Excellence Award, 111
DocEdge Communicator, 173–176
Drop-down menus, for electronic health record, 162
Due dates, on CDI workplan, 226–227

EDI 837, 123
Edits, 179. *See also* claims edit
Education, CDI. *See* clinical documentation improvement education
Efficiency, as quality measure, 99
835 file, 227–228
837 file, 123, 227–228
837i form, 51
837p form, 50
Electronic health record (EHR)
 Advancing Care Information, 107–108
 AHIMA Standards of Ethical Coding and, 92–93
 alerts for, 162
 benefits of, 4
 CDS assessment of, 53
 certified, 102–103
 clinical documentation improvement and, 13, 161–163
 clinical documentation risks with, 163–165
 common systems of, 51
 communication tools in, 165
 computer-assisted coding software and, 168
 description of, 4
 DocEdge Communicator interface with, 173
 drop-down menus for, 162
 evaluation and management coding in, 75–76
 functionality, 161–165
 hard-copy documentation and, 51
 hybrid health records, 15
 incorrect documentation with, 164
 inline documentation functionality, 162–163
 insufficient documentation with, 164
 interoperability of, 52–53, 121, 160
 natural language processing and, 165–167
 outpatient records by settings in, 35–36
 overdocumentation with, 164–165
 problem list and, 33–34
 prompts for, 162
 risks with, 4, 163–165
 semantic reasoning in, 166
 standards for, 22–23
 templates for, 161–162
 timeliness and, 17
 unstructured data from, 165
 workflow redesign and, 152–153
Emergency department (ED)
 admission documentation for, 350–351
 charge capture, 352–353
 coding in, 74–76, 353
 critical care documentation, 351–352
 E/M codes in, 72, 74–75, 353–355
 E/M level benchmarking, 355–358
 observation services and, 358
 outpatient record categories at, 36
 Type A, 74–75
 Type B, 75
Emergency department (ED) record, 28–29
 attending physician and, 37
Emergency medicine query example, 341
Emergency Severity Index (ESI), E/M code frequency data compared with, 356–358
Encoder, 50
Encounter summary, 31, 36
Endocrinology, nutritional disease query example, 342
EPIC, 51
Evaluation, as higher-order thinking, 277–278, 281–282
Evaluation and Management Codes by Specialty file, 147
Evaluation and management (E/M) coding
 ACEP and, 75–76
 benchmarking for, 355–358
 EHRs and inappropriate automatic assignment of, 164
 in emergency department, 72, 74–75, 353–355
 Emergency Severity Index compared with, 356–358
 modifier -25, 353
 in physician practice, 63–65
Evidence-based clinical practice guidelines, 6
Evidence-based medicine
 guidelines for, 6
 promotion of, 11
Examination. *See* physical examination
Executive sponsor, 215
External records and reports, 27–28, 36

Facility-specific standards, 24
Federal compliance guidance for CDI programs
 analysis and remediation of underlying misconduct, 88–89
 autonomy and resources, 89–90
 CMS guidance, 87
 confidential reporting and investigation, 91–92
 continuous improvement, periodic testing, and review, 92
 DOJ compliance memorandum, 87–92
 Office of Inspector General guidance, 83–87
 OIG guidance for hospitals, 83–84
 OIG guidance for individual and small group practices, 84–85
 OIG guidance for third-party medical billing companies, 84–85
 OIG Work Plan, 86–87
 operational integration, 91
 policies and procedures for, 90
 senior and middle management, 89
 training and communications, 91
Fee-for-service payment methodology, 8–9
Fee schedule–based payments, 97
Fellows. *See* house staff
Financial resources, for CDI program, 195
Foundational interoperability, 52
Fraud prevention and detection, with outpatient clinical documentation, 10
Frequency limits, claims edits and, 141

General industry-standard edits, 141–142
General practice providers, national percentage utilization of E/M codes, 64–65

388 Index

Geographic practice cost index (GPCI), in relative value units calculation, 65
Glasgow coma scale, 29
Global period, claims edits and, 141
Goals, of CDI program, 199–201
Governance
 of CDI program, 193–197
 as CDI workplan task, 231–232
Government agencies, clinical data use by, 5–6
Greenway, 51
Group health plan, 68

HCC suspecting
 Patient HCC Capture report, 169–170
 Patient HCC Profile report, 171
 Physician HCC Capture report, 171–172
 process of, 168–169
HCPCS Procedure Modifier Codes, 42
Healthcare
 critical thinking in, 276–277
 government agencies regulating, 94
Healthcare Common Procedure Coding System (HCPCS)
 for ambulatory facility setting, 72
 application of, 50
 CDI and accurate assignment of, 119
 CDI assessment program and errors in, 125, 127, 130–131
 CDS expertise in, 261
 CDS training in, 268
 for clinical documentation analysis, 138–140
 clinical documentation specialists and, 51
 clinical editors and, 180
 code sets of, 9
 coding guidelines for, 57–62
 colonoscopy example for, 57–59
 Current Procedural Terminology and, 57–58
 in emergency department, 74–75
 evaluation and management coding with, 63–65
 guidelines and specifications for, 51
 levels of, 42, 57–58
 medically unlikely edits and, 142–143
 in Medicare Physician Fee schedule, 65
 for observation services, 360
 OPPS and, 73
 in outpatient settings, 41–42
 pilot program review of, 149
 quality of care and, 10
 research identifiable files and, 144–145
 top 200 Level I and II codes for, 146–147
Healthcare consulting, CDS experience in, 262
Healthcare costs, HCCs for, 68
Healthcare delivery system, transformation of, 4
Healthcare organizations
 clinical data use by, 5
 identifying CDI team members within, 211–214
 staffing considerations in, 246–248
Healthcare record. *See* clinical documentation
Healthgrades, 11, 82, 99, 110–112
Health information, importance of, 4
Health information management (HIM)
 coding audit reports of, 143
 compliance plan for, 82
 professional competencies for, 275
 recruiting professionals trained in, 249
Health Information Management (HIM) apprenticeships, 254–255

Health information management (HIM) director
 in CDI program creation, 192–193
 as CDI team member, 212–216, 218
Health Information Technology for Economic and Clinical Health (HITECH) Act, 22, 98
Health Insurance Portability and Accountability Act of 1996 (HIPAA), 96
 deidentification, 26
 electronic health records and, 22
 protected health information, 25
Health IT Standards Committee (HITSC), 22
Health Level Seven (HL7), 22–23, 173
Health maintenance organization, 68
Health plan, types of, 68
Health record. *See* clinical documentation
Health systems and facilities, clinical data use by, 5–6
Hierarchical Condition Categories (HCCs)
 in annual Medicare Advantage payment calculation, 69
 CDI assessment program and, 125–127, 129
 CDS expertise in, 262
 CDS training in, 268
 for chronic illnesses, 71
 code sets of, 9
 ICD-10-CM HCCs mapped to, 68–69
 inline documentation functionality for, 162–163
 MEAT requirements for, 70
 medical coder education on, 316–318, 320–321, 323, 328
 in Medicare Advantage program, 68
 in outpatient settings, 41
 pilot program and monitoring capture of, 149
 provider and clinical staff education on, 304
 quality of care and, 10
 reports and audits of, 143–144
 review of, 151–152
 for risk-adjusted payment, 68–71
 Risk Adjustment Factor score and, 68–69
High-level technology assessment, as CDI workplan task, 234–235
High risk, 148
History. *See* patient history
Hospital chargemaster, medical coder education on, 326
Hospital Outpatient Quality Reporting (OQR) Program, 99–101, 144
Hospital Readmissions Reduction Program (HRRP), 351
Hospitals
 chargemaster of. *See* charge description master
 OIG guidance for, 83–84
House staff, clinical documentation by, 37
Hybrid health records, 15, 23–24

ICD-10-CM Official Guidelines for Coding and Reporting, 56
Indian Health Services, 68
Individual practice, OIG guidance for, 84–85
Infectious disease query example, 342
Injections and infusions, 363
Inline documentation functionality, 162–163
 speech recognition with, 167
Inpatient CDI programs
 staffing for outpatient programs integrated with, 247
 staffing for outpatient programs separate from, 247–248
Inpatient Prospective Payment System (IPPS), 42–43
 readmissions and, 351
Insurance plan, reimbursement claims submission to, 9

Interdisciplinary CDI team
  characteristics of good teams, 219
  definition of, 210
  fostering collaboration among, 218–219
  identifying organizational leaders to be members of, 211–214
  need for, 210–211
  selection and roles of members of, 215–218
Internal audits, 92. *See also* coding audit reports
Internal medicine query example, 343
International Classification of Diseases, Tenth Revision, Clinical Modification (ICD-10-CM)
  application of, 50
  CDI and accurate assignment of, 119
  CDS expertise in, 261
  CDS training in, 268
  clinical documentation specialists and, 51
  code sets of, 9
  coding guidelines for, 56–57
  colonoscopy example for, 57–59
  EHRs and incorrect assignment of, 163–164
  in emergency department, 74–75
  guidelines and specifications for, 51
  HCCs mapped to, 68–69
  medical necessity and, 142
  in outpatient settings, 41–42
  quality of care and, 10
International Classification of Diseases, Tenth Revision, Procedure Coding System (ICD-10-PCS)
  application of, 50
  code sets of, 9
  quality of care and, 10
International Classification of Functioning, Disability and Health (ICF), 56
Interns. *See* house staff
Interoperability, 52–53, 121, 160
InterQual admission criteria, 350
Interviews, as CDI workplan task, 228, 230
IT director, as CDI team member, 216
Item code, 140–141

The Joint Commission, 10–11, 99

Key performance indicator (KPI), 124
Kickoff meeting, as CDI workplan task, 228, 230
Knowledge, as lower-order thinking, 277–279

Leaders, 211
  on CDI steering committee, 212–216
  on CDI taskforce, 212–214, 216–218
Leapfrog Group, 11, 82, 99, 108–109
Leapfrog Hospital Safety Grade, 109
Leapfrog Hospital Survey, 108–109
Learning process
  in CME, 290–292
  critical thinking and, 277–279
Legal health record
  clinical records in, 27–28
  contents of, 24–25
Legibility
  in clinical documentation, 15
  of patient history and physical examination, 31
  of progress notes, 34
  query for, 334
Licensed practical nurses (LPNs), 294

Licensure requirements, 24
Limited data set (LDS) files, 98
Local coverage determinations (LCDs)
  CDS expertise in, 262
  claims denial and, 126–128
  claims edits and, 141
  clinical editors and, 180
  medical necessity and, 44

Malpractice coverage, in relative value units calculation, 65
McKesson, 51
Meaningful Use requirements, 34, 102–103, 107
MedeAnalytics, 128–129
  Revenue Integrity, 169–172, 181–184
Medicaid program, 68, 96
Medical coding professionals
  CDI education for. *See* coder educational programs
  educational and training background of, 311
  job responsibilities of, 312
  required competencies of, 310–311
Medical decision making, evaluation and management coding and, 64
Medically Unlikely Edit (MUE), 124, 142–143
Medical necessity
  admission documentation and, 350
  claims scrubbers and, 142
  EHRs and denials of, 164
  two-midnight rule, 361
Medical staff
  CDI education for. *See* clinical documentation improvement education
  CDI program support by, 194
  communicating about CDI program with, 201–203
Medicare Access and CHIP Reauthorization Act of 2015 (MACRA)
  Meaningful Use requirements and, 34
  physician practice Medicare payments and, 66–67
  quality measures of, 144
  Quality Payment Program of, 102
Medicare Administrative Contractors (MACs), 97
Medicare Advantage (MA) plans, risk-adjustment coding for, 310
Medicare Advantage program
  annual payment determination for, 69–71
  case reviews for, 151–152
  chronic illnesses and, 71
  Hierarchical Condition Categories in, 68
  per-payment, per-month contract rate of, 69
  return on investment with, 69
Medicare Claims Processing Manual, 9
Medicare Fee for Service claims, CMS 1500 form for, 50, 141
Medicare Learning Network, on evaluation and management coding, 63
Medicare Physician Fee schedule (MPFS)
  application of, 65
  development of, 66
Medicare program
  observation services and, 360
  Part A of, 68, 94
  Part B of, 68, 94, 96
  Part C of, 96
  Part D of, 96
  Quality Payment Program and, 102

Medicare Provider and Analysis Review (MedPAR), 98
Medication administration record (MAR), 32, 36
Meditech, 51
Meeting frequency, of CDI taskforce, 196–197
Merit-Based Incentive Payment System (MIPS), 66
    electronic health records and, 164
    payment adjustments under, 104–105
    performance categories of, 102–103
    providers included in, 103–104
    quality scores and, 123, 144
Metrics
    for CDI program assessment, 195–196
    CDS training in, 270–273
    medical coder education on, 328–329
Midlevel practitioners (MLPs), clinical documentation by, 39
Mid-level providers. *See* nonphysician providers
Milliman admission criteria, 350
Missing charges revenue risks, 128–129, 181–182
Mission statement, of CDI program, 198–199
Modifier -25, 353
Modifiers, multiple codes requiring, 142
Monitoring, evaluation, assess/address, and treat (MEAT) requirements
    for clinical records, 70
    HCC suspecting and, 168–169
Multiple codes requiring modifiers, 142

Nail plate coding example, 59–60
National Committee for Quality Assurance (NCQA), 99
National Correct Coding Initiative (NCCI)
    claims edits and, 124, 141
    guidelines of, 59
National coverage determinations (NCDs)
    CDS expertise in, 262
    claims denial and, 126–128
    claims edits and, 141
    clinical editors and, 180
    medical necessity and, 44
National Uniform Billing Committee (NUBC)
    revenue codes by, 140
    UB-04 of, 51
National Uniform Claim Committee (NUCC), CMS 1500 form by, 51
Nationwide interoperability, 52–53
Natural language processing (NLP)
    big data, 166
    CAC applications of, 167–168
    CDI applications of, 167
    data types and, 165
    HCC suspecting with, 168
    query template and, 337
    semantic reasoning and, 166
Needs assessment, 119
Neurology query example, 344
NextGen, 51
Next Generation ACO Model, 106
Noncovered service revenue risks, 128–129
Nonphysician practitioners, 39
Nonphysician providers (NPPs), CDI education for, 292–295
Nonprovider clinicians (NPCx), CDI education for, 294–296
Notes, in electronic health records, 165
Nurse practitioners (NPs), 293
Nurses
    clinical documentation by, 39
    clinical specialists, 293
    licensed practical, 294
    practitioners, 293
    registered, 294
    utilization review, 350, 361
Nutritionists, clinical documentation by, 39–40

Objectives, of CDI program, 199–201
Observation services
    CDI for, 358–359
    dates and times, 359–360
    other documentation for, 363
    provider orders and documentation in, 360–362
Obstetrical (OB) billing and care revenue risks, 128–129
Office of Family Assistance (OFA), 96
Office of Inspector General (OIG)
    CDI program guidance from, 83
    HHS program oversight by, 10
    hospital guidance from, 83–84
    individual and small group practice guidance from, 84–85
    OIG Work Plan, 86–87
    risk-adjustment data validation audit by, 319–320
    third-party medical billing company guidance from, 84–85
Office of the National Coordinator for Health Information Technology (ONC)
    electronic health records and, 22
    nationwide interoperability and, 52–53
OIG Work Plan, 83, 86–87
Oncology Care Model (OCM), 106
Oncology query example, 343
Ongoing program monitoring, as CDI workplan task, 239, 242
Online training, for physician CDI education, 292
Operational integration, 91
Operative and procedure reports, 32, 36
    house staff responsibility for, 37
    surgeon responsibility for, 37
Orthopedics and pain management query example, 344
Outcome, as quality measure, 99
Outpatient assessment report, as CDI workplan task, 234, 236
Outpatient clinic
    claims submittal at, 51
    interoperability at, 52–53
    outpatient record categories at, 36
Outpatient clinical documentation
    CDS training in, 268–269
    challenges of, 12–14, 40–44
    evidence-based medicine promotion with, 11
    fraud, waste, and abuse prevention and detection with, 10
    population health improvement with, 12
    quality criteria for, 14–18
    quality of care measurement and marketing with, 10–11
    for regulatory requirements, 7–8
    reimbursement maximization with, 8–10
    by settings, 35–36
    users of, 5
    uses of, 6–7
Outpatient coding experts, 42–43
Outpatient facility case review, as CDI workplan task, 231, 233
Outpatient Prospective Payment System (OPPS), 41–42, 138
    Addendum B, 72–73
    for ambulatory facility setting, 71
    ambulatory payment categories and, 72–73
    HCPCS codes and, 73
    payment methodologies of, 73
    SIs of, 60–62

Outpatient records by settings, 35–36
Outsourcing
    of CDI program staff, 251–255
    permanent, 253
    planned conversion to internal project management model of, 255
Overcoding, 84
Overdocumentation, 164–165
Oversight, as CDI workplan task, 231–232

Paper records, 23–24
Part B National Summary Data File, 355–356
Partners in Information Access for the Public Health Workforce, 99
Passive dissemination, physician CDI education using, 292
Passive learning, 277
    in CME, 290–292
Patient-centered medical home, 66
Patient HCC Capture report, 169–170
Patient HCC Profile report, 171
Patient history
    in clinical record, 31
    evaluation and management coding and, 64
    house staff responsibility for, 37
    settings for, 36
Patient severity, 354
Payers, clinical data use by, 5
Payer-specific edits, 142
Per-patient-per-month (PPPM) contract rate
    calculation of, 69
    case review and, 152
Personal mobile devices
    communication with, 172–173
    DocEdge Communicator, 173–176
Pharmaceutical companies, clinical data use by, 5
Physical examination
    in clinical record, 31
    evaluation and management coding and, 64
    house staff responsibility for, 37
    settings for, 36
Physician advisor role, CDS training about, 270
Physician advisors, CDI program staffing and, 249–251
Physician assistants (PAs), 293
Physician buy-in, 121
Physician collaboration, as CDI workplan task, 237, 239–240
Physician education, about CDI
    recommended approaches to, 291–294
Physician executives, clinical documentation by, 38
Physician Fee Schedule (PFS)
    for CDI assessment program, 123
    CMS revisions to, 65–66
    medical coder education on, 325
    pilot program review of, 149
    search tool for, 66–67
Physician HCC Capture report, 171–172
Physician orders, 33, 36
    for observation services, 360
Physician practice
    alternative payment models for, 66
    chronic illness identification by, 71
    coding in, 63
    837p form for, 50
    evaluation and management coding in, 63–65
    Hierarchical Condition Category codes in, 68–71
    interoperability at, 52–53
    OIG guidance for, 84–85

    outpatient record categories at, 36
    relative value units and fee schedule for, 65–68
Physician Quality Reporting System (PQRS), 102–103
Physician query. See query process
Physicians
    CDI education for, 290–292, 295–296
    CDI program adoption by, 194, 196
    CDI program communication for, 201–203
    CDI program training for, 196
Physician Value-Based Modifier program. See Value Modifier program
Physician work, in relative value units calculation, 65
Pilot clinic, rapid redesign of workflow at, 234, 237–238
Population health, improvement of, 12
Postencounter case review, 153, 160
Posttraining evaluation, of CDS training, 274–275
Practice expenses, in relative value units calculation, 65
Practice plan administrator, as CDI team member, 216
Preauthorization, 126
Preceptorship, CDS training with, 254
Precertification, 126
Precision
    in clinical documentation, 16
    consultation reports and, 30
    operative and procedure reports and, 32
    of progress notes, 34
    query for, 334
Pre-encounter case review, 151–153, 160
Pretraining assessment, for CDS training, 262–263
Price point, as staff outsourcing consideration, 251–252
Prior indications, 88
Problem list, 33–34, 36
Problem resolution
    with critical thinking, 280–282
    without critical thinking, 279
Procedure Modifier Codes, HCPCS, 42
Procedure-related revenue risks, 128–129
Procedures, for observation services, 363
Process, as quality measure, 99
Professional practice case review, as CDI workplan task, 231, 233
Professional revenue risks report, 183
Program monitoring, as CDI workplan task, 239, 242
Progress notes, 34–36
    house staff responsibility for, 37
    surgeon responsibility for, 37
Project kickoff meeting, as CDI workplan task, 228, 230
Project management
    for CDI program, 224–225
    CDS skills in, 262
    process of, 224
    workplan for. See project workplan
Project manager (PM)
    outsourcing and employed staff options for, 251–255
    outsourcing considerations for, 252
    responsibilities of, 224
    selection of, 224
    steps followed by, 225
Project timeline, on CDI workplan, 226–227
Project workplan, 225–227
    clinical documentation assessment, 234, 236
    data analytics, 227–229
    high-level technology assessment, 234–235
    ongoing program monitoring, 239, 242
    on-site kickoff meeting and interviews, 228, 230
    outpatient and professional practice case review, 231, 233
    physician collaboration and education, 237, 239–240

Project workplan (*Continued*)
    program governance and oversight, 231–232
    rapid redesign of clinical documentation workflow at pilot clinics, 234, 237–238
    rapid redesign of clinical documentation workflow in remaining clinics, 239, 241
Prompts, for electronic health record, 162
Prospective payment system (PPS), 97
    DRG categories and, 73
Protected health information (PHI), 25–26, 96, 98
Provident, 173
Provider collaboration
    CDI and improved, 120
    clinical records for, 6
Provider practice manager, as CDI team member, 217
Providers
    buy-in by, 121
    CDI education for. *See* clinical documentation improvement education
    clinical data use by, 5
    observation services and, 360
    outpatient clinical documentation improvement and, 12–13
Public data, 98–99
Public health agencies, clinical data use by, 5
Public health and safety, 97
Public speaking, CDS skills in, 262

Quality, in MIPS, 103
Quality and compliance director, as CDI team member, 216
Quality measure scores, 144
Quality of care
    CDI and accurate scores of, 119
    clinical data for, 6
    measurement and marketing of, 10–11
    reimbursement and revenue generation and, 122–123
    reporting for, 98–99
Quality Payment Program (QPP)
    advanced APMs of, 105–107
    Advancing Care Information Performance Measure, 107–108
    Merit-Based Incentive Payment System of, 102–105
    participation in, 104–105
    privately held hospital compare organizations, 108–112
Query metrics, 337–339
Query process
    CDS training in, 269–270
    in clinical documentation improvement process, 334
    criteria for submission of, 334–335
    guidelines for, 335–337
    improvements to, 339–340
    medical coder education on, 317–318
    physician education on, 300–302
    specialty-specific diagnosis, 340–344
    timing of, 334
Query templates, 336–337
    specialty-specific, 341–344
Query Toolkit, of AHIMA, 334, 336–337

Radiation oncology, work RVUs in, 66
Rapid redesign, as CDI workplan task, 234, 237–239, 241
Readmissions, 351
Real-time computerized reminders, physician CDI education using, 292

Recommended Approaches to Physician Education about CDI, 291–294
Redesign
    as CDI workplan task, 234, 237–239, 241
    of existing CDI program, 205
    medical coder education on, 323–324
    provider and clinical staff education on, 304–305
Registered nurses (RNs), 294
Regulatory requirements, outpatient clinical documentation for, 7–8
Reimbursement
    CDI and accurate, 119
    outpatient clinical documentation for maximization of, 8–10
    outpatient systems for, 40–41
    quality scores and cash-flow issues and, 122–123
Relative value units (RVUs), 40–41
    application of, 42
    calculation of, 65
    CMS revisions to, 65–66
    CPT codes and, 65
    in radiation oncology, 66
Reliability
    in clinical documentation, 15–16
    problem list and, 33
    query for, 334
Remediation, 89
Reporting mechanism effectiveness, 91–92
Research, 97
Research Data Assistance Center (ResDAC), 98
Research identifiable files (RIFs), 144–145
Research institutions, clinical data use by, 5
Residents. *See* house staff
Resource use, in MIPS, 103
Responsibility for integration, 91
Return on investment (ROI)
    of CDI program, 192, 195, 211, 319
    claims edits and, 128–129
    for clinical documentation improvement, 118, 129–131
    Medicare Advantage program and, 69
    technology landscape and, 161
Revenue code, 140
Revenue generation
    quality scores and cash-flow issues and, 122–123
    risks to, 128–129, 181–183
Revenue Integrity (RI), 169–172, 181–184
Revenue risks, 128–129, 181–183
Risk-adjustment coding
    medical coder education on, 318
    for Medicare plans, 310
Risk adjustment data validation (RADV) audit, of clinical documentation, 70
Risk Adjustment Factor (RAF) score
    in annual Medicare Advantage payment calculation, 69–71
    calculation of, 68–69
    CDI assessment program and, 129
Risk-based payment methodology, 9
Risk-based training, 91
Risk of mortality (ROM), 111–112, 267
Risk scores
    medical coder education on, 319
    provider and clinical staff education on, 303–304

Risk target dashboard, 183–184
Root cause analysis, 88

Scope of work (SOW), as staff outsourcing consideration, 251–252
Self-evaluation, for CDS training, 265–266
Semantic interoperability, 52
Semantic reasoning, 166
Semantics, 166
Senior vice presidents (SVPs), as CDI team members, 212–214
Sepsis care, 111–112
Severity of illness (SI, SOI), 111–112, 267
Shared Commitment, 89
Shared Nationwide Interoperability Roadmap, 53
Shared Savings Program, 106
Slide presentation, for CDI educational sessions, 297–305
Small group practice, OIG guidance for, 84–85
SMART mnemonic, 200
Social services, 96
Specific, measurable, attainable, relevant, time-bound (SMART), 200
Speech recognition with in-line documentation prompts, 167
Staffing
    availability of qualified program staff for, 248–249
    cash flow issues affecting, 249
    issues with, 120
    organizational considerations and, 246–248
    outsourcing and employed staff options for, 251–255
    physician leaders and, 249–251
    selection of model for, 248
Staff interventions/point system, 354
Stakeholder interviews, as CDI workplan task, 228, 230
Stakeholders
    CDI assessment program and buy-in by, 134
    CDI expansion adoption by, 348–349
    CDI pilot program and interviews of, 150
    in CDI program creation, 192–193
    program data report for, 153–154
Standard analytical files (SAFs), 145
Standards of conduct, for third-party medical billing companies, 85
Start dates, on CDI workplan, 226–227
State Medicaid Provider Manual, 9
Status indicator (SI) codes, 60–62
Status notes, on CDI workplan, 226–227
Steering committee
    CDI expansion and, 348–349
    as CDI workplan task, 231–232
    DOJ memorandum on, 89
    goals and objectives developed by, 199–201
    members of, 194, 212–216
    mission statement development by, 198–199
    phases in discussions of, 195
    program communication by, 201–203
    responsibilities of, 194–195
    vision statement development by, 197–199
Structural interoperability, 52
Structure, as quality measure, 99
Structured data, 165–166
Structured query language (SQL), 145
Subtasks, on CDI workplan, 225–226
Success barriers, critical thinking for surmounting, 282–285

Succession planning, for CDI team leaders, 215
Surgeons, clinical documentation by, 37–38
Surgical procedure, documentation for, 32
Sustainability, of CDI program, 195, 273–274
Sustainable growth rate (SGR) program
    MPFS methodology and, 66
    repeal of, 67, 102
Synthesis, as higher-order thinking, 280–282

Tabular List, of ICD-10-CM, 56
Taskforce
    as CDI workplan task, 231–232
    DOJ memorandum on, 89
    establishment of, 122
    meeting frequency of, 196–197
    members of, 194, 212–214, 216–218
    responsibilities of, 196–197
Taskforce chair, 215, 217
Tasks
    on CDI workplan, 225–226
    in electronic health records, 165
Team. *See* interdisciplinary CDI team
Technology assessment, as CDI workplan task, 234–235
Technology landscape for outpatient clinical documentation, 160–161
    CAC applications, 167–168
    clinical editors, 179–185
    denials tracking, 176–178
    electronic health record functionality, 161–165
    HCC suspecting, 168–172
    natural language processing, 165–167
    personal mobile device query options, 172–176
Templates, for electronic health record, 161–162
Temporary Assistance for Needy Families (TANF), 96
Therapists, clinical documentation by, 40
Third-party medical billing companies, OIG guidance for, 84–85
Timeline, on CDI workplan, 226–227
Timeliness
    in clinical documentation, 17–18
    of patient history and physical examination, 31
    of progress notes, 34
    query for, 334
Time spent with patient, 354
Top 200 Level I HCPCS/CPT codes, 146–147
Top 200 Level II HCPCS/CPT codes, 146–147
Training, CDS. *See* clinical documentation specialist training
Treating providers, 38
Trending
    CDS training in, 270–273
    medical coder education on, 328–329
Two-midnight rule, 361–362
Type A emergency departments, 74–75
Type B emergency departments, 75

UB-04 Uniform Bill format, 51, 141
Unbundling, 59, 84, 86
Underlying misconduct, analysis and remediation of, 88–89
Uniform Claim Form Task Force, 51
Unit count revenue risks, 128–129
Unstructured data, 165–166
Upcoding, 83–84, 86

Urgent care center, outpatient record categories at, 36
Utilization review (UR) nurse, 350, 361

Value-based programs, 97
Value Modifier (VM) program, 97, 102–103
Vendors, CDI
    preceptorship options offered by, 254
    selection of, 251–253
Virtual private network (VPN), 22
Vision statement, of CDI program, 197–199
Vital signs flowsheet, 35–36

Waste prevention and detection, with outpatient clinical
    documentation, 10
Wellington Group
    Ambulatory Revenue Manager, 179–181
    DenialsNavigator, 176–178
Workflow redesign
    for clinical documentation, 148, 152–153
    medical coder education on, 323–324
    provider and clinical staff education on, 304–305
Workplan. *See* project workplan
World Health Organization (WHO), 56